ROUTLEDGE LIBRARY EDITIONS:
HISTORY OF MEDICINE

Volume 9

MEDICAL THEORY, SURGICAL PRACTICE

MEDICAL THEORY, SURGICAL PRACTICE

Studies in the History of Surgery

Edited by
CHRISTOPHER LAWRENCE

Routledge
Taylor & Francis Group
LONDON AND NEW YORK

First published in 1992 by Routledge

This edition first published in 2019
by Routledge
2 Park Square, Milton Park, Abingdon, Oxon OX14 4RN

and by Routledge
52 Vanderbilt Avenue, New York, NY 10017

Routledge is an imprint of the Taylor & Francis Group, an informa business

British Library Cataloguing in Publication Data
A catalogue record for this book is available from the British Library

ISBN: 978-0-367-08576-6 (Set)
ISBN: 978-0-429-02312-5 (Set) (ebk)
ISBN: 978-0-367-03019-3 (Volume 9) (hbk)
ISBN: 978-0-429-02009-4 (Volume 9) (ebk)

Publisher's Note
The publisher has gone to great lengths to ensure the quality of this reprint but points out that some imperfections in the original copies may be apparent.

Disclaimer
The publisher has made every effort to trace copyright holders and would welcome correspondence from those they have been unable to trace.

MEDICAL THEORY, SURGICAL PRACTICE

STUDIES IN THE HISTORY OF SURGERY

Edited by Christopher Lawrence

ROUTLEDGE

London and New York

First published in 1992
by Routledge
11 New Fetter Lane, London EC4P 4EE

Simultaneously published in the USA and Canada
by Routledge
a division of Routledge, Chapman and Hall Inc.
29 West 35th Street, New York, NY 10001

Typeset by LaserScript, Mitcham, Surrey
Printed in Great Britain by
Biddles Ltd, Guildford and King's Lynn

British Library Cataloguing in Publication Data
Medical theory, surgical practice: studies in the
history of surgery. – (The Wellcome Institute series
in the history of medicine)
I. Lawrence, Christopher II. Series
617.09

Library of Congress Cataloging in Publication Data
Medical theory, surgical practice: studies in the history of surgery/
edited by Christopher Lawrence
p. cm. – (Wellcome Institute series in the history of medicine)
Includes bibliographical references and index.
1. Surgery – history. I. Lawrence, Christopher, 1947– .
II. Series.
[DNLM: 1. Surgery – history. Wo 11.1 M489]
RD27.M44 1992
617'.09 – dc20
DNLM/DLC
for Library of Congress 91-32852
CIP

ISBN 0–415–00046–7

Contents

Figures

Acknowledgements

This book began as a symposium of the same title at the Wellcome Institute for the History of Medicine in 1985. In addition to the participants, I invited contributions to the volume from other historians working on the history of surgery. A version of Lucinda Beier's paper appeared as chapter 3 of her book *Sufferers and Healers* (1987). That essay contained so much of relevance to the themes of this volume – the relation of surgical practice to medical theories about the body – that I encouraged her to adapt it. The long period between conception and production of the present book must be the source of a number of thanks and apologies. To those contributors who delivered early, many thanks, and my apologies for the long wait. I am particularly grateful to Roger French for his patience with my editorial urge to interfere. To the publishers too, my apologies and thanks for waiting. Since I am relatively technologically illiterate, various people helped with the really hard work. Sally Bragg put much of the material on disc. More recently Jacqui Canning has been of immense assistance endlessly retyping my work and bringing the other papers into a single format. Many thanks.

1

Democratic, divine and heroic: the history and historiography of surgery

Christopher Lawrence

> Whether an operation was performed or not depended not so much on whether the surgeons were able to perform such an operation technically or not as on the medical theories prevailing at the time.[1]

Popular mythologies

In 1904 Frederick Dennis, Professor of Clinical Surgery at Cornell University, addressed the International Congress of Arts and Science at St Louis. Surveying the previous century, and chronicling what he described as 'the victories gained in every field' he said,

> But while the other sciences have indeed thrilling stories to relate, and can point with just pride to excellent deeds performed, the science of surgery stands out in bold relief, and conspicuous grandeur, apart from and above the others, in that it deals directly with human life, that most precious of mortal possessions, often lending to it not only a helping, but a saving hand. At the same time, its story is so simple and yet so grand, that the child and the savant may alike participate in the pleasure which the wonderful narrative is fitted to convey.[2]

Dennis's claims for the triumph of surgery were echoed in print by many other writers, by no means all of whom were surgeons. By 1900, in Europe and America the lesser of the healing arts, surgery, had, in the eyes of its practitioners and the public, eclipsed its more dignified superior, physic, in its therapeutic power. Late Victorians and Edwardians identified it with exploration and engineering as being among the great accomplishments of nineteenth-century civilisation.[3] Surgeons became national heroes. Crowds thronged to Waterloo Station to dispatch Frederick Treves to the Boer War.[4] Lister's public funeral service packed Westminster Abbey with dignitaries from all over the world.[5]

Dennis's simple and grand story utilised elements familiar to many Victorian tales: the march of science, the progress of civilisation and individual heroism. These ingredients remain essential to current popular histories of surgery in which the nineteenth century is represented as 'the age of miracles' and the long and simple history is seen as one of 'the courage to fail'.[6] Although Dennis's story is much like the popular one told today, his story had been given that shape only in the last two decades of the nineteenth century. Prior to that, surgery's history had been shaped and reshaped several times as surgeons in different epochs fashioned it to suit their particular ends and to define the enemies of their discipline. I examine here some of the ways in which the story was shaped in the Anglo-American world. Then I review works which suggest alternative approaches to surgical history. Finally I outline how it is possible to use Owsei Temkin's work to construct a model for writing the history of surgery. Continental matters have, of course, been central to the creation of the history and historiography of surgery but will only be considered here in so far as they relate to the rather more parochial tale of British and American surgical affairs.

Much of the history of medieval, Renaissance and post-Renaissance surgery and thus of surgeons' accounts of themselves has been written in the light of relations between medicine and surgery in the nineteenth century. More recent work has begun to change the view of the surgical past as merely a rags to riches, barber-surgeon to brain surgeon tale, a view which has eclipsed a possible history of surgery since the Middle Ages as an elite, socially successful, and theoretically informed occupation, often hostile to manual labour. In a revision of the received view of humanist surgery Vivian Nutton has argued that the distinction often (correctly) made by historians between Renaissance physician and surgeon has obscured the common cause of the learned men in these occupations and ignored the principal object of humanist medical polemic: barbers, barber-surgeons and vulgar practitioners.[7] There are certainly plenty of medieval and Renaissance examples to show that some practising surgeons were thoroughly conversant with the theory of medicine and saw themselves as the equals (or better) of physicians. In the early fourteenth century Henri de Mondeville was proclaiming that he was, and any other surgeon should be, an *artifex scientificus*.[8] As part of their claim to eminence medieval surgeons also told stories about themselves which were 'secular parallels' of narratives of miraculous cures.[9] Throughout Europe in the sixteenth century, medical scholars (both physicians and surgeons) found in Galenic tracts with their wealth of surgical learning not an authority for dividing the healing arts but 'a model for the integration of medicine'.[10] The vision of surgery as a learned profession and its enemies being ignorant interlopers rather than physicians can be found in the works of the London surgeons of the period. Thus Thomas Gale in 1563 averred surgery was 'a longe arte, and requireth longe tyme in lernynge, and also exercising: as both the princes of physicke Hippocrates & Galen do testifie'.[11] Gale thanked the physician William Cunnyngham for help in composing his argument and savaged those who 'under the name of chirurgions be nothynge else but open murtherers . . . and rude Empirikes'.[12] Similarly the Paris-trained Scottish surgeon, Peter Lowe, averred, invoking Plato, that there was 'nothing harder than Chirurgie'.[13] It was a learned science and art, of high antiquity, esteemed by all men and yet also practised by deceivers 'with their charmes, heartes full of poison and false promises'.[14] Significantly Lowe was instrumental in the establishment in Glasgow of a Faculty of Physicians *and* Surgeons.[15] Margaret Pelling and Charles Webster have argued that, up until the third quarter of the sixteenth century, these English surgeons viewed the physician as 'their mentor and senior partner'. However, the generation which flowered at the end of the century, and which included William Clowes, George Baker, John Bannister and John Reed, quoted Galen 'to undermine the traditional division between physic and surgery'.[16] Clowes, indeed, argued that surgery had been practised by the great spiritual leaders of antiquity.[17]

In comparison with the relative profusion of elegant, learned and self-assured English surgical texts of the late sixteenth century there is a scarcity of seventeenth-century work and a lack of any consistent account of surgery's place in the healing order.[18] Translation rather than domestic stock was the textual base of English surgery. In both England and France the physician's voice was more prominent. Alexander Read, author of a number of surgical works, was a physician who lectured to the Barber-Surgeons Company. Read's works invoke much the same image of surgery as that of the late sixteenth-century writers: its antiquity, dignity and its great textual tradition. But there was no suggestion of it being united with physic.[19] In the seventeenth century, the accounts which physicians and surgeons gave of each other began to be inflected with the language of experience. In this regard, surgeons (and physicians) began to find in Ambroise Paré the epitome of the surgeon as the experienced practitioner. One of his translators, Thomas Johnson (a physician), noted that Paré was 'well versed in the writings of the antient and moderne physitians, and surgeons', but added 'his experience or practice (the chief help to attaine the highest perfection in this Art) it was wonderfull great'.[20] With Richard Wiseman, writing in the 1670s, the new historical and programmatic possibilities of this view were thoroughly developed. Wiseman argued that his fellow practitioners should compare 'the Empirical part of the Profession with the Rationall', and although not contemptuous of renowned surgical texts, argued that 'judgement and experience' were worth more than the reading of 'eminent chirurgicall Authors' which simply amounted to 'other mens [*sic*] authority'. Progress lay not in scrutinising the ancients but in adding 'Observations to the bulk of what hath been heretofore heaped up'.[21] For the seventeenth-century surgeon, the 'Common Enemy' as Daniel Turner called him remained the unlicensed practitioner.[22] Wiseman's outline of a new historical script for surgery, an independent discipline, growing cumulatively through empirical enquiry, lay relatively unnoticed until it was seized upon by the self-confident English surgical community of the late eighteenth century.

It seems to have been the polemical literature of these surgeons which first identified the early practice of surgery as crude and subservient to physic, a view which permitted them to stress that, within the very recent past, the 'art' of surgery, as they usually called it, had undergone a vast transformation and was now the equal, in status and therapeutic power, of physic.[23] Where Renaissance surgeons found the source of their self-esteem and identity in newly translated ancient texts, English surgeons of the Enlightenment grounded their claims for recognition in their recent empirically acquired knowledge of anatomy, of operative techniques and of instrument design. Improvement was the key word used to describe these changes. In 1750 the London surgeon Samuel Sharp wrote that 'Perhaps there never was a Period of Time in which any Art was more cultivated than Surgery has been for these last thirty years.'[24] Discussing amputation he noted that the disadvantages under which the ancients laboured when amputating 'have been gradually removed by a succession of Improvements'.[25] Similarly, in 1767 Benjamin Gooch, in his *Historical Account of the Rise and Progress of Surgery and Anatomy*, noted how surgery had lately received 'great improvements' mainly because 'Anatomy is more universally known, and better understood' and thus 'the world must consequently have abler Surgeons than in former ages'.[26] In 1789 John Justamond, surgeon to the Westminster Hospital, outlined the history of surgery in a similar manner. He identified its meteoric progress with his own century and reckoned the 'father of surgery in this Kingdom' to be William Cheselden, a man who had died only thirty-seven years previously.[27] The origin of this progress, Justamond observed, lay in the recognition that anatomy and surgery were 'sister arts'. That surgery was empirically based in anatomy did not mean that it was a rule-of-thumb art. Knowledge of anatomy had 'reduced the practice of Surgery as well as Physic to fixed and rational principles'.[28] Similarly Percivall Pott, one of the most cited hospital surgeons of the late eighteenth century, noted 'Many and great are the improvements which the chirurgic art has received within these last fifty years.'[29] The origin of this improvement lay in anatomy, 'which kind of knowledge has been so cultivated in our times as to convert ignorance into a vice'.[30] Ancient surgery, the source of inspiration for late sixteenth-century English surgeons, Pott now perceived as 'coarse' and 'encumbered with a multitude of awkward unmanageable instruments'.[31]

Coupled with the English surgeons' account of the role of empirical discovery in the recent history of their art was their designation of the surgeon's personal attributes. Not surprisingly the emphasis lay on the surgeon's senses. Gooch cited Celsus, on the necessity for 'a strong, steady hand, a clear sight, with calmness and fortitude of mind'.[32] Justamond found the qualities to be 'Youth, firmness, dexterity, acute sensation, sound judgement, and humanity'.[33] The public seemingly shared this image of the good surgeon. Campbell, in his *London Tradesman*, observed that it was vulgarly said that a surgeon should have 'a Lion's heart, a Hawk's eye, and a Lady's Hand'.[34]

During the years of the French wars British surgeons gradually changed the tone of their histories and began to introduce new themes. Whereas the previous generation had written of surgery as equal to but distinct from physic, surgeons now began to write of both physic and surgery as equal branches of a new and wider body of knowledge, identified with experimentally derived physiology and general pathology. In spite of international conflict, British surgeons who had previously applauded the endeavours of their own countrymen, increasingly cited France as having had a more distinguished history of surgery than Britain, and the French government as having an enlightened view of the value of surgeons. Britain, they admitted, remained the home of technical improvement. The French, however, had distinguished their surgeons with the honours due to them, notably creating professorial chairs in the subject. Thus in 1797 the London surgeon Thomas Chevalier noted how it was in emulation of the rank which the French surgeons had achieved during the early eighteenth century that the English surgeons had broken off their 'vile' connection with the barbers in 1745.[35]

Besides this comparison with France there was also a change of emphasis in the surgical histories of these years. Surgeons talked less and less about the 'art' of surgery and increasingly referred instead to what Chevalier called the 'science of surgery'.[36] From the extramural classes of the University of Edinburgh and from the London schools and hospitals, surgeons began to proclaim the existence of a synthetic, new science which embraced both physic and surgery. In his *Lectures on Inflammation*, delivered in Edinburgh in the early nineteenth century, John Thomson, like Chevalier, applauded the institutional progress of surgery in France. Unlike Chevalier, however, Thomson argued that the historical origins of the distinction between surgery and physic demonstrated not that there should be two separate disciplines but that a reconciliation was appropriate. This was necessary, he claimed, because both physic and surgery were based on the same basic science: general pathology.[37] In Edinburgh Thomson drew on a university-generated model of general pathology, that of William Cullen. In London, however, hospital surgeons such as Sir Astley Cooper and John Abernethy turned to the texts and teaching of John Hunter as providing the fundamental science of all rational healing.[38] Hunter self-consciously promoted the view that surgery was a discipline with experimentally generated foundations or 'principles'. Hunter lectured on the 'principles' of surgery, as well as the operations. These physiological principles were used by Hunter to define surgery as a discipline whose proper history had only just begun. Surgery was a procedure in which the operator employed his knowledge of the body's preservative powers to cure disease rather than simply extirpate it. In some instances, as L. S. Jacyna shows here, his use of physiological principles accompanied a change in practice.[39]

During the nineteenth century British surgeons gradually became ambivalent about their eighteenth-century ancestors and their self-styled era of operative and instrumental improvement. On the one hand Victorian surgeons recited their lineage and the advances of the previous century, reeling off the names of Cheselden, Sharp, Pott and Monro. On the other, they began to cut themselves off from their forefathers and endorsed John Hunter's account of himself as having inaugurated an entirely new era in surgical history (Hunter had spurned history as a legitimising resource). What for eighteenth-century surgeons had been a golden age began to become for nineteenth-century surgeons, and for us, 'the age of agony'.[40] Hunter was now the 'father' of a new discipline, 'scientific surgery'. As L. S. Jacyna has shown, however, the scientific surgery of which Hunter was the putative father changed its definition with subsequent generations of surgeons.[41]

During the nineteenth century, histories of surgery written by surgeons and, later, their biographers, exploited new literary resources. Victorian histories of surgery began to use the Romantic language of heroic, individual struggle which had increasingly appeared in the literature of science. The surgical 'genius' made his appearance as a historical figure.[42] These new histories also began to suggest not merely surgery's equality with physic, but its superiority. In this respect the introduction of anaesthesia and Listerian antisepsis were eventually singled out as crucial circumscribed episodes which virtually transformed surgery overnight. It is arguable, however, that it was not until the 1860s that surgeons began creating the introduction of anaesthesia as a significant *historical* moment. Although some surgeons praised the virtues of anaesthesia from the first, other surgeons in the 1850s paid no great attention to it, or merely regarded it as a valuable way of subduing the uncooperative patient. In 1853 James Syme surveyed 'improvements' in surgery over the previous thirty years. First he noted the increasing simplicity of technique in operating and dressing and the current 'confident expectation' of primary healing.[43] Of amputations he noted gratefully that chloroform had abolished the pain but, 'more important', the increasing use of the skinflap technique had vastly increased the success of the operation.[44] Nearly ten years later the Dublin surgeon Maurice Collis identified the 'progress of surgery' with 'advances' in physiology which had led to a 'proportionate increase in our knowledge of the principles on which we must combat disease'.[45] As with Syme, Collis did not draw particular attention to anaesthesia. Indeed, in the case of lithotomy he noted, 'If the chloroform is to be used, the old plan of fastening the hands to the feet must be given up.'[46] By the mid-1860s, surgeons began to make anaesthesia's introduction a heroic landmark. In 1864 William Fergusson, surgeon to King's College Hospital, suggested a history of surgery should be written on the lines of Samuel Smiles's *Lives of the Engineers*. 'Within the present century', he noted, 'volumes might be written.'[47] Like Syme he found few things more remarkable in modern surgery than 'simplicity of appliances and dressings'.[48] However, he also noted that 'nothing . . . has transpired in the present century which, in magnitude or importance, can compare in our annals with anaesthesia'.[49] In the same year the Addenbrooke's surgeon G. M. Humphry declared that surgery had become a 'true science', and he too extolled the discovery of anaesthesia.[50] Humphry declared that chloroform had widened the range of 'tentative and conservative surgery' and he exemplified the treatment of wounds, based on 'a gradual increase of knowledge and an improvement in practice', as one of the great advances made by nineteenth-century surgery.[51] By now the voice of American surgeons began to be heard. In Boston, also in 1864, J. Mason Warren surveyed the previous thirty years which were, he noted, 'ever memorable for great practical inventions and great scientific discoveries'.[52] Within three decades of this an identical language was to be used by surgeons who stigmatized the 1860s as the surgical dark ages and an era of barbaric wound treatment.

By the end of the 1870s surgeons were affirming their superiority over physicians. 'Surgery', George MacLeod, Regius Professor of Surgery at Glasgow, declared in 1877, 'is, I hold, medicine and something more. It is medicine with an additional arm.'[53] Surgeons perceived themselves the equals of, or greater than, physicians, not only in therapeutic power. The American surgeon, J. Ewing Mears, averred that the surgeon had climbed from being 'bleeder and barber' to being 'pathologist [and] diagnostician' and was now 'crowned above all as the refined and cultured gentleman'.[54] We are, the Philadelphia surgeon W. W. Keen noted, 'possibly more than respectable'.[55] The enemy of surgery was no longer intra- or extra-professional competition. It was anything, including religion, which questioned its power and the new god of science. In his *Four Apostles of Surgery*, which extolled science over religion, Macleod condemned the priesthood of the past for obstructing the progress of scientific surgery. Using the language of heroic individual struggle and genius he eulogised the men who had escaped sacerdotal bondage, noting that 'Every great epoch in the history of medicine has been signalised by the advent of a man of genius.' In the past seventy-five years 'our science' had seen 'every department . . . benefited by the light reflected from the collateral branches of medical and other sciences'.[56] He added, 'Of all the improvements or discoveries made, however, one can compare to anaesthetics and antiseptics, which have done more to diminish suffering and save human life than the united inventions of two thousand years.'[57] A similar denunciation of clerical hands in surgical places was made by an American surgeon, George Jackson Fisher, in 1886. He noted, 'During all the ages that the healing art was held and practised by the priest-physicians, its degradation was extreme and disgraceful to the last degree.' Clerics had been guilty of the 'invasion of a profession to which they had no claims and for which they had no scientific affinity or adaptability'.[58] Although surgeons denounced the obstructive force of religion in history they could also represent themselves as the new divine healers (see below).

The last significant element in the creation of the modern account of the history of surgery was the identification of antisepsis as the final breakthrough. Significantly antisepsis was represented not as a corporate achievement but as the heroic discovery of one man, Joseph Lister; the man whose name, as one surgeon explained, it was 'hardly necessary to utter'.[59] Yet, just as surgeons took time to construe and represent anaesthesia as an event which, overnight, transformed the shape and direction of their practice, so too, many years of antiseptic and aseptic experimentation were retrospectively compressed into a brief Listerian revolution. By 1890 the manufacture of this was virtually complete. Surgeons flattened out the brilliant peak of the 1850s from which they once surveyed the benighted past. The bright revolutionary world of mid-century was simply part of the long dismal history of surgical darkness. Deploying the language of victorious generals, surgeons looked only to the 'enormous advances and magnificent triumphs of surgery' during the preceding twenty-five years.[60] When, in 1895, a surgeon compared surgery at the Leeds General Infirmary then with the practices of a quarter-century previously, he found nothing but uninterrupted progress. The primary healing of wounds, which Syme had welcomed as a common occurrence in the 1850s, was now remembered as a rare gratification.[61] In America, in 1904, William Halsted surveyed the 'wondrous period' of the previous thirty years with equal satisfaction.[62]

Serious histories

This version of surgical history was Dennis's simple and grand story of 1904, a story with which many historians in the twentieth century seem to have concurred. Given the major position in modern medicine of surgery, its practice, technology, anatomy and pathology, the serious historical attention which surgery and particularly surgical concepts of disease have received is surprisingly scant. This neglect is obvious both in the older literature on pathological ideas and surgical techniques and, until very recently, in the newer social historical accounts of medicine. This relative dearth of interest in surgical ideas and their relation to practice is very odd since, on a head-counting basis alone, surgical practice of the simplest sort must have been one of the commonest encounters in the history of medicine. For instance, on a day-to-day basis the taking of blood and the dressing of leg ulcers were, as Irvine Loudon has shown, the staple of most eighteenth-century surgical incomes.[63] Surgical texts, particularly medieval ones, have been made visible by bibliophiles, and surgical instruments, notably those of the ancients, have been the subject of a number of monographs.[64] There are, of course, some fine nineteenth-century German studies of surgery.[65] There are also a number of excellent bibliographies, notably that by John Shaw Billings.[66] Aspects of the surgical trade or profession, individual surgeons and surgical institutions have often been investigated. However, first-rate scholarly studies of the substance of surgery and the wider historical issues this raises are less common.

In Britain the origin of this neglect may well have lain with the distinguished physician- and surgeon-historians (such as D'Arcy Power, Clifford Allbutt and William Osler) whose interests encouraged investigation of certain aspects of surgery rather than others. For example, their emphasis on medicine's relation to the humanities generated a number of fine bibliographical studies and their stress on the moral qualities of the physician drew them to biography. In addition, professional interests directed their perceptions to the institutional relations of medicine and surgery in the past. Thus Clifford Allbutt's valuable *The Historical Relation of Medicine and Surgery to the End of the Sixteenth Century* was a description of what he saw as the historical origins of an unfortunate and continuing intellectual separation of two branches of the same tree.[67] Similarly Sir D'Arcy Power's erudite *A Short History of Surgery*, published in 1933, used historical examples to construct an image of the sempiternal surgeon. Henri de Mondeville, wrote Power, switching from past to present tense, 'describes the ideal surgeon' when he says (and the reader needs to bear in mind the surgeons of the great London voluntary hospitals here),

> A surgeon ought to be fairly bold. He should not quarrel before the laity and . . . should not undertake any dangerous operation unless he is sure that it is the only way to avoid a greater danger. His limbs, and especially his hands, should be well-shaped with long, delicate and supple fingers which must not be tremulous. He ought to promise a cure to every patient but should tell the parents or friends if there is any danger. He should refuse as far as possible all difficult cases and never interfere with desperate ones. He may give advice to the poor for the love of God only, but the rich should be made to pay well. He should neither praise himself nor blame others and he

> should not hate any of his colleagues. He ought to sympathise with his patients in their distress and fall in with their lawful requests so far as they do not interfere with the treatment.

Likewise Power invoked Mondeville on the responsibilities of patients and assistants:

> Patients, on the other hand, should obey their surgeon implicitly in everything appertaining to their cure. The surgeon's assistants must be loyal to their master and friendly to his patients. They ought not to tell the patient what the surgeon says unless the news is pleasant and they should always appear cheerful. They should not be constantly grumbling, because this inspires fear and doubt in the patient.[68]

Physicians and surgeons, therefore, have had occasion to investigate the bibliographical and institutional aspects of surgery but rarely the historical construction of surgical knowledge and practice. Curiously, surgeons interested in history have often been overawed by physic. Indeed, one of the greatest surgeons of this century – Harvey Cushing – wrote a best-selling life of the archetypal scholar physician, William Osler.[69] Owen Wangensteen has been one of the few practising surgeons to have persistently examined the social relations of surgical theory and practice.[70] There have been, of course, a small number of useful in-depth technical studies, particularly of the specialities.[71] Studies in this vein, however, very often encompass a vast time span and tendentiously beg the question of whether, say, gynaecology, could have 'a history' before the speciality was created in the nineteenth century.[72] In this particular case Ornella Moscucci has now localised this timeless surgical discipline to a specific historical moment – post-Enlightenment culture.[73] Like speciality histories national histories are not uncommon.[74] Occasionally, as in Ronnie Beth Bush's study of lithotomy in America, national and speciality histories have been successfully blended.[75]

A relative indifference to surgical knowledge and operative practice can also be found among professional medical historians. Where the practice of surgery has been re-evaluated it has been because it has been marginal to other concerns. This has been most noticeable in women's history.[76] We are still very far from what might, paradoxically perhaps, be called an intellectual history of surgical practice. Indeed, surgery remains so far beyond the pale that, in 1983, neither Charles Webster nor Margaret Pelling describe any literature on its history in their essays in *Information Sources in the History of Science and Medicine.*[77] Only Indian surgery in the eighteenth century and surgical instruments appear in the index of this work.

This apparent neglect is surprising considering the possible wider significance of surgery in history. With the increasing acknowledgement by historians of the wider cultural uses of ideas of the body, a bodily representation which is used as the basis of internal, manual intervention in disease seems to cry out for analysis at a deeper level.[78] Two studies have obviously grasped this nettle; Marie Christine Pouchelle's contentious account of Henri de Mondeville and Ludmilla Jordanova's provocative *Sexual Visions.*[79] That the surgical body might have other political meanings besides those of gender is a possibility I shall raise below. The surgical past offers a vast resource to the historian. A detailed history of the theory and practice of, for instance, wound healing and amputation could be used as a means to explore ideas about life, organisation, putrefaction and decay and, in turn perhaps, order and disorder in society.[80] Local versus general pathology offers the opportunity of examining intra-professional relations. More prosaically, biographies of major figures, for example Cheselden, Pott, Liston, Lister, Billroth, could be used to map surgeons on to a wider or different social canvas. Models now exist for this; in the case of William Hunter, Roy Porter has shown how the activities of an eighteenth-century teacher of surgery can be illuminated by turning to the constraints and opportunities of an emerging consumer society.[81]

There is, of course, a continuous history of exceptions to this neglect of the serious study of surgery. The polymathic Leipzig students who trained in the 1920s and 1930s and established history of medicine as an academic discipline in America inevitably, in their global vision of the medical past, took a broad interest in the social relations of surgical ideas. Erwin Ackerknecht's studies in anthropology, to which I shall return, are perhaps the best example of this sort of scholarship. Henry Sigerist produced an edition of a Salernitan text and wrote several articles on surgery. There were some critical pieces too, although his writings on surgery were mostly bibliographical. The theory-bound relations of surgery were not lost on him however.[82] Owsei Temkin, however, remains the most prominent exception to the rule of neglect, for throughout his work problems about the nature of surgery recur, of which more below.

More recently a number of other historians have begun to indicate the ways in which surgical ideas can be fruitfully explored. Vivian Nutton, Margaret Pelling, Jerome J. Bylebyl and Lucinda Beier have illuminated the Renaissance, and the studies of Irvine Loudon, Stephen Jacyna and Russell Maulitz on the years of the French wars have all expanded the horizons of surgical history.[83] Further, work on disciplines pertinent to surgery, notably anatomy, has begun to reassess the meanings of dissection and display in different contexts.[84] In this respect a study of nineteenth-century surgery through an examination of the transition from the teaching of anatomy by systems to teaching by topography would be invaluable.

These promising re-evaluations aside, there is perhaps a further reason why surgery has remained in the twilight of serious scholarship – the practical nature of surgical intervention. Because it is a practice, surgery has been easily accommodated to empirical and positivist philosophies of medical progress. (Or, more subtly, the creators of those philosophies were the intellectual kin of the creators of modern surgery.) Surgery, as John Shaw Billings put it, is an art with 'discoverers, improvers, and inventors'.[85] Historians seem to have been unwilling to question this perception, which represents surgery as having a simple and determined technological history in which human ingenuity is the sole motor of change.[86] Working on these lines, historians have not viewed surgical concepts of disease as puzzling. Anatomy has been taken as an unproblematical given, as has abnormal morphology; the historical problem is how surgeons discovered, improved or invented techniques for extirpation. It might, however, be promising to consider how the knowledge, created by surgeons, of body parts and their diseases, has built into it the possibility, indeed the desirability, of surgical intervention. How, in other words, is surgical knowledge not objective, not the sole possible way of describing the body, but constituted by the goals and interests of the surgeons? New approaches being developed with the history of technology itself might be profitably applied here. For example, how were problems defined or redefined as surgical, and can their solution by one route rather than another be construed in terms of conflict between different communities with differing interests? For instance, can standard surgical operations or instruments be viewed as socially sanctioned compromises between a number of alternative solutions rather than simply the best tools for the job?[87] Detailed historical studies of current conflict, and not simply of the distant past, could be valuable here. How, for example, did modern surgical practitioners construct and maintain polarised positions over the value or otherwise of drainage after cholecystectomy?[88] More broadly the success of surgery as a whole in the nineteenth century can be construed as the attainment of social and institutional power achieved partly by the redefinition of internal disease as a surgical problem. Such an approach might well work at a finer level, in describing, say, competition between radical and conservative treatment for limb injuries. From the new history of technology, but possibly less helpful, also comes the systems approach. Within this view technological success is explained in terms of the triumphant individual or group having successfully manipulated and integrated into a system a range of recalcitrant social, natural and technical factors.[89] Suggestions as to how new approaches might be applied to surgical instruments are explored here by Ghislaine Lawrence.[90]

Surgical practices, it is arguable, are never mere empirical procedures. Even the most simple of them employ a theory of the body and disease, either explicit or implicit. After all, pulling a tooth implies a theory of the local origin of pain and the relative harmlessness of removing a body part. In the Middle Ages some texts emphasised that tooth extraction should be a procedure of last resort.[91] In the eighteenth century physicians considered toothache the result of systemic disorder and the object of general therapy.[92] That the simplest of surgical procedures are complex cultural phenomena was, in many ways, the lesson of Ackerknecht's ethnographical studies of the 1930s and 1940s. In 'Surgery and its paradoxes' Ackerknecht described a number of very familiar forms of manual intervention among non-western peoples justified by what seem to us utterly strange reasons. Likewise, he described the absence of intervention in situations where we might expect that empirically (or even 'naturally') a simple procedure might be used. Further, he showed that in some contexts quite different manual procedures from our own, such as the breaking and binding of the legs of a chicken, might be employed in wound healing. In general, Ackerknecht pointed to the arbitrariness of the term surgery. Many of the peoples he had studied had no such concept. They certainly did not distinguish between manipulative interference with the body which was medical and that which was non-medical.[93]

In spite of such work as this, modern conjectural historians continue attributing universality to complex human actions, discovering twentieth-century therapeutic aims in, for example, neolithic trephination, which is often interpreted as a cure for epilepsy or headache. Naturalising surgery dies hard, as one recent history of medicine demonstrates:

> Primitive medicine-men . . . must have been able to cope with many varieties of injury. Broken bones obviously need straightening and to be held still by splinting and bandaging for the relief of pain. In the 1970s in Australia an Aborigine woman was partially buried in sand to immobilize her broken thigh. It is interesting too that there are many examples of healed fractures in apes, such as gorillas, chimpanzees, orangutans, gibbons, and in monkeys and other animals.[94]

A exemplary corrective to the view that surgery is, by definition, concerned with timeless, life-threatening events is to be found in Margaret Pelling's illuminating study of the barber-surgeons of sixteenth-century London. By paying close attention to the local context Pelling argues that the Tudor identification of ugliness and deformity as mirrors of morals and metaphors of social order shaped the goals and techniques of surgical practice.[95]

Temkin's view

As suggested above, one historian who has consistently worried about the intellectual nature of the object of surgical practice is Owsei Temkin. In a paper published in 1953 Temkin traced a transition in Greek medicine from craft to 'science', which he saw as a move from the use of traditional or unreflexive medical practices to the employment of more explicit theories about the body's function. The shift was effected as Greek physicians drew on the doctrines of contemporary philosophical sects.[96] This was a change which, as Temkin described it, permitted intervention at an individual level rather than formulaic treatment. Following Edelstein, Temkin related this change to the rise of dietetic medicine and the individualisation of Greek life. The result of the change was that 'Greek medicine became split into sects not over preferences for one or the other drug or one or the other surgical technique, but over different explanations of diseases or the very need for such explanations'.[97] The sects, that is, had different ways of individualising the body. Within these different but rational accounts of the body, whether empiric, methodic or dogmatic (including its own sub-sects), surgery had a place, albeit somewhat limited. Surgical practice was not tied to a single account of the body, but was carried out within the framework of a number of rather different medical theories. Surgery, however, was an essential part of medicine; the *medicus* could be referred to as a *chirurgus* while performing a manual operation.[98]

Temkin added an epilogue to his account which was a synopsis of the history of western medicine from Galen to the early sixteenth century:

> By the middle of the fourth century Galen has emerged as the great medical authority next only to Hippocrates, and his true heir. From now on there is only one medical science [dogmatism], based on just those parts of philosophy which Galen accepted. And since, moreover, this science at an increasing rate is acquired from books, the break is prepared between the mere craftsman, the mechanic, and the learned doctor . . . The transmittal of that tradition to the West transformed the physician of 400 B.C. into a physicus in the literal sense, while the craftsman found his own way of life in the guild.[99]

Quite how the creation of surgeon *qua* craftsman and physician *qua* theoretician, and the concurrent designation of surgical diseases as external occurred in the medieval world is a vexed historical question. What was involved was not the separation of a pre-existing manual part of medicine from a theoretical part; no such parts existed. In early twelfth-century treatises, surgery did not comprehend all manual medical acts. Nor did the *physicus* as theoretician exist.[100] Relating these changes to the creation of the medieval universities and the broader currents of medieval economic and social change is, at present, a distant goal.

The surgery of the Middle Ages and Renaissance has been a prime target for bibliophiles and antiquarians and their editions of surgical texts and their researches into the creation and functioning of early medical institutions are invaluable source material. The most notable challenge to conventional views of medieval surgery has been Marie Christine Pouchelle's account of the metaphorical world of the sacred craftsman Henri de Mondeville. In Pouchelle's account the surgeon is metaphorically linked to butchers, executioners and Christ; the body to the political order of society; disease to animality and sin; and dissection is identified as a fundamentally sacrilegious act. The study remains unparalleled and problematic.[101] Elsewhere studies of the uses of surgical ideas in Renaissance and medieval society are few.[102] As Vivian Nutton has described it, 'The modern historiography of renaissance surgery resembles a moral fable concocted out of ignorance and tralatician prejudice.'[103] Nutton's essay also underlines the need for a comparative history of European surgery. Conditions were quite different in different countries. It does seem increasingly clear, however, that nineteenth-century histories, which always invoked surgery's connexions with barbering in order to emphasise its humble origins and to tell a heroic success story, were eclipsing a major part of surgical history. Since the very early Middle Ages there has always been an elite class of highly specialised, theoretically sophisticated and technically accomplished surgical practitioners. Menial activities such as blood-letting may never have been within the orbit of surgeons who belonged to this group.[104]

How the various medical groupings of the Renaissance created and employed disease concepts in their differing social contexts remains largely unexplored.[105] Once again, however, it is Temkin who has shed some light on this darkness, in two essays on syphilis. In these essays he pointed to the social relations of medical and surgical therapy. Temkin claimed that during the Renaissance, barbers, pox-doctors and the humbler surgeons were the healers of the masses, and physicians the therapists of the aristocracy. These humbler surgeons used mercury relatively indiscriminately as a specific and although physicians also used mercury, they tailored their prescriptions to their patients. Temkin then pointed to the social role of such therapy: 'The common people accepted the terror of the mercurial cure as a punishment for their sins. The nobility were less inclined to seek moral improvement from their physicians and preferred a treatment that was less severe.'[106] Physicians used what Temkin, elsewhere, reckoned a physiological or individual concept of disease and surgeons an ontological or disease-entity model.[107]

Temkin drew a broad conclusion from these observations and, as usual, it was an unusual one: 'It is by no means true that treatment is always adapted to the nature of the disease. Treatment can determine how disease should be considered'.[108] The ontological or disease-specific perceptions of surgeons were embodied in their treatment and the physiological perceptions of physicians in theirs. These distinctions were further sanctioned by the familiar division of labour in which diseases treated by surgeons were external and, as one seventeenth-century surgeon put it, 'internal, so far as Hand or Instruments may reach'.[109] It is quite clear, of course, that in many contexts such injunctions did not deter surgeons from dealing with systemic matters on an individual basis. For example, as Lucinda Beier shows, the seventeenth-century surgeon Joseph Binns regularly ministered to the particular and hidden, intangible features of his patients' acknowledged external complaints.[110] Besides this, as Temkin argues, surgeon and physician shared the treatment of many diseases: 'scurvy, diseases of the eyes and ears, skin diseases, and venereal diseases'.[111] To which might be added scrophula, the stone, cancer and toothache. Thus, on different occasions and in different arenas disease could change its character – being predominantly ontological or physiological – according to who treated it and how. Roger French's study of scrophula explores the changing meaning of this term in different contexts.[112]

Renaissance and post-Renaissance surgery, like so many other subjects in the current history of science and medicine, raise the problem of the local and the general. Local studies of surgery in context are badly needed, yet the general question also remains. How, from a diverse past in Europe and America, did modern, relatively uniform, surgical theory and practice arise? In the seventeenth and eighteenth centuries historical scrutiny can exhibit both similarity and difference. In parts of continental Europe, notably Italy and Germany, medicine and surgery still conversed as equals in the universities.[113] At Göttingen, Albrecht von Haller taught anatomy, surgery and medicine from the same chair. In the Netherlands surgery was confined to the guilds but many guild members had medical degrees. In France a dynamic, Paris-centred school grew up and, with its own academic apparatus, controlled surgical teaching and practice. The continuing continental recognition of surgery's historical association with learning was demonstrated by the production of impressive bibliographical surveys of surgical history.[114] In Scotland different relations pertained in different places. In Edinburgh, in the seventeenth century, the city's surgeons, incorporated in a college, displayed a vigorous independence of physic. They valued book-learning and were proud of their all-round skills.[115] During the eighteenth century they had to compete with the rather different account of surgery fashioned by the Monro dynasty ensconced within the town's university. The establishment at the university of a chair of anatomy and surgery, which was successively occupied by three Monros, could be interpreted as a positive valuation of surgery. But, when teaching at least, the Monros employed the physician's stereotypic designation of surgery as a practical art, concerned merely with external disorders.[116] The model seems continental, based on the idea of educated, university teachers, who might be physicians or surgeons, and a lower class of artisans, such as the *feldschers* of German medicine, a class of practitioner in existence until the end of the eighteenth century.[117] As noted above, in England during the seventeenth century surgery appears relatively beleaguered. In the eighteenth century, especially in London, surgeons used the hospitals and private medical schools to make a power base for themselves and created a robust model of surgical individualism as the Company of Surgeons fell into relative decline.

Oddly enough, what might have been the conclusions of Temkin's work on the history of surgery were contained in an early and now much cited paper, 'The role of surgery in the rise of medical thought', a paper which begins to tackle the general issue of the surgeon's success by way of the local French context. In it, Temkin claimed an important role for what he called 'the surgical point of view', an anatomical and local pathological approach to disease, in the rise of modern medicine.[118] Temkin claimed that this view had been gaining ground during the eighteenth century, especially in France, an observation later explored and expanded by Toby Gelfand.[119] Temkin also made a subtle linkage between medical knowledge and medical power. He argued that when, at the end of the eighteenth century, French surgeons gained power and prestige they, and the aspiring physicians they taught, employed the ancient concept of *anatomical* reasoning, coupled with their familiar nosography of external diseases (ontological in Temkin's sense), to explore and give shape to the internal disorders of the body. The intellectual possibilities inherent in ancient medicine had been given social flesh.[120] Temkin's approach suggests that the historian might consider how 'the surgical point of view' was not a timeless, or value-free way of describing the body and disease but a partial or interested perception, which shaped bodily knowledge in a particular way. Temkin argued, however, that there was more to the intellectual invasion of the body by surgeons than the use of local pathology. In Temkin's opinion the surgical point of view was not the only intellectual 'determining factor in the reorientation of medicine'. Chemistry and physiology were important and above all 'localized pathology was in need of general pathology'.[121]

Temkin's observation pointedly raises the issue of the significance of attempts to localise disease in the eighteenth century both through post-mortems and at the bedside. This approach, as Malcolm Nicolson shows here, was not simply confined to surgeons; Morgagni often attempted to identify the physical limits of disorders in the living.[122] It remains debatable, however, whether eighteenth-century localism can be equated with that of the nineteenth century. Eighteenth-century practitioners recognised diseases such as arterial ossification and aneurysm, with their seats in the parts. Yet most diseases, by nature of their history or by good or bad management, could change their bodily site.[123] This rather obvious point has been eloquently laboured by Foucault, who insists that the local pathology of the Paris clinic is epistemically distinct from that of Enlightenment medicine.[124] It is the gulf that separates Morgagni from Bichat, not their proximity, that is striking. For Morgagni, according to Foucault, 'Morbid kinship rested on a principle of organic proximity.' Thus 'asthma, pleuropneumonia, and haemoptysis formed related species in that they were all three localized in the chest'.[125] For Bichat, famously, 'Since every organized tissue has everywhere a general arrangement, and, whatever its situation may be, retains the same structure and properties, &c, its disease must unquestionably be every where the same.'[126] The difference between this and the pathological model employed thirty years earlier by Alexander Monro *secundus* is striking:

> our several organs are supported from, and in a great measure composed of branches of the same hydraulic system, so that a disease primarily influencing a single organ may in various degrees be communicated to others or to the whole.[127]

Historians, while absorbing Foucault, have been relatively loath to address themselves directly to the epistemic issues he raises.[128] None the less, Foucault's claims coincide with Temkin's assertion that a new general pathology was required to make localism of the eighteenth-century sort the basis of a new medicine. More recently Russell Maulitz's work can be read as elaboration of this position. Maulitz has argued that the establishment of Bichat's membrane or tissue pathology was based on its value as intellectual cement to the medical and surgical communities in France, thrown together by the Revolution.[129] Maulitz argues that the membrane pathology employed by early nineteenth-century French physicians and surgeons is not to be construed, as histories of pathology and surgery have often done, as simply a refinement of the organ pathology of the eighteenth century. Echoing Foucault, Maulitz calls this earlier surgical pathology 'natural historical'.[130] Maulitz thus cuts the thread, spun in the nineteenth century and employed by historians of ideas ever since, that provides intellectual continuity between Morgagni and Bichat and between Bichat and Virchow. For different reasons, however, John Pickstone had earlier cut the same thread in a different place, arguing that the epistemological assumptions of Bichat's tissue pathology were fundamentally different from those of Virchow's cell theory.[131] Pickstone seated Bichat firmly back in the Enlightenment where, presumably, he shared his assumptions with Morgagni. It is to be regretted that Maulitz does not address Pickstone's claim.

Resolution of these difficulties must certainly take account of a significant element in the general pathology of the nineteenth century: the view that each and every part of the body, whether tissue or cell, was living. Only when physicians and surgeons used this concept was pathology made synonymous both with altered functioning and, crucially, with the changed appearance of the ultimate units of life itself.[132] A further question now arises: how far were developments elsewhere identical to those in France? In particular, were the intellectual refashionings taking place in London and Edinburgh only superficially similar to those occurring in Paris? At first sight there seem to be great similarities. In both British cities there was a limited coalescence of medicine and surgery. Physicians were proclaiming the value of local pathology and surgeons were showing interest in reshaping theories of general disease.[133] Yet recent work on London suggests that the Channel separated rather different orientations. Maulitz has argued that 'John Hunter folded enough physiological theory into his surgical system to make clear to all professional comers the elevated, esoteric status of surgical science.' Hunter and his work were invoked by his illustrious successors anxious to establish their status as scientific practitioners. Yet that 'did not *necessarily* translate . . . into the further step, taken in France . . . by which surgical theory might methodically be integrated into medical theory.'[134] Maulitz invokes the work of L. S. Jacyna and Susan Lawrence to support this position.[135] In Maulitz's account John Hunter, Matthew Baillie and their circle were eighteenth-century taxonomists and natural historians.[136] Only in the 1830s with the work of, for example, Bright, Hodgkin and Carswell, did French pathology enter English medicine.[137] In Edinburgh, where the tight hold of the grandees of the medical school and the College of Physicians collapsed during the Revolutionary years, French pathology seems to have had an earlier reception. Outsiders, such as John Thomson, who were seeking to create a new general pathology seem to have used French ideas in part to attack the Tory establishment.[138]

The surgeon as democratic hero

The significance of the rise of 'the surgical point of view' is not simply that physicians now viewed internal pathology as local (which is the usual, and perfectly acceptable inference) but that the interior of the body was now a surgical object *in potentia.* Once surgeons had defined the interior of the body as their rightful domain and their social status was assured, practice eventually followed. As noted earlier, surgeons reflecting on this change identified anaesthesia and Listerian antisepsis as the crucial inventions making internal intervention practical. If, however, we abandon the notion of the 'moment of discovery' it becomes possible to jettison the technological determinism inherent in this concept. Sigerist made this point in a curiously teleological way in 1935:

> Surgery became great, not because anesthesia and antisepsis were introduced, but anesthesia and antisepsis were found because surgery was to become great; because surgery was the anatomical method of therapy.[139]

The making of these two innovations into historical landmarks was itself an historical process. It took time for the use of anaesthesia to be created as a monumental surgical event and, as Alison Winter has shown, the introduction of ether in England was closely coupled with attempts to suppress the radical politics of the mesmerists.[140] The little work that has been done on everyday surgery in the 1840s and 1850s suggests that anaesthesia made less impact than is sometimes claimed. Contrary to the usual assertion, it seems that the use of anaesthesia made little or no difference in the short term to the types of operation being performed.[141] Similarly, in spite of claims that anaesthesia made all surgery painless at a stroke, it is certain that, until the twentieth century, many surgeons and general practitioners performing routine minor surgery, for instance tonsillectomy, often did not use anaesthesia at all.[142] In addition, the saltatory history of surgery has usually represented the deep anaesthesia that was attained in the late nineteenth century to have been the norm immediately after 1846. In fact, in the first years after its introduction, most anaesthesia was very light indeed, surgeons being told not to be surprised if patients talked and sang during operations.[143] Further, the whole issue of the cultural meanings of pain, except in relation to anaesthesia and obstetrics, have been little explored.[144] It is salutary to remember that in the Middle Ages, according to one source, the more pain an operator produced, the better surgeon he was considered to be. A similar sentiment was expressed in the late nineteenth century.[145]

Finally, as Martin Pernick has shown, much of the public

prominence of anaesthesia in the 1850s was owing to its place in an ideological conflict. Anaesthesia in childbirth was singled out to champion the cause of secularism, science and progress over superstition, conservatism and religiosity.[146] The battle over anaesthetics was part of that broader struggle in Victorian culture in which teleological and theological accounts were losing ground to the technically rational, and a religious clergy losing social and ideological control to a scientific clerisy. Pain was ceasing to have cosmic significance, it was increasingly construed as a natural (eventually naturally evolved) physiological and pathological mechanism. If it had a purpose it was to teach people, especially poor people, to be grateful to medicine, not God. When the party of technical rationality finally won the ideological battle, anaesthetics became an exemplary statement of its position and power.

It is quite clear that, regardless of its introduction, early nineteenth-century surgeons were expanding their operative skills without the use of an anaesthetic. Many were also developing a brash theatricality which others deplored.[147] During the first half of the nineteenth century surgeons (increasingly including American surgeons) created a range of complicated operations, many of which required a protracted period at the operating bench. These included ligature of major blood vessels, operations on ankylosed joints (including hips), the extension of trepanation to diseases such as epilepsy, amputation in non-life-threatening conditions, excision of diseased bones and joints, excision of the upper or lower jaw, oesophagectomy and amputation of the tongue.[148] Paradoxically, as Gert Brieger shows, surgeons of the time increasingly began to designate their era as one of 'conservative surgery'.[149] Conservative meant, however, not limited surgical intervention, but preservative; an early operation now saved tissue from excision later. A complicated operation of joint resection today saved the patient from heroic amputation tomorrow. The conclusion seems inescapable; early nineteenth-century surgeons were making their assault on the body with or without pain relief or, put less crudely, so great was the determination to invade by the 1840s that, in retrospect, the invention of technologies to facilitate this invasion seems inevitable.

Similarly, it is argued by Lawrence and Dixey that Listerism, like anaesthesia, was made retrospectively into a revolution.[150] The triumphant surgeons of the early twentieth century, the proponents of asepsis (itself a complicated creation), represented Lister's practice, antisepsis, as the progenitor of their aseptic technique. Such an acknowledgement of fatherhood served a number of causes: laboratory science, surgical heroism and individual therapeutic intervention.[151] It also silenced the voices of alternative reform. But Listerism and the possibility of surgical invasion of the body cavities was a construction after the fact. By the 1860s surgeons, notably the ovariotomists, had begun to enter the abdomen. By harnessing a technology of cleanliness, the isolation of the operating field and chemical purification into an integrated system they were able to perform internal surgery. John Erichsen in 1881 saw the origin of this not in Listerism but in obstetrics: 'Surgery is most indebted to obstetricians for great improvements in operative surgery, for it is to them we owe the great precautions which independently of antiseptic or Listerian method, tended to lower the mortality of ordinary surgical cases.'[152] By the 1870s non-Listerians, such as Lawson Tait, had a technology at their disposal which allowed them to remove gall-bladders safely.[153] The germ theory and the creation of Lister as its prophet sanctioned an enterprise that was well underway.

By the 1880s surgeons were developing a variety of measures to make safe the handling of the viscera; antisepsis and asepsis were not determining concepts that carried within themselves clear definitions of operating technology. There were many different types of antiseptic and aseptic routines, many different ways of achieving the desired operative result. The modern aseptic ritual and the modern image of surgery were only created slowly, as surgeons began to perceive themselves 'apart from and above' their colleagues, as Dennis put it.[154] Frederick Treves, an antiseptic surgeon, identified what he regarded as this undesirable process in 1896:

> In this practical country we have been fortunately spared the extravagances which have brought certain Continental operating theatres into ridicule. Those who come after us will read with interest of the operating theatre built like a diving tank, of the glass table for the patient, of the exquisite ceremonial of washing on the part of the operator, of the rites attending the ostentatious cleansing of the patient, of the surgeon in his robes of white mackintosh and his india-rubber fishing boots, and

> of the onlookers beyond the pale who are excluded with infinite solicitude, from the sacred circle as septic outlaws. This exhibition may be scientific, but it is no part of surgery.[155]

In fact it was Treves, still operating in conditions resembling those of a domestic setting, who was becoming the anachronism. The quote, however, serves to make the point that the apparent simple functionalism of, for example, surgical clothing, theatre architecture and operative ritual was not determined by germ theory. This is an explanation, however, which historians seem to have found unproblematical.[156] In the light of the recognition that the operating practices of modern surgery were contingent on, but not determined by, the germ theory, the historian needs to ask how the surgical community came to perceive (in all senses, including the literal) itself as different and how those perceptions were transformed into a new model of practice.[157]

Courting their various versions of sterility, by the late nineteenth century surgeons had entered the body with a vengeance. The rise of surgery was the rise of the surgical point of view, the disease-specific view, which was, as Temkin suggested in at least two contexts, associated historically with practice among the many, not the few.[158] If physic had once been the medicine of aristocracy, surgery had become the medicine of democracy. The surgical concept of disease, in this sense, was democratic and indeed the organisation of surgery itself was, as Treves described it, 'an earnest democracy . . . precisely in accord with the spirit of the times'.[159] Yet, also in accord with 'the spirit of the times', surgeons were heroes, models of the Victorian cult of manliness, possessing the Carlylean virtues singled out in *Past and Present* as 'sheer obstinate toughness of muscles and much more what we call toughness of heart'. This modelling of surgery as democratic heroism, Elizabeth Johns has suggested, lay with the men who, in the Revolutionary years, created surgery as a medicine of the interior: 'French surgeons put themselves forward . . . as the very embodiment of Enlightenment values and egalitarian opportunities taken seriously – as heroes of modern life'.[160] Americans who flocked to Paris to learn surgery in the 1830s took this model home. They admired men who, like Velpeau, who had climbed from humble origins to the peak of their profession and cited them as examples of talent and industry justly rewarded.[161] Historically, Paré, who 'began life as a humble barber-surgeon, and ended as the greatest surgical authority in Europe', was chosen to exemplify similar virtues.[162] In Thomas Eakins's 'The Gross Clinic' the surgeon is both solid democratic citizen and singular hero.[163] Courage ('the courage to fail') was the virtue most frequently ascribed to these 'daring and brilliant' operators.[164] Surgeons, said William Keen, were a 'noble array of generous men battling for life . . . [a] serried phalanx of unselfish heroes'. But surgeons were also a secular priesthood, they were the humble inheritors of Christ's healing mission:

> [It is] the province of the surgeon, in imitation of Him who went about doing good, to restore to health and happiness. Even where life can not be prolonged, the agonies of death itself can be soothed by his gentle hand and his fruitful skill.

Keen was not afraid to draw the appropriate conclusion. The end of the nineteenth century 'vouchsafed . . . magical nay . . . almost divine power to the modern surgeon'.[165] By 1900 the theatricalism which had been observed at operations in the 1850s had been replaced by a hushed ritual. Surgical intervention could be viewed as a sacred event. The British surgeon, Berkeley Moynihan, was said to have approached every operation as a 'religious rite or sacrament'.[166]

Not surprisingly, perhaps, the ascribing of democratic and heroic virtues to surgeons and surgery was most evident in America. By the 1870s American surgeons, who had long depended on foreign tutelage and texts, began to extol their national products. 'American surgical literature', Richard J. Levis announced in 1888, 'is entitled to our almost exclusive patronage'. It was simply 'prejudice' on the part of American medical colleges to 'recommend works of foreign origin'.[167] The American instrument making company, George Tiemann and Co., prefaced its first catalogue of 1872 with the note that 'most of the instruments represented are American *improvements*, very many of them *American inventions*, and all of them modern'.[168] Frederick Dennis, after extolling the role of surgery in the making of modernity, turned his attention to America's 'illustrious height in the surgical world'. Dennis equated America's political power with her surgical power:

> It goes without saying, gentlemen, that within the past decade, America, without any effort of her own, without the least self-seeking, but through the force of her national greatness – moral, intellectual, physical – has come to the front as a world power among the nations of the earth. She now ranks second to none as an important and controlling factor in the congress of nations, and when she speaks, her voice commands the attention of a listening world. In this regard her science of surgery has kept even pace with her political advancement upon the powers. At the present time her surgeons are not outclassed by those of any other country, while in her contributions to the general literature of surgery, she stands unsurpassed.[169]

American surgeons were taking revenge for Sydney Smith's famous jibe in the Edinburgh Review of 1820, 'In the four quarters of the globe, who reads an American book? or goes to an American play? or looks at an American picture or statue? What does the world yet owe to American Physicians or Surgeons?'[170]

That surgery was celebrated as a great American triumph is hardly surprising, for it was invested with all those qualities which Americans were celebrating in themselves. If, in Europe, the surgeon's identity was akin to that of the imperial explorer, in America his cognate was the frontiersman. American surgical writing of this time employed many of the themes, assumptions and metaphors found in contemporary celebrations of democracy, of which the most famous was Frederick Jackson Turner's frontier hypothesis. Turner's works celebrated the rise of what he perceived as individualism, a vigorous, healthy democracy and the end of the 'reign of Aristocracy'. For Turner democracy, although analysable as an 'absolute system' in political thought, was very much a product of the particular 'conditions and forces' of time and place.[171]

The source of American democracy for Turner was the frontier encounter, 'the meeting point between savagery and civilization'.[172] American surgeons, too, saw their theory and practices as democratic, the product of their ongoing intervention. As William Keen put it in 1897,

> Surgery is one and the same the world over. Whether in the frozen north or under the equator, in civilised America or

> barbaric Africa, be the patient white Caucasian, swarthy Negro, red Indian or yellow Malay, the same accidents and diseases assail him, the same remedies save him, identical operations cure him; a new remedy discovered in Japan is equally efficacious in Philadelphia; a new operation devised in America is equally applicable in Egypt.[173]

The source of this surgical democracy was the frontier of the body where, surgeons declared, darkness was giving way to light and civilisation was taming the 'primary terrors' of pain and suffering. In the body surgeons had 'conquered' the 'inaccessible'.[174] For Turner American democracy had been produced by 'frontier individualism' and, in turn, it was to the frontier the American intellect owed its characteristics which Turner described as follows:

> That coarseness and strength combined with acuteness and inquisitiveness; that practical, inventive turn of mind, quick to find expedients; that masterful grasp of material things, lacking in the artistic but powerful to effect great ends; that restless, nervous energy; that dominant individualism, working for good and for evil, and withal that buoyancy and exuberance which comes with freedom – these are traits of the frontier.[175]

Likewise cultured east-coast surgeons found the virtues of American surgeons were those same rugged virtues which had made America. As Dennis put it,

> There is no science that calls for greater fearlessness, courage, and nerve than that of surgery, none that demands more of self-reliance, principle, independence and the determination in the man. These were the characteristics which were chiefly conspicuous in the early settlers of this country. And it is these old-time Puritan qualities, which, descending to them in succeeding generations, have passed into surgeons of America, giving them boldness in their art, and enabling them to win that success in surgery, which now commands the admiration of the civilized world.[176]

The surgeon's explanation for the rise of American surgery was inherited by the historians. Sigerist observed in 1934, 'the technical skill of Americans made them especially fitted to be surgeons'.[177]

At times in the late nineteenth century the frontier and the west were the source of explicit metaphors for surgeons. As the Philadelphia operator Richard Levis observed,

> It is said that the ploughman, tilling the fields of the western slope of our continent, who keeps his eyes intently on the furrow, may occasionally find nuggets of gold; and so the faithful toiler amidst human ills is liable to unearth jewels of fact, which, garnered and recorded, will add to the wealth of surgical knowledge.[178]

These similarities between the language of the frontier and the language of surgery were sustained by investing both surgery and American life with a number of virtues. The surgical body and the west were also related in another way. In 1959 Henry Nash Smith asked an interesting question of the following passage in Turner's work:

> Into this vast shaggy continent of ours poured the first feeble tide of European settlement. European men, institutions, and ideas were lodged in the American wilderness, and this great American West took them to her bosom . . . and ever as society on her eastern border grew . . . she [the West] opened new provinces, and dowered new democracies in her most distant domains with her material treasures.[179]

Of this Smith asked, 'Is it wholly meaningless, for example, that the West, the region close to nature, is feminine, while the East, with its remoteness from nature and its propensity for aping Europe, is neuter?'[180] Not neuter, but masculine; the language of late nineteenth century surgery and the language of the frontier are replete with gendered associations of power, penetration and pleasure; of nature being unveiled, revealed, known and conquered. A culturally specific, gendered account of nature and, by extension, the surgical body permeates these two discourses.[181]

From being the treatment of last resort surgery was establishing itself as the therapy of choice. Perhaps more than any other group of healers it was surgeons who identified medical progress, overwhelmingly, with intervention at the individual level. In surgery the fiction that medicine had nothing to do with politics reached its purest expression. Surgical intervention could be represented as the inevitable, scientific solution to disease, in comparison to which alternative solutions seemed inferior. In 1917 for instance Rickman Godlee looking back to the continental solution to the 'hospitalism' of the 1870s – the building of countryside hospitals – remarked that such institutions were

> needlessly extravagant . . . They still stand as an outward and visible sign of the stages by which scientific thought advances, but they are no more healthy than many an old hospital that escaped the pick, but set its house in order by revolutionizing treatment.[182]

The generation of surgeons which flourished around the Edwardian era changed public perceptions about what was possible or desirable with regard to the treatment of disease. Halsted, Billroth, Horsley and a galaxy of other famous names created a new, radical surgery which was seen as the ultimate conservative treatment. Massive dissections for breast and neck cancer, thyroid extirpation, prostatectomy and herniorrhaphy were now deemed more likely than any alternatives to conserve the patient's life. Like their predecessors this generation also represented themselves as the first to practise surgery as a true science. Watson Cheyne identified their era as that of the 'scientific surgeon' and the foregoing one as that of the 'practical surgeon'.[183]

Even if many of the generation before Cheyne would have been surprised to hear that they were not scientific there were differences. The science of the Edwardian surgeons was not simply that of the surgeons themselves. It was the science of, for example, the physiologist and the bacteriologist and it was a science generated in a new area, the laboratory. It was also different in content; it was overwhelmingly experimental. Experimental or physiological surgery, as it was also called, introduced a new dimension to surgical practice. With the exception of dissection and the practising of operations on corpses the new sciences were the first disciplines to attack surgical problems away from the operating table. Shock was one of the first problems to fall to this new approach.[184] The establishment of scientific surgery in the Edwardian era, however, must not be overstated. Many surgeons continued to hold that their clinical judgements, and not the pronouncements of laboratory scientists, were the ultimate arbiters of practice.[185] Only, perhaps, when surgeons were sure that laboratory science was subservient to surgery was that science designated the basis of surgical practice. Professional scientists could, after all, have a totally different perspective on the object of surgical attention. As Lindsay Granshaw shows, rectal anatomy looked different to pedagogical anatomists from how it looked to surgeons.[186] Similarly, anaesthetists could find laboratory experiments less relevant to their discipline than others suggested they were.[187]

As the whole history of surgery demonstrates, making a part of the body into a surgical object was a long, piecemeal process. The twentieth century has witnessed a continuation, and to some extent an acceleration of this process. The rise of cardiovascular surgery is often described as though the only obstacles to operating on the heart were technical.[188] I have argued elsewhere, however, that during the first decades of this century a generation of self-styled 'new cardiologists' created an account of the heart in which its mechanical deformities were usually considered relatively unimportant and not the proper object of therapy.[189] The cardiologists themselves recognised that this made the heart an inappropriate object of surgical intervention.[190]

Such intellectual obstacles to heart surgery were eventually overcome as were similar obstacles obstructing the surgical assault on a whole range of other anatomical elements. Indeed lobotomy demonstrated that the mind itself was not, in certain respects, beyond falling within the 'surgical point of view'. More recently, however, there has been some questioning of whether, in certain contexts, the breast, the uterus and other body parts are appropriately considered as surgical objects. Such questioning usually employs a local comparative therapeutic framework; for instance it denies that surgery has any effect on mortality in breast cancer, or argues that hysterectomy does more psychological harm than good in menorrhagia. A more historically informed questioning, however, might provoke a different query. What is the relation between the rise of surgery and the constitution of the body as an array of objects of surgical knowledge? After all the *way* in which we know the body in western medicine to a great extent implies the possibility of surgical intervention. Surgical practice is not simply the result of bodily knowledge. Bodily knowledge made by surgeons has built into it the possibility of surgical practice.

Acknowledgements

I should like to thank Jerome Bylebyl, Bill Bynum, Cathy Crawford, Russell Maulitz, Vivian Nutton, John Pickstone and Roy Porter for their comments on an earlier draft of this paper.

Notes and references

1. Henry E. Sigerist, 'Surgery at the time of the introduction of antisepsis', *Journal of the Missouri State Medical Assocation*, vol. 32 (1935), pp. 169–76: 171.

2. F. S. Dennis, *The History and Development of Surgery during the Past Century* (Philadelphia, 1905), p. 2 (repr. from *American Medicine*, vol. 9 (1905), pp. 139–46, 181–7, 227–34, 265–71).

3. *Chambers's Encyclopaedia* of 1901 described surgery's 'present position [as] one of the greatest triumphs of human intellect, energy and resource', vol. 9, p. 819.

4. Stephen Trombley, *Sir Frederick Treves: the Extra-Ordinary Edwardian* (Routledge, London, 1989), p. 86.

5. Rickman John Godlee, *Lord Lister* (Macmillan, London, 1917), p. 593.

6. Renée C. Fox and Judith P. Swazey, *The Courage to Fail: A Social View of Organ Transplants and Dialysis* (The University of Chicago Press, Chicago, 1974). The short title of Fox and Swazey's sensitive study was used in a popular television series on the history of surgery first screened in 1988. Fox and Swazey intended their title to apply to both patients and surgeons. See also Guy R. Williams, *The Age of Miracles: Medicine and Surgery in the Nineteenth Century* (Constable, London, 1981).

7. V. Nutton, 'Humanist surgery', in A. Wear, R. K. French and I. M. Lonie (eds), *The Medical Renaissance of the Sixteenth Century* (Cambridge University Press, Cambridge, 1985), pp. 75–99.

8. Marie Christine Pouchelle, *The Body and Surgery in the Middle Ages*, translated by Rosemary Morris (Rutgers University Press, New Brunswick, N.J., 1990), p. 15.

9. Nancy Siraisi, *Medieval and Early Renaissance Medicine* (University of Chicago Press, Chicago, 1990), p. 171.

10. Nutton, 'Humanist surgery', p. 79.

11. Thomas Gale, *Certaine Workes of Chirurgerie Newly Compiled and Published* (Thomas Gale, London, 1563), Salutations.

12. Ibid., p. 8. In particular: 'hosiers, taylours, fletchers, mynstrelles, souters, horsheches, juglers, wiches, sorcerers, baudes!'

Cunningham (or Keningham) was admitted MB at Cambridge and created MD at Heidelberg. He was appointed public lecturer at Surgeons' Hall in 1563. See *Dictionary of National Biography.*

13. Peter Lowe, *A Discourse of the Whole Art of Chirurgerie,* 2nd edn (Thomas Purfoot, London, 1612), p. 3.

14. Ibid.

15. A College of Physicians and Surgeons briefly existed in London in 1423–4. Sidney Young, *The Annals of the Barber-Surgeons of London* (Blades, East & Blades, London, 1890), p. 42; Jessie Dobson, *Barbers and Barber-Surgeons of London* (Blackwell Scientific Publications, Oxford, 1979), pp. 25–8.

16. Margaret Pelling and Charles Webster, 'Medical practitioners', in Charles Webster (ed.), *Health, Medicine and Mortality in the Sixteenth Century* (Cambridge University Press, Cambridge, 1979), pp. 165–235: 177.

17. Nutton, 'Humanist surgery', p. 98; on Clowes see Margaret Pelling, 'Appearance and reality: barber-surgeons, the body and disease', in A. L. Beir and Roger Finlay (eds), *London 1500–1700: the Making of the Metropolis* (Longman, London, 1985), pp. 82–112.

18. John Woodall's text was aimed only at surgeon's mates and gives no account of the place of surgery in the healing order. John Woodall, *The Surgions Mate* (Edward Griffin for Laurence Lisle, London, 1617). The relative paucity of seventeenth-century English surgical treatises can be gauged from Leo M. Zimmerman, 'Surgery' in Allen G. Debus (ed.), *Medicine in Seventeenth Century England* (University of California Press, Berkeley, 1974), pp. 49–69.

19. Read, however, still perceived a danger to surgery to lie among 'empirical knaves, filthy bauds and bold queanes'. Alexander Read, *The Works,* 2nd edn (Richard Thrale, London, 1650), p. 7.

20. Ambroise Paré, *The Workes,* translated by Thomas Johnson (T. Cotes & R. Young, London, 1634), To the Reader.

21. Richard Wiseman, *Severall Chirurgicall Treatises* (R. Royston, London, 1676), Epistle to the Reader.

22. Daniel Turner, *Apologica Chyrirgica. A Vindication of the Noble Art of Chyrurgery from the Gross Abuses Offer'd thereunto by Montebanks, Quacks; Barbers, Pretending Bone-setters, etc.* (J. Whitlook, London, 1695), p. 25. I am grateful to Philip Wilson for this reference.

23. Physicians did not necessarily concur, nor did laymen. In his review of London trades Campbell noted surgery as the second branch of the Medical Art, 'very little inferior to the first in point of Utility, but founded upon Principles much more certain'. R. Campbell, *The London Tradesman* (London, [1747], reprinted by David & Charles, London 1969), see p. 47.

24. Samuel Sharp, *A Critical Enquiry into the Present State of Surgery,* 2nd edn (J. & R. Tonson, London, 1750), Preface.

25. Ibid., p. 264.

26. Benjamin Gooch, *A Practical Treatise on Wounds and other Chirurgical Subjects to which is Prefixed a Short Historical Account of the Rise and Progress of Surgery and Anatomy,* 3 vols. (Printed for the author by W. Chase, Norwich, 1767), vol. 1, p. 62. This same argument was used by

London physicians who regarded the surgeons as allies in the fight against the privileges of the Royal College of Physicians. William Black, for instance, was a licentiate of the College, and his *Historical Sketch of Medicine and Surgery* was devoted to attacking the 'monkish abuse' whereby the Fellows had turned the College into 'a very small club'. Of the surgeons, he noted the 'great superiority of the moderns above the ancients' which was the consequence of 'the knowledge of Anatomy; and the superiority . . . in the construction and workmanship of their instruments', two factors which necessarily 'render all their operations much more safe and prosperous'. William Black, *An Historical Sketch of Medicine and Surgery* (J. Johnson, London, 1782), pp. 162, 293. Physicians did not necessarily concur. On the subservience of surgery and its place as a manual skill see John Gregory, *Lectures on the Duties and Qualifications of a Physician* (W. Strahan & T. Cadell, London, 1772), p. 47.

27. J. O. Justamond, *Surgical Tracts Consisting of 1. Outlines of the History of Surgery* (T. Cadell, London, 1789), p. 49.

28. Ibid., p. 52. Anatomy in this context is best understood as animated or functional.

29. Percival Pott, *The Chirurgical Works*, 3 vols. (J. Johnson, London, 1790), vol. 3, p. 209.

30. Ibid., vol. 2, p. 5.

31. Ibid.

32. Gooch, *Treatise*, p. xv.

33. Justamond, *Surgical Tracts*, p. 54.

34. Campbell, *Tradesmen*, p. 47.

35. Thomas Chevalier, *Observations in Defence of a Bill . . . Including a History of Surgery in England* (J. Johnson & J. Debrett, London, 1797), p. 52. French surgery had been approvingly cited earlier, but not to the disparagement of British surgery: see Gooch, *Treatise*; Sharp, *Critical Enquiry*.

36. Chevalier, *Observations*, p. 32. It was not new to call it a science. The emphasis was changing: 'Some call *Surgery* a *Science* others an *Art*', Laurence [*sic*] Heister, *A General System of Surgery . . . Translated from the Author's Last Edition*, 7th edn (J. Clarke, London, 1763), p. 2, would have been unremarkable to English readers.

37. John Thomson, *Lectures on Inflammation* (William Blackwood, Edinburgh, 1813), ch. 1, 'On the division of medicine into physic and surgery – history of the origin of this division'.

38. Robert Lee Kilpatrick, 'Nature's schools: the Hunterian revolution in London hospital medicine 1780–1825', unpublished PhD thesis, Cambridge University, 1988.

39. L. S. Jacyna, this volume. See also G. Lawrence, this volume. Heister, *General System*, observed that the 'science' of surgery or 'medical surgery' comprehended the 'Rules . . . which teach the best methods of treating disorders', p. 3. Hunter presented his 'principles' as something quite different.

40. Guy R. Williams, *The Age of Agony: the Art of Healing c. 1700–1800* (Constable, London, 1975).

41. L. S. Jacyna, 'Images of John Hunter in the nineteenth century', *History of Science*, vol. 21 (1983), pp. 85–108.

42. On romanticism and the scientific genius see Simon Schaffer, 'Genius in romantic natural philosophy', in A. Cunningham and N. Jardine (eds), *Romanticism and the Sciences* (Cambridge University Press, Cambridge, 1990) pp. 82–98; Ludmilla Jordanova, *Sexual Visions: Images of Gender in Science and Medicine between the Eighteenth and the Twentieth Centuries* (Harvester Wheatsheaf, New York, 1989), pp. 74–5.

43. James Syme, *On the Improvements which have been Introduced into the Practice of Surgery in Great Britain within the Last Thirty Years*, p. 3. (reprinted from *The Monthly Journal of Medical Science*, April 1853).

44. Ibid., p. 4.

45. Maurice Henry Collis, *Retrospect of the Progress of Surgery during the Last Decade* (Fannin & Co., Dublin, 1862), p. 3 (reprinted from the *Dublin Quarterly Journal of Medical Science*, May 1862).

46. Ibid, p. 36.

47. William Fergusson, 'A course of lectures on the progress of anatomy and surgery during the present century', *The Lancet*, vol. ii (1864), p. 662.

48. Ibid., p. 663.

49. Ibid., p. 665.

50. G. M. Humphry, 'Address on surgery', *The Lancet*, vol. ii (1864), p. 142.

51. Ibid., p. 143.

52. J. Mason Warren, *Recent Progress in Surgery* (Boston, 1864), p. 4.

53. George MacLeod, *The Four Apostles of Surgery: an Historical Sketch* (Glasgow University Press, Glasgow, 1877), p. 4.

54. J. Ewing Mears, *The Evolution of Surgery* (W. J. Dornan, Philadelphia, 1904), p. 16. See 'refined and cultured' also as the ideal in S. D. Gross, 'A century of American medicine 1776–1878. II–Surgery', *American Journal of Medical Science*, n.s., part 71 (1876), p. 431.

55. William W. Keen, 'Address in surgery', *Journal of the American Medical Association*, vol. 28 (1897), pp. 1102–10.

56. Macleod, *Four Apostles*, pp. 5, 34–5.

57. Ibid., p. 35. Surgeons may sometimes have stretched public credibility in their efforts to link their practice to basic science. In 1877 the President of the Royal College of Surgeons in Ireland called attention to experimental physiology as the cornerstone of the surgical revolution, and he noted, 'First, as regards anaesthetics, I may observe that chloroform was in fact discovered through experimentation on a low form of animal – the ant.' Robert McDonnell, *What has Experimental Physiology done for the Advancement of the Practice of Surgery?* (Fannin & Co., Dublin, 1878), p. 13.

58. George Jackson Fisher, 'A history of surgery', in John Ashhurst, *The International Encyclopedia of Surgery*, 7 vols. (Macmillan & Co., London, 1886), vol. 6, p. 1181.

59. William Anderson, *Introductory Address Delivered at St. Thomas's Hospital* (Adlard & Son, London, 1889), p. 35 (reprinted from *St. Thomas's Hospital Reports*, vol. 18).

60. Nelson C. Dobson, *Some Advances in Modern Surgery* (1894?), p. 4.

61. A. W. Mayo Robson, 'An address on the surgery of to-day as compared with that of twenty-five years ago', *The Lancet*, vol. ii (1895), p. 1095.

62. William Stewart Halsted,'The training of the surgeon', *Bulletin of the Johns Hopkins Hospital*, vol. 15, no. 162 (1904), p. 267.

63. I. S. L. Loudon, 'Leg ulcers in the eighteenth and early nineteenth centuries', *Journal of the Royal College of General Practitioners*, part I, vol. 31 (1981), pp. 263–73, part II, 'Treatment', vol. 32 (1982), pp. 301–9. See also the study by Robert Jütte, 'A seventeenth-century German barber-surgeon and his patients', *Medical History*, vol. 33 (1989), pp. 184–98.

64. See for example John Stewart Milne, *Surgical Instruments in Greek and Roman Times* (Clarendon Press, Oxford, 1907); Vilhelm Møller-Christensen, *The History of the Forceps* (Levin & Munksgaard, Copenhagen, 1938).

65. Notably Ernst Julius Gurlt, *Geschichte der Chirurgie und ihrer Ausübung*, 3 vols. (A. Hirschwald, Berlin, 1898), a history of surgery to the end of the sixteenth century (reprinted 1964). For other studies see Leslie T. Morton, *A Medical Bibliography*, 4th edn (Gower, Aldershot, 1983), pp. 789–92.

66. John Shaw Billings, 'The history and literature of surgery', in Frederick S. Dennis (ed.), *System of Surgery* (Lea Brothers, Philadelphia, 1895), vol. 1 (reprinted Argosy, New York, 1970).

67. T. C. Allbutt, *The Historical Relation of Medicine and Surgery to the End of the Sixteenth Century* (Macmillan, London, 1905). The insight into Allbutt's aim can be found in Owsei Temkin, 'The role of surgery in the rise of modern medical thought', *Bulletin of the History of Medicine*, vol. 25 (1951), p. 248. Usefully found in Owsei Temkin, *The Double Face of Janus and other Essays in the History of Medicine* (Johns Hopkins University Press, Baltimore, 1977), pp. 487–96. There is a valuable study of this generation of physician historians by Charles Webster, 'Medicine as social history: changing ideas on doctors and patients in the age of Shakespeare', in Lloyd S. Stevenson (ed.), *A Celebration of Medical History* (Johns Hopkins University Press, Baltimore, 1982), pp. 103–26.

68. Sir D'Arcy Power, *A Short History of Surgery* (John Bale, London, 1933), pp. 18–19. Power's essays are full of rewards for the historian of surgery. See those collected in *Selected Writings 1877–1930* (Clarendon Press, Oxford, 1931) which also contains a complete bibliography.

69. Harvey Cushing, *The Life of William Osler*, 2 vols (Clarendon Press, Oxford, 1925).

70. Owen H. and Sara D. Wangensteen, *The Rise of Surgery* (Dawson, Folkestone, 1975). For Owen Wangensteen's papers see the bibliography.

71. Two useful specialist studies are Lew A. Hochberg, *Thoracic Surgery before the Twentieth Century* (Vantage Press, New York, 1960); Richard H. Meade, *A History of Thoracic Surgery* (Charles C. Thomas, Springfield, Ill., 1961).

72. For example, W. J. Stewart McKay, *The History of Ancient Gynaecology* (Ballière, Tindall & Cox, London, 1901).

73. Ornella Moscucci, *The Science of Woman* (Cambridge University Press, Cambridge, 1990).

74. On America see the very useful bibliographical/historical work by Ira M. Rutkow, *The History of Surgery in the United States* (Norman Publishing, San Francisco, 1988). See also the useful Mark M. Ravitch, *A Century of Surgery: the History of the American Surgical Association*, 2 vols. (J. B. Lippincott Co., Philadelphia, 1981).

75. Ronnie Beth Bush, *Lithotomy, its Practice and Practitioners in Philadelphia during the Colonial and Early Republican Period*, unpublished PhD thesis (University Microfilms International, Ann Arbor, Michigan, 1976).

76. See for example G. Barker-Benfield, *The Horrors of the Half-Known Life* (Harper Colophon, New York, 1976); Elaine Showalter, *The Female Malady: Women, Madness, and English Culture, 1830–1980* (Pantheon, New York, 1985), esp. pp. 74–98; Moscucci, *Science of Woman*; see Jordanova, *Sexual Visions*, for a feminist account of the gendered nature of surgical practice.

77. Charles Webster, 'The historiography of medicine'; Margaret Pelling, 'Medicine since 1500', in Pietro Corsi and Paul Weindling (eds), *Information Sources in the History of Science and Medicine* (Butterworth Scientific, London, 1983), pp. 29–43, 116–33.

78. For an important study of medicine and the body see Dorinda Outram, *The Body and the French Revolution* (Yale University Press, New Haven, Conn., 1989). Outram's account does not deal with surgery in detail.

79. Pouchelle, *Body and Surgery*; Jordanova, *Sexual Visions*, p. 104.

80. Allen O. Whipple, *The Story of Wound Healing and Repair* (Charles C. Thomas, Springfield, Ill. [1956]) is an older history unredeemed by anything. Much more thorough, but equally presentist in its interpretation is Guido Majno, *The Healing Hand: Man and Wound in the Ancient World* (Harvard University Press, Cambridge, Mass., 1975). For a suggestive study relating theories of the social order and accounts of bodily decay see John V. Pickstone, 'Ferriar's fever to Kay's cholera: disease and social structure in Cottonopolis', *History of Science*, vol. 22 (1984), pp. 401–19.

81. Roy Porter, 'William Hunter: a surgeon and a gentleman', in W. F. Bynum and Roy Porter (eds), *William Hunter and the Eighteenth-Century Medical World* (Cambridge University Press, Cambridge, 1985), pp. 7–34.

82. For this last point see Sigerist, 'Surgery'. See also Genevieve Miller (ed.), *A Bibliography of the Writings of Henry E. Sigerist* (McGill University Press, Montreal, 1966).

83. Nutton, 'Humanist surgery'; M. Pelling, 'Occupational diversity: barber-surgeons and the trades of Norwich, 1550–1640', *Bulletin of the History of Medicine*, vol. 56 (1982), pp. 484–511; Pelling, 'Appearance and reality'; M. Pelling and C. Webster, 'Medical practitioners'; Jerome J. Bylebyl, 'The School of Padua: humanistic medicine in the sixteenth century', in Webster, *Health, Medicine and Mortality*, pp. 335–370; Lucinda Beier, *Sufferers and Healers: the Experience of Illness in Seventeenth Century England* (Routledge & Kegan

Paul, London, 1987) and this volume; Irvine Loudon, *Medical Care and the General Practitioner 1750–1850* (Clarendon Press, Oxford, 1986); Russell C. Maulitz, *Morbid Appearances: the Anatomy of Pathology in the Early Nineteenth Century* (Cambridge University Press, Cambridge, 1987); L. S. Jacyna, 'Au lit des malades: A. F. Chomel's clinic at the Charité, 1828–9', *Medical History*, vol. 33 (1989) pp. 420–49; *A Tale of Three Cities: the Correspondence of Allen Thomson and William Sharpey*, *Medical History*, Supplement 9 (1989). On the more recent surgical past see Roger Cooter, 'The meaning of fractures: orthopaedics and the reform of British hospitals in the inter-war period', *Medical History*, vol. 31 (1987), pp. 306–32; L. S. Jacyna, 'The laboratory and the clinic: the impact of pathology on surgical diagnosis in the Glasgow Western Infirmary, 1875–1910', *Bulletin of the History of Medicine*, vol. 62 (1988), pp. 386–406.

84. See for example Toby Gelfand, 'The "Paris Manner" of dissection: student anatomical dissection in early eighteenth century Paris', *Bulletin of the History of Medicine*, vol. 46 (1972), pp. 99–130; A. Cunningham, 'Fabricius and the "Aristotle Project" in anatomical teaching and research in Padua', in Wear, *Medical Renaissance*, pp. 195–222; Ruth Richardson, *Death, Dissection and the Destitute* (Routledge & Kegan Paul, London, 1987); Christopher Lawrence, 'Alexander Monro *primus* and the Edinburgh manner of anatomy', *Bulletin of the History of Medicine*, vol. 62 (1988), pp. 193–214.

85. Billings, *History*, p. 17.

86. But see Nutton, 'Humanist surgery' on the importance of translation as a generator of surgical innovation.

87. For the use of this model in another context see Trevor J. Pinch and Wiebe E. Bijker, 'The social construction of facts and artifacts: or how the sociology of science and the sociology of technology, might benefit each other', in Wiebe E. Bijker, Thomas P. Hughes and Trevor J. Pinch (eds), *The Social Construction of Technological Systems* (The MIT Press, Cambridge, Mass., 1987), pp. 17–50.

88. J. Alexander Williams, 'Cholecystectomy: ironmasters and eggheads', *Journal of the Royal Society of Medicine*, vol. 81, no. 10 (1988), pp. 560–1.

89. Bijker, *Technological Systems*, esp. John Law 'Technology and heterogeneous engineering: the case of Portuguese expansion', pp. 111–34. For a variant of this model, which raises interesting methodological questions for writing the history of antiseptic and aseptic surgery, see Bruno Latour, *The Pasteurization of France* (Harvard University Press, Cambridge, Mass., 1988).

90. Ghislaine Lawrence, this volume.

91. Siraisi, *Medieval Medicine*, p. 157.

92. 'A Central African will not consent to an operation (not even tooth extraction), as it conflicts with the anticipation of his dismembered spirit', in James Johnson, *Reality Versus Romance in South Central Africa* (New York, 1893), cited in E. Ackerknecht, 'Surgery and its paradoxes' in *Medicine and Ethnology: Selected Essays* (Johns Hopkins Press, Baltimore, 1971), pp. 95–113; 111; see the description of the

toothache by the eighteenth-century author William Buchan who, in nearly all cases, considered it a symptom of a systemic disorder, *Domestic Medicine*, 3rd edn (W. Strahan, London, 1774), pp. 388–91.

93. Ackerknecht, *Ethnography*. See the other essays in this volume, esp. 'Incubator and Taboo', pp. 162–6.

94. Philip Rhodes, *An Outline History of Medicine* (Butterworth, London, 1985), p. 6. See also John Kirkup who posits a 'surgical like instinctive response' in 'Surgery before general anaesthesia', in Ronald D. Mann (ed.), *The History of the Management of Pain* (The Parthenon Publishing Group, Carnforth, Lancs., 1988), pp. 15–30: 16. The paper itself is a sensitive survey of pre-modern responses to surgery.

95. Pelling, 'Appearance and reality'.

96. Owsei Temkin, 'Greek medicine as science and craft', *Isis*, vol. 44 (1953), pp. 213–25 and *Janus*, pp. 137–53.

97. Temkin, *Janus*, p. 148. The expression 'but over' in this quote is an interesting one since it turns the whole argument into an idealist form. It suggests that differences in philosophical theory were the *cause* of division into sects, whereas earlier the argument seems to have been that the 'competitive character of Greek Medicine certainly induced many leeches to borrow from the philosophers', ibid., p. 147. That is, the cognitive changes were the consequence of social change. A similar idealism is to be found in Ludwig Edelstein's 'The relation of ancient philosophy to medicine', *Bulletin of the History of Medicine*, vol. 26 (1952), pp. 299–316, which is all the more curious since Edelstein himself was the originator of a rather more social historical account of Greek medical ideas in 'The Hippocratic physician'. See Ludwig Edelstein, *Ancient Medicine, Edited by Owsei and C. Lilian Temkin* (Johns Hopkins University Press, Baltimore, 1967), pp. 87–110.

98. Darrel W. Amundsen, 'Medicine and surgery as art or craft: the role of schematic literature in the separation of medicine and surgery in the late Middle Ages', *Transactions and Studies of the College of Physicians of Philadelphia*, series V, vol. 1 (1979), pp. 43–57.

99. Temkin, *Janus*, p. 153.

100. The best survey is in Amundsen, 'Surgery as art'; see also Jerome J. Bylebyl, 'The medical meaning of *Physica*', *Osiris*, vol. 6 (1990), pp. 16–41.

101. Pouchelle, *Body and Surgery*; for the problems see a review of the original, Toby Gelfand, 'Imagining the body', *Bulletin of the History of Medicine*, vol. 60 (1986), pp. 109–13.

102. One recent attempt to rewrite the history of surgeons and surgery in medieval England has been almost universally condemned: Robert F. Gottfried, *Doctors and Medicine in Medieval England, 1340–1530* (Princeton University Press, Princeton, NJ, 1986). One reviewer called it 'unintelligible nonsense' Martha Carlin, *Medical History*, vol. 31 (1987), pp. 360–2. See also Carole Rawcliffe, *Social History of Medicine*, vol. 1 (1988), pp. 93–5.

103. Nutton, 'Humanist surgery', p. 75.

104. See for example, Siraisi, *Medieval Medicine*, pp. 153–86.

105. One recent interesting development is the exploration of the

use by surgeons of Paracelsian ideas; see, for example, Allen G. Debus, 'John Woodall, Paracelsian surgeon', *Ambix*, vol. 10 (1962), pp. 108–18. More especially see the works cited by Charles Webster in his critical review of this literature in 'Alchemical and Paracelsian medicine', in Webster, *Health, Medicine and Mortality*, pp. 300–36.

106. Owsei Temkin, 'Therapeutic trends and the treatment of syphilis before 1900', *Bulletin of the History of Medicine*, vol. 29 (1955), pp. 309–16 and *Janus*, pp. 518–24: 524; see also 'On the history of "Morality and Syphilis"', *Janus*, pp. 472–84.

107. Owsei Temkin 'The scientific approach to disease: specific entity and individual sickness', in A. C. Crombie (ed.), *Scientific Change* (Basic Books, New York, 1963), pp. 629–47 and *Janus*, pp. 441–55. As Temkin recognises, there are difficulties associated with employing the term ontological but I employ it here, as he does, to mean identifying disease with a specific entity which might be clinical, pathological, or aetiological but not necessarily all of these at once. It is important to stress the context-dependent nature of these perceptions. Physicians were quite capable of discussing diseases as entities, just as surgeons could construe diseases as individual disturbances. It is in the area of therapy among rich and poor that these distinctions prove most useful. The ontological physiological distinction is, actually, an early nineteenth–century one, and would have been unrecognisable in that form to physicians and surgeons prior to this period. I am grateful to Dr J. Bylebyl for his discussion on this point.

108. Temkin, *Janus*, p. 454.

109. James Cooke, *Mellificium Chirgurgiae: or the Marrow of Chirurgery*, (Benj. Shirley, London, 1676), p. 443.

110. Beier, this volume.

111. *Janus*, p. 490.

112. This volume.

113. For a brief synopsis and a guide to sources see Temkin, 'Role of surgery'. A quite useful comparative account, which centres on Dutch material, is Daniel de Moulin, *A History of Surgery* (Martinus Nijhoff, Dordrecht, 1988).

114. F. Dujardin and B. Peyrilhe, *Histoire de la chirurgie*, 2 vols (Paris, 1774–80); Albrecht von Haller, *Bibliotheca Chirurgica*, 2 vols (J. Schweighauser, Basle, 1774–5); Stephenus Vigilis von Creutzenfeld, *Bibliotheca Chirurgica* 2 vols (J. T. Trattner, Vienna, 1781).

115. See Rosalie Mary Stott, 'The origins of the Edinburgh Medical School 1696–1755', unpublished PhD thesis, University of Edinburgh, 1984. Stott's material on the seventeenth-century corporation is invaluable but I cannot accept her argument that William Cullen's concepts of disease owed much to the Edinburgh surgeons.

116. Like their continental counterparts the Monros were authors of bibliographically learned texts on anatomical and surgical history. The history of anatomy, by Alexander Monro *primus*, can be found prefixed to most of the manuscripts containing his anatomical lectures. For details see D. W. Taylor, 'The manuscript lecture notes of Alexander Monro *primus* (1697–1767)', *Medical History*, vol. 30 (1986), pp. 444–67. The history was plagiarised and published almost verbatim

as, William Northcote, *A Concise History of Anatomy, from the Earliest Ages of Antiquity* (T. Evans, London, 1772). See K. F. Russell, *British Anatomy 1525–1800* (Melbourne University Press, Melbourne, 1963), p. 174. On Monro's history of surgery see R. E. Wright-St Clair, 'History of surgery and introduction to surgical lectures, by Monro Primus', *Medical History*, vol. 5 (1961), pp. 286–90. On Monro *secundus* on the history of anatomy, see Douglass W. Taylor, *The Monro Collection in the Medical Library of the University of Otago* (University of Otago Press, Dunedin, 1979), M185.

117. In Württemburg at least, the surgeon-artisans were prosperous, well-educated members of the middle class. See Sabine Sander, *Handwerkschirurgen: Sozialgeschichte einer Verdrängten Berufsgruppe* (Vandenhoeck & Ruprecht, Göttingen, 1989).

118. Temkin, *Janus*, p. 493.

119. Toby Gelfand, *Professionalising Modern Medicine* (Greenwood Press, Westport, Conn., 1980), p. 187.

120. These possibilities included the anatomical reasoning of the dogmatists, the clinical approach of the Empiricks and the ontological view of the Methodists. See Temkin, 'Scientific approach'. The anatomical argument had been adumbrated by Sigerist in 1935, 'Surgery'.

121. Temkin, *Janus*, p. 496. The teleological tone of this quote is unusual.

122. Nicolson, this volume.

123. For a series of examples see Malcolm Nicolson, 'The metastatic theory of pathogenesis and the professional interests of the eighteenth-century physician', *Medical History*, vol. 32 (1988), pp. 277–300.

124. Michel Foucault, *Birth of the Clinic* (Tavistock, London, 1973).

125. Ibid., p. 127.

126. X. Bichat, *General Anatomy Applied to Physiology and the Practice of Medicine*, 2 vols (S. Highley, London, 1824), vol. 1, p. lxvii.

127. Alexander Monro *secundus*, [Lectures in Anatomy], *c.*1770, Pybus Collection, University of Newcastle upon Tyne, MS PYB L. iii 6–10, vol. 1, Lecture 1.

128. Toby Gelfand seems to agree that there was a fundamental epistemic reorientation in Paris, but like Temkin he has called attention to the preconditions of that change, 'Gestation of the clinic', *Medical History*, vol. 25 (1981), pp. 169–80. Othmar Keel, however, seems to adopt a much more continuist position although agreeing there was a Paris 'Problématique': 'The politics of health and the institutionalization of clinical practices in Europe in the second half of the eighteenth century', in Bynum and Porter, *William Hunter*, pp. 207–58.

129. Maulitz, *Morbid Appearances.*

130. Ibid., p. 114. For Maulitz's stress on how different Bichat's pathology was from the local pathology of other surgeons see pp. 62, 75, 82.

131. John Pickstone, 'Bureaucracy, liberalism and the body in post-Revolutionary France: Bichat's physiology and the Paris School of medicine', *History of Science*, vol. 19 (1981), pp. 115–42. For a concise

summary of this position see L. S. Jacyna, 'Romantic thought and the origins of cell theory', in Cunningham and Jardine, *Romanticism*, pp. 161–8.

132. This argument, essentially correct it seems to me, is in a way implicit in Foucault's analysis. Yet Foucault chooses to identify the new science of life not with an ontology, the tissue, but with organisation, as found for example in the work of Cuvier. Using this criterion William Albury who has employed a Foucauldian model, has, like Pickstone, found Bichat to lie on the eighteenth-century side of the epistemic divide. Michel Foucault, *The Order of Things* (Tavistock, London, 1970), Ch. 8, 'Cuvier'; William Randall Albury, 'Experiment and explanation in the physiology of Bichat and Magendie', *Studies in the History of Biology*, vol. 1 (1977), pp. 47–131. On varying definitions of the science of life see Joseph A. Caron, '"Biology" in the life sciences: an historiographical contribution', *History of Science*, vol. 26 (1988), pp. 223–68.

133. On London see Susan Lawrence, 'Science and medicine at the London hospitals: the development of teaching and research, 1750–1815', unpublished PhD thesis, University of Toronto, 1985. There is no comparable study of Edinburgh at this time. For a speculative survey see Christopher Lawrence, 'The Edinburgh Medical School and the end of the "Old Thing"', *History of Universities*, vol. 7 (1988), pp. 259–86.

134. Maulitz, *Morbid Appearances*, p. 116.

135. Jacyna, 'Images'; Lawrence, 'Science and medicine'. For the contrary view see Keel, 'Politics of health' and *La Généalogie de L'Histopathologie, une Révision Dechirante: Philippe Pinel, Lecteur Discret de J. C. Smyth (1741–1821)* (Vrin, Paris, 1979).

136. Maulitz, *Morbid Appearances*, p. 176. For a Foucauldian analysis of Hunter which finds elements of a modern or proto-biological problematic in his work on organisation yet finally consigns it to eighteenth-century natural history see Stephen J. Cross, 'John Hunter, the animal oeconomy, and late eighteenth-century physiological discourse', *Studies in the History of Biology*, vol. 5 (1981), pp. 1–116.

137. Maulitz, *Morbid Appearances*, pp. 112, 177. On Hodgkin see Amalie M. Kass and Edward H. Kass, *Perfecting the World: the Life and Times of Dr. Thomas Hodgkin 1798–1866* (Harcourt Brace Jovanovich, Boston, 1988).

138. Maulitz, *Morbid Appearances*, p. 143; Lawrence, 'Old Thing'.

139. Sigerist, 'Surgery', p. 171.

140. Alison Winter, 'Ethereal epidemic: Mesmerism and the introduction of inhalation anaesthesia to early Victorian London', *Social History of Medicine*, vol. 4 (1991), pp. 1–28.

141. Nicholas M. Greene, 'Anesthesis and the development of surgery', *Anesthesia and Analgesia*, vol. 58, no. 1 (1979), pp. 5–12 and Martin S. Pernick, *A Calculus of Suffering: Pain Professionalism and Anesthesia in Nineteenth Century America* (Columbia University Press, New York, 1985), pp. 192–3. See also Christopher Lawrence and Ghislaine Lawrence, *No Laughing Matter: Historical Aspects of Anaesthesia* (Wellcome Institute/Science Museum, London, 1987), pp. 24–5.

142. See for example W. Stanley Sykes, *Essays on the First Hundred Years of Anaesthesia, Edited by Richard Ellis* (Churchill Livingstone, Edinburgh, 1982), p. 111. Conversely surgeons were not deterred from major operations by the absence of anaesthesia. In 1867 James Syme was not inhibited from performing a massive resection of the jaw simply because anaesthetic could not be given. James Syme, 'Excision of the tongue', *The Lancet* (1865), i, p. 115. See also Joseph Lister on the incision of a carbuncle in one of James Syme's clinics in 1854, 'The patient was not under chloroform', *The Collected Papers of Joseph, Baron Lister*, 2 vols (Clarendon Press, Oxford, 1909), vol. 1, p. 206. See also Granshaw, this volume.

143. A. E. Sansom, *Chloroform: its Action and Administration* (John Churchill & Sons, London, 1865), pp. 19–31.

144. See the complementary essays, Helen King, 'The early anodynes: pain in the ancient world', and Wendy Savage, 'The management of obstetric pain', in Mann, *Pain*, pp. 51–62, 187–200.

145. Pouchelle, *Body and Surgery*, p. 76; see Lawrence, 'Artifact', this volume, her note 58.

146. Pernick, *Calculus.*

147. Brieger, this volume. Brieger deals with the American case, but it is possible the Americans learnt it from the French. Dupuytren's theatricality when operating and interviewing patients was notorious. See *The Parisian Education of an American Surgeon. Letters of Jonathan Mason Warren (1832–1835)*, with Notes and Introduction by Russel M. Jones (The American Philosophical Society, Philadelphia, 1978) pp. 89, 108.

148. For a catalogue of operations and American surgeons' representations of their role in creating them see J. Mason Warren, *Recent Progress in Surgery* (Boston, 1864); Gross, 'American surgery', pp. 431–84. For a graphic example of the range and complexity of pre-anaesthetic surgery see the text by the American surgeon Joseph Pancoast, *A Treatise on Operative Surgery* (Carey & Hart, Philadelphia, 1846). Pancoast borrowed heavily from French sources for his arrangement and illustration.

149. Brieger, this volume. See also Peter C. English, *Shock, Physiological Surgery, and George Washington Crile* (Greenwood Press, Westport, Conn., 1980), Ch. 2; also the quote from Humphry, note 50 above.

150. Lawrence and Dixey, this volume.

151. Nicholas J. Fox, 'Scientific theory choice and social structure: the case of Joseph Lister's antisepsis, humoral theory and asepsis', *History of Science*, vol. 26 (1988), pp. 367–97.

152. *The Lancet* (1881), vol. i, p. 332.

153. Tait performed his first gall-bladder removal in 1879. W. J. Stewart McKay, *Lawson Tait: his Life and Work* (Ballière, Tindall & Cox, London, 1922), p. 397.

154. Dennis, *History and Development of Surgery*, p. 2.

155. Frederick Treves, 'A review of the surgery of the peritoneum', *British Medical Journal*, vol. ii (1896), p. 1305.

156. See for example, James M. Edmondson, *Surgical Garb 1870–1920* (The Cleveland Health Sciences Library, Ohio, 1982).

157. See the attempt to deal with the changing visual aspects of surgery as constitutive of a change in the social relations of surgery rather than a technologically determined event in Daniel M. Fox and Christopher Lawrence, *Photographing Medicine: Images and Power in Britain and America since 1840* (Greenwood Press, New York, 1988).

158. Among the common people of the Renaissance, see above note 106. See also his observation that the Methodists' ontological conception of disease, 'was popular in the Roman Empire, and it would be of interest to find out whether it had its social roots among military surgeons and in the latifundia, since such hospitals (*valetudinaria*) as existed in Antiquity were for soldiers and slaves', 'Scientific approach' in *Janus*, p. 446.

159. Cited in Trombley, *Treves*, p. 83. Treves was referring to the organisation of the profession but the invocation of democracy and surgery is new.

160. Elizabeth Johns, *Thomas Eakins: the Heroism of Modern Life* (Princeton, Princeton University Press, 1983), p. 58.

161. *Parisian Education*, p. 29.

162. James Gregory Mumford, 'Narrative of surgery; a historical sketch', in William Williams Keen (ed.), *Surgery: its Principles and Practice* (W. B. Saunders, Philadelphia, 1906), vol. 1., pp. 17–78: 32.

163. Johns, *Thomas Eakins*; 'The Gross Clinic' is, of course, a much more complex picture than this, see Michael Fried, *Realism, Writing, Disfiguration: on Thomas Eakins and Stephen Crane* (University of Chicago Press, Chicago, 1987).

164. Gross, 'American surgery', p. 443.

165. Keen, 'Address', pp. 1105, 1109, 1103.

166. D'Arcy Power and W. E. Le Fanu, *Lives of the Fellows of the Royal College of Surgeons of England 1930–1951* (RCS, London, 1953), p. 567. See also Brieger, this volume.

167. Richard J. Levis, *The Traditional Errors of Surgery* (W. J. Dornan, Philadelphia, 1888), pp. 2–3.

168. Tiemann & Co., *American Armanentarium Chirugicum* (1872), preface. Cited in ibid., 1889, *The Centennial Edition*, reprinted with an introduction by James M. Edmondson and F. Terry Hambrecht (Norman Publishing, Boston, 1989), p. 32. Curiously this edition dropped the claim.

169. Dennis, *History*, p. 84. American surgery, said another, 'stands for the best work being done in the world'. James Gregory Mumford, 'Narrative of surgery; a historical sketch', in Keen (ed.), *Surgery*, p. 65. For a splendidly written and scholarly review of the history of surgery and its role in creating the American hospital, see Charles Rosenberg, *The Care of Strangers: the Rise of America's Hospital System* (Basic Books, New York, 1987). Rosenberg's text is full of suggestions about why surgery was congenial to the American doctor. Rosenberg, however, never quite grasps the epistemological nettle of the status and role of germ theory.

170. See Edward B. Krumbhaar, 'The early days of the American Journal of the Medical Sciences', *Medical Life*, vol. 36 (1929), pp. 240–56.

171. Cited in Henry Nash Smith, *Virgin Land: the American West as Symbol and Myth* (Vintage Books, New York, 1959), p. 294.

172. Frederick Jackson Turner, *The Frontier in American History* (Henry Holt & Co., New York, 1921), pp. 3, 243.

173. Keen, 'Address', p. 1104.

174. Keen, 'Address', p. 1109.

175. Turner, *The Frontier*, pp. 30, 37. The apparently unresolved contradiction between the qualities brought to the frontier and those produced by it were pointed out in William Coleman, 'Science and symbol in the Turner frontier hypothesis', *American Historical Review*, vol. 72 (1966), pp. 22–49. Coleman also brilliantly analyses the scientific borrowings of Turner's thesis.

176. Dennis, *History*, p. 84.

177. Henry Sigerist, *American Medicine*, translated by Hildegard Nagel (W. W. Norton, New York, 1934), p. 270.

178. Richard J. Levis, *The Traditional Errors of Surgery* (W. J. Dornan, Philadelphia, 1888), p. 4.

179. Turner, *The Frontier*, p. 267.

180. Nash, *Virgin Land*, p. 298.

181. Jordanova has argued that the practice of anatomy (and by implication surgery) is 'quintessentially gendered'. See *Sexual Visions*, esp. pp. 149–53. By the 1930s the small group of men who were creating neurosurgery were using another gendered account. So intricate was their craft, they designated it as woman's work. I am grateful to Jack Pressman for this point.

182. Godlee, *Lister*, p. 137.

183. William Watson Cheyne, *Lister and his Achievement* (Longmans Green & Co., London, 1925), p. 34.

184. English, *Shock*.

185. Jacyna, 'The laboratory'.

186. Granshaw, this volume.

187. See Lawrence, 'Levy', this volume.

188. See the extremely useful Stephen L. Johnson, *The History of Cardiac Surgery, 1896–1955* (Johns Hopkins Press, Baltimore, 1970). Johnson attributes the growth of cardiac surgery to 'improvement in techniques', p. xiv.

189. Christopher Lawrence, 'Moderns and Ancients: the "New Cardiology" in Britain 1880–1930', in W. F. Bynum, C. Lawrence and V. Nutton (eds), *The Emergence of Modern Cardiology, Medical History*, Supplement 5 (1985), pp. 1–33.

190. Maurice Campbell, a 'new cardiologist', remembered 'Modern cardiology was only just starting out and two of its principles were not helpful to the operation [for mitral stenosis]'. 'The early operations for mitral stenosis', *British Heart Journal*, vol. 27 (1965), pp. 670–3. See also James Mackenzie's ridiculing of the operation in Sir John McMichael, 'A transition in cardiology: the Mackenzie Lewis era', *The Harveian Oration, 1975* (Royal College of Physicians, London, 1976), p. 11.

2

Seventeenth-century English surgery: the casebook of Joseph Binns

Lucinda McCray Beier

Joseph Binns

A full discussion of seventeenth-century surgery is beyond the scope of this or any paper. Rather than attempting to place the wide variety of seventeenth-century surgeons in their social, cultural or economic context, this paper is concerned with a subject which has hitherto attracted little attention from historians of medicine – the day-to-day practice of surgery. The discussion will centre on the experience and methods of one mid-seventeenth-century London surgeon, Joseph Binns (d. 1664). Much of the material included in this paper also appears in my book *Sufferers and Healers: the Experience of Illness in Seventeenth-Century England* (1987). As in the book, the types of conditions Binns treated and the therapeutic methods he employed will be described. However, here comparisons will be drawn between the ways he dealt with his cases and the recommendations made in the sixteenth- and seventeenth-century surgical literature, principally those offered by Richard Wiseman, surgeon to Charles II, in order to investigate the difference, if any, between literary and actual practice. It is hoped that such comparisons will serve to broaden the perspective from which Binns's casebook can be viewed.

It cannot be argued that Binns was a typical seventeenth-century English surgeon. He was a full-time practitioner who neither barbered nor kept a shop. He knew some Latin, belonged to the Barber-Surgeons' Company, was attached to a great hospital, rubbed shoulders with London's medical and surgical luminaries and wrote a casebook describing many of the cases with which he dealt during a career spanning the years

1633 to 1663.[1] These factors combine to identify him as quite unusual. However, unlike a number of his colleagues, Binns achieved no fame, lasting or otherwise. In his own time, he was respectable, but unremarkable. Thus he may be viewed as an ordinary member of London's surgical community, a group which was fairly large. Pelling reminds us that the Barber-Surgeons' Company of London numbered 293 freeman householders in 1641, of whom approximately half were surgeons.[2] Even though it cannot be assumed that all the surgeons belonging to the company were as successful as Binns, his casebook leaves the clear impression that he was a relatively small fish in a relatively large pool.

Joseph Binns was born in Derbyshire. He served his apprenticeship with the prominent London surgeon Joseph Fenton, and was made free of the Company of Barber-Surgeons on 28 March 1637. Binns was elected as one of the three surgeons to St Bartholomew's Hospital on 12 November 1647, a position which he occupied until his death on 18 May 1664. He was paid £30 a year by the hospital. In addition to his attendance at St Bartholomew's, Binns had an active private practice, the details of which are recorded in his casebook. He finished his career as a warden of the Barber-Surgeon's Company in 1662 and 1663.[3] He married Mary Holland whose father, Master Richard Holland, was named as one of the executors of Binns's will.[4] At the time of his death he had at least three living children, none of whom had reached the age of 21. During his working life, Binns leased a house on Butchers Hall Lane in Christchurch parish.

At the end of his life, Binns was in an enviably solid financial position. He was receiving income from properties in Berkshire, Oxfordshire and Middlesex. In 1664 he had loaned two gentlemen £800 and £500 respectively. He left his eldest son Fenton £100 in cash, and his daughter Mary £125 set out in East India Company shares. He left £5 apiece to the poor of the parish of Christchurch and the Barber-Surgeons' Company. He left £10 apiece to his executors. His will provides for mourning clothes for his two executors, the minister who was to preach his funeral sermon, his wife and children, his sister and brother-in-law and his servants. In addition, he bequeathed between 10 and 40 shillings apiece to 17 friends and relations to be used to purchase rings.

Binns had wide contacts within medical and surgical circles. His cousin and executor, Joseph Colston, was a physician. His casebook mentions approximately 40 physicians and surgeons with whom he had dealings of one kind or another. Some, like the surgeon John Woodall and the physician Charles Scarborough, are well known to historians. Others, like Joseph Fenton, William and Edward Molins, Edward Arris and William Clowes, Jr, Sergeant Surgeon to Charles I, were leading members of the Barber-Surgeons' Company in their own day, meriting repeated references in Sidney Young's useful *The Annals of the Barber-Surgeons of London.*[5] Most have been as totally forgotten as Binns himself. Binns apparently had a regular arrangement with at least one physician, Dr John Bathurst, whose patients he treated at the physician's house.

Unlike his son Fenton, who became a surgeon, and was accused in 1690 by the Royal College of Physicians of prescribing internal medicines, Joseph Binns got on reasonably well with both medical and surgical colleagues.[6] He expressed none of the contempt for his colleagues so amply displayed by elite surgical authors such as Thomas Gale, William Clowes and Richard Wiseman, although he did disparage some non-surgeons for lack of skill. In an age riddled with occupational wrangles and disputes between patients and surgeons about the proper delivery of surgical care, Binns apparently completed a lengthy career without ever appearing before the Master and Wardens of his Company upon charges of misbehaviour. This is not to say that he completely avoided disputes. In two cases involving members of the Molins family, he expressed doubts about both therapeutic judgement and personal integrity. In the first case, he consulted with Edward Molins about the treatment of a lawyer suffering from mouth cancer. Binns left the case because 'Ed Molins pretended he could do him good (though he said to me he did not desire to deal with it for no good could be done in it) but did not for he died in 14 days after'. In the second case,

> 6 June 1643 7 o'clock at night on the backside of the Red Lion in Holborn one Samuel Ward, an old Gardener near 80 years of age, asking an alms of one Sergeant Major Jenkins, he refused to give, the old man replied some words, Jenkins drew his sword and thrust him into the belly . . . with a broad sword. I put my finger as I conceive into the cavity, the wound went somewhat upward toward the liver. He had a puncture behind close to the left

> shoulder, bruised about the head and arm, dressed him up to stay blood, next morn his pulse high and he hot . . . 4th day, some digestion & they [*sic*] friends of Jenkins desired that Will: Molins might join with me he goes with them next day (without me) and reports the patient afore the Justice to be past danger, so Major Jenkins was discharged out of prison upon bail. Next day Molins dresses the patient without me, and leaves word that I must meddle no further.[7]

Molins was obviously exercising, not surgical, but social judgement. In addition, he took over a case originally belonging to another member of his own Company – a breach of occupational etiquette and ethics. Had Binns not been peaceably inclined, he would certainly have had grounds for complaint before the Court of the Barber-Surgeons' Company.

Binns's stature within the surgical community is demonstrated in the thirty cases in which he acted as a consultant rather than the initial or the sole healer involved. Small by today's standards, this figure reflects the medical and surgical climate of the period. Healers were chosen by sufferers according to their symptoms, their pocketbooks and their opinions about the merits of various types of practitioners. Thus, surgeons competed with each other for the opportunity to treat the self-selected group of patients who chose to consult surgeons. Their incomes and reputations were based on the size of their practices, the social status of their patients and reports of their success in curing. Consultations were resorted to either in very unusual or difficult cases where the surgeon in charge wanted to make sure he was doing everything possible for the patient, or in cases where the patient had a high social status. In addition, a consultation involving senior members of the Barber-Surgeons' Company was required in cases where the patient seemed likely to die. Failure to present such cases to the court could result in either a fine or the loss of the right to practise.[8] Consultants of choice were those who could give expert advice and, at the same time, be relied upon not to try to steal the patient. Binns's colleagues must have both respected his skill and trusted his honour to have consulted with him as often as they did.

The practice of surgery

Binns's casebook mentions approximately 671 patients. This number is necessarily approximate because some case-notes are incomplete, some illegible, and some duplicates. Out of the total, only 616 are detailed enough to make any sort of analysis possible. These case-notes, while they vary enormously in quality, provide information about the conditions Binns treated, the therapies he applied, the names, addresses and social status of his patients and the dates and periods during which they consulted him. I have given a brief analysis of the social profile of Binns's patients elsewhere.[9] Here, I will summarise by saying that they came from all social backgrounds, although the middling orders predominated. While most were Londoners, 30 came from further afield. He treated at least 368 men and 217 women; the sex of 31 of his patients is unknown.[10]

Binns's practice was largely local. Although information is sparse, it seems that he visited his patients rather than expecting them to visit him. He often saw a patient once or twice a day. This fact might explain why he apparently treated so few patients during his career and perhaps suggests one major way in which surgeons' practices differed from those of physicians. Michael MacDonald reported that the early seventeenth-century astrological physician Richard Napier, in a practice spanning thirty-seven years, 'treated tens of thousands of patients for every kind of malady'. Napier's patients visited him, thus making it possible for him to treat 'between five and fifteen patients a day, repeating with each of them a ritual of interrogation and annotation that invoked the axioms of astrological medicine'.[11] Binns's therapeutic routine, which involved lengthy discussions of the patient's history, condition and regimen, repeated examinations, the application of medicines and dressings and a variety of surgical procedures, was too time-consuming to allow for a practice on the scale of Napier's.[12] Not all of Binns's patients about whom the necessary information exists required long-term care; 184 consulted him during a period of less than a week, many simply obtaining a prescription or two. Most, however, needed more complicated treatment. Binns treated 211 patients for between one week and one month, 164 patients for between one and six months, 28 patients for between six months and one year, and 13 patients for over a year.

Binns identified nearly 100 symptoms or disorders which patients brought to him for treatment. For most of these (often quite specific, such as 'lip ulcer' or 'gored by a bull') he treated very few people; in most cases, less than five during his entire career. In the more general categories the numbers are larger. He treated at least 77 cases of apostems (matter-filled swellings). However, a numerical breakdown of his cases also reveals that Binns had a minor speciality in the treatment of venereal diseases. Of his patients, 196 complained of gonorrhoea, 'whites' or syphilitic symptoms. In addition, he treated numerous cases of hernia and urinary retention in men. Unlike another London surgeon, Thomas Hollier, who was lithotomist to both St Thomas's and St Bartholomew's hospitals during the mid-seventeenth century, Binns did not cut for the stone. Nor did he assist at difficult childbirths, as did some contemporary surgeons.

Most of the disorders Binns treated would have been considered specifically surgical problems in his own time. These included wounds, fractures and dislocations, ulcers, fistulae, herniae, apostems, tumours, skin rashes and venereal diseases. Such ills provided the subject matter for the general works on surgery published during the early modern period. However, unlike surgical writers such as William Clowes, John Woodall and Richard Wiseman, Binns was a civil rather than primarily a naval or military surgeon and, therefore, less concerned about gunshot wounds and those inflicted by other weapons used in battle than he was about the illnesses and injuries encountered in the course of daily social and industrial life.[13]

In addition to these disorders, sixty-one of Binns's case-notes refer to 'medical' problems, such as ague, stomach-ache, headache, insomnia, diarrhoea and epilepsy. Some of these patients, including two who were apparently given prophylactic purges, were the surgeon's relatives who may have received free treatment. According to one entry, Binns dosed himself for ague. However, he gave internal medicines to non-relatives as well. These cases show that to some extent Binns was operating as a general practitioner, despite the monopoly granted to the Royal College of Physicians over the prescribing of internal medicines. Thus Binns daily committed technical violations of the conventional and legal distinction between surgery and physic. He was not exceptional. The sixteenth-century surgeon Thomas Gale wrote, 'Chirurgery is the art, which cureth those infirmities, and griefs of man's body, which are to be done by right use, and application of the hand.' He went on to say, however,

> Also it is to be understand [*sic*], though in the definition is put no other ways of curing those griefs, but by the right use of the hand, yet chirurgery hath need both of that part which cureth by diet, and of that which helpeth by medicine.[14]

For legal purposes, surgery was defined less by the disorders which surgeons treated than by the therapeutic methods they used. Surface applications of remedies and the use of instruments were appropriate surgical treatments; prescription of internal medicines was the physician's province. Yet the humoral theory which was employed by both physicians and surgeons required that surgical patients be placed under the regimen appropriate to their conditions. Binns's practice demonstrates not the familiar historical axiom about conflict between medicine and surgery, but the shared theoretical assumptions according to which both were practised.

Whatever the disorder, internal or external, the cure depended upon the humoral principle of maintaining or restoring the body's internal balance, often through evacuation. Ideally, the patient consulted a physician, a surgeon and an apothecary who organised treatment among themselves. However, in practice most patients consulted one healer at a time. Thus, Binns dosed his patients with a large variety of purgatives and emetics. He undoubtedly made up many of these remedies himself (thus acting as an apothecary). One strong laxative, his 'pill fortis', may have been a secret recipe of his own, since he never gave details of its ingredients. Other medicines were compounded of the herbal and metallic substances commonly mentioned in both medical works and diaries of the period. Binns also prescribed diets which were expected to prevent or reduce apostemation and thus help in the healing process.

Was this overlap with the physician's sphere typical of seventeenth-century English surgeons? From the information provided by R. S. Roberts and Sir George Clark, it is clear that early modern London physicians, in their effort to protect their monopoly over the prescription of internal remedies, fought a losing battle against surgeons, apothecaries, and unlicensed healers.[15] Nonetheless, published surgical works of the sixteenth and seventeenth centuries, perhaps understandably, keep a low profile regarding this point. Although he gave details of many of the cases he had dealt with in his *Several Chirurgical Treatises* of 1676, Richard Wiseman, a slightly younger contemporary of Binns, confined his specific descriptions to wound management and the application of surgical instruments. Indeed, in the case of 'a sedentary young gentleman, of an ill habit of body' who 'was wounded by a penknife in the inside of the calf of his leg into the sural artery', Wiseman exercised his skill in dealing with the wound, but carefully reported sending the patient to a 'Doctor W.' for treatment of 'his ill habit of body, he being highly scorbutical, and subject to fainting, loss of appetite, and pituitous swellings on his Feet'. While it is possible that Wiseman, a royal surgeon with a well-heeled clientele, may simply have found it more convenient to leave the prescribing of internal remedies to his medical colleagues, it is equally possible that he dosed his patients more often than his published reports lead us to believe. Consider, for instance, his comment, regarding the cure of fistulae, that the surgeon should 'in the first place . . . proceed by evacuation of those humours which may disturb you in your work; and that is done by purging and bleeding, good traumatick decoctions, with observation of diet, etc.'[16] Although Wiseman gave no recipes for purges or 'good traumatick decoctions', and never indicated that these should be administered by a surgeon, he undoubtedly was competent to apply the measures he recommended. Certainly, Binns would have found no difficulty in dealing with the young gentleman's ill habit of body. Equally certainly, the great majority of Binns's patients required that he, as the healer of choice, take over total management of their illness. Most of his patients would simply have lacked the means to consult several practitioners at once.

Binns's case-notes thus reveal that his therapeutic routine was governed by rarely stated humoral theory. Regardless of the patient's disorder, a careful record was kept of the number, and sometimes the consistency, of his or her daily and nightly bowel movements. These were controlled by laxatives, enemas, and suppositories. The prescription given depended upon the patient's age and his or her 'habit of body' as well as upon the ailment. The 80-year-old gardener, mentioned above, was given clysters and suppositories (specifically 'surgical' treatments) rather than laxatives because he was elderly and weak. Binns routinely began any sort of treatment by prescribing a laxative. This might be given on its own or as one ingredient (such as rhubarb or senna) in a general-purpose 'diet drink' or 'bolus'.

In addition, and sometimes in preference to purges, Binns prescribed emetics or 'vomits'. The most frequently used ingredients were cream of tartar and antimony. Vomits were used for prophylactic as well as curative purposes. It was common for the English to take physic at least once a year, usually in the spring, whether or not they were in poor health. In one instance, Binns prescribed vomits, laxatives and 'stomach' pills to five members of his cousin Edward Griffing's family: Griffing, his wife, his daughter, his maid and the maid's mother.[17] Vomits were also used as the preferred treatment for agues. In one case, Binns prescribed a vomit for a maid-servant with ague; the preparation produced fifteen or sixteen vomits. There is no record of whether or not the maid recovered.[18] Like laxatives, emetics were used to prepare patients for further treatment. Binns routinely prescribed vomits before operating on cases of hernia aquosa (a collection of fluid in the scrotum).[19]

While laxatives and emetics were the common currency of all medical practitioners, other means of evacuation were performed chiefly by surgeons, barber-surgeons and barbers. Letting blood, cupping, scarifying, blistering and making issues or using setons (to produce ulcers which were not allowed to heal), were specifically surgical methods used to help the body void unnecessary or evil humours. Blood-letting, like vomiting and purging, could be either curative or prophylactic. Binns, however, did not record a single case of prophylactic phlebotomy, but used the procedure only under specific circumstances. He routinely let blood in cases of head injuries, and, indeed, criticised the St Bartholomew's Hospital staff for neither letting blood nor administering a purge or clyster in the case of one patient who died of a head wound. Richard Wiseman would have agreed with Binns, for he advised that once a head wound had been dressed, 'let him [the patient] blood in the arm or neck of the same side, and some hours after let a clyster be administered'.[20] Binns also let blood in other cases where wounds appeared to be apostemating.[21] He drew blood for headaches. He also let blood when humoral tradition specifically required such treatment, such as in a case of amenorrhoea, where Binns drew blood from the saphenous vein (in the foot) in order to draw the menses downward. In a case of a matter-filled swelling of the arm Binns also opened a vein in the foot.[22] Binns used phlebotomy when the circumstances seemed to warrant it, even though he did not normally let blood for the condition being treated. He only occasionally bled his syphilis patients, which represents a change from the routine bleeding recommended by William Clowes in 1597.[23] In one desperate case of a gunshot wound which had bled much initially, Binns let blood after the wound was dressed, and again the next day. Unfortunately, the patient died that evening.[24]

Cupping, which Binns referred to as the application of boxing glasses, was another means the surgeon occasionally used to bleed patients (through suction rather than incision). He employed this method for ailments of the head and eye, and appeared to apply it when counter-irritation was in order. In one case of an ulceration in the eye he applied boxing glasses, blistered the patient's neck, and made an issue in her arm, all on the first day of treatment. He repeated the blistering and applied boxing glasses every day for about six weeks thereafter.[25] Cupping was sometimes combined with scarification. This increased the flow of blood through a number of shallow incisions. Such treatment was usually applied to the shoulders or neck. Binns also used scarification on its own. In the case of a syphilitic patient whose foreskin was becoming gangrenous, Binns cut away the mortified flesh and scarified the remaining foreskin. This was apparently the approved means to stave off further mortification.[26]

Blistering and the making of issues were the methods of counter-irritation Binns used most frequently. These were expected to provide alternative means of evacuation for the surplus or peccant humours causing the patient's discomfort. They were also expected to draw such humours away from the primary location of the disorder, thus giving relief. Patients themselves requested issues. In one case, that of a serving-maid who had burned the left side of her face, the patient did not feel completely well until Binns had made an issue in her left arm. In the case of another patient who was suffering from leg ulcers, Binns removed and cured an issue which was not helping the patient, and then made a new issue in her arm three months later. The patient recovered.[27]

Injuries, repairs and venereal disease

Like his colleagues, Binns mainly named and treated symptoms rather than specific diseases. This is not surprising, since according to humoral theory it was quite possible for collections of symptoms to alter, becoming more or less serious depending upon the individual sufferer's 'complexion'. Thus, although healers identified specific diseases as well as symptoms, the symptoms were the main targets for treatment. This therapeutic approach and the way it was described presents obvious problems for the historian. For purposes of convenience, the symptoms Binns treated will be discussed within three major groups: conditions resulting from recent injuries, long-standing disorders requiring repair work, and the collections of symptoms produced by venereal disease.

Injuries

Binns's thirty years of practice spanned a particularly violent and dangerous period of English history, including the years of the Civil War. A number of his patients – possibly as many as 15 – were wounded in battle. However, his case-notes show that London streets, shops and taverns were as dangerous as battlefields. While 14 of his patients were injured in the course of their occupations and 19 hurt by horses or coaches, some 41 were wounded by personal violence. Weapons varied. Binns treated nine gunshot wounds. Twelve people were injured with such instruments as rapiers, broadswords and a pack-needle. One husband broke his wife's nose with his fist. Several head and face injuries were dealt with pint pots. Binns treated three wounds caused by human bites. (He also treated three cases of dog-bite).[28] Often these violent injuries were crimes of passion, perpetrated when one or both of the participants were drunk. For example, on 25 February 1638, at 9 p.m.,

> One Mr. Robert Peyton of Donnington received a wound (by one Captain Nayle) with a pottle pot intercilium from the right eyebrow to the left, upon the very edge of the os frontis, the which fractured the cranium and depressed the lower part . . . . He was much in drink. With to do I dressed up the wound and stayed the bleeding & forced to

> hold on the medicines all night otherwise he would have plucked all off.[29]

Certainly, passion, with or without the aid of alcohol, provoked the following assault:

> May 10 1643 at night Mr. Ashberry (a lutanist) was bitten by Gottier the French lutanist in Covent Garden had a piece of his cheek bitten out the breadth of an inch & longer on the left side from the corner of his mouth & nether lip down to the lower parts of his jaw, and as much tore up toward his cheek.[30]

Drunkenness and passion help to explain these violent acts, but a number of the injuries Binns treated are harder to understand. It would be interesting to know why Mrs Chayre, a butcher's wife, was stabbed in the belly with a pack-needle by the porter. And an almost modern impression of anonymous urban violence is given in the case of a servant of a trunk-maker who 'was shot in the shoulderblade through the bone with a pistol out of Pauls through two thick deals & he standing in the shop at work'.[31] The man died two days later, presumably without ever having seen his murderer.

Binns also dealt with wounds received in battle. He treated three soldiers wounded at the battle of Newbury, fought on 20 September 1643. One, Captain Broomfield, was 'shot . . . with a brace of bullets', one passing through the left shoulder, the other entering the same armpit and lodging in the scapula. Major Manwaring was more fortunate, merely having been 'shot through his gorget [a piece of armor protecting the throat] & so did but bruise his neck where the bullet lay'. Binns's cousin, Edward Green, who served under the major, had both bones of his right arm broken by a splinter, just above the wrist.[32]

Of course, many people were hurt accidentally. Binns described eleven cases where patients were injured in the course of their occupations. The most dangerous trades he came into contact with were associated with construction. The carpenter Mr Day and his 'man' both injured themselves with tools. Thomas Johnson, a joiner, fell off a ladder breaking both bones of his left leg below the knee. A glazier, Launcelott Derrick, fell two storeys into a courtyard, breaking his left leg. A bricklayer called Myllis was either unlucky or clumsy. On 27 November 1639, he

> had a severe fall near upon 3 storeys in the inside of a new building from the timber of one floor to another taken up speechless but within an hour spoke but not sensibly no hurt about him but his left clavicle broken close to the sternum & a little place contused in the occiput or pole behind his head.

Binns reported laconically, 'Afterwards was killed in the same work, no one knows how, found under a great window'.[33]

Of course, other occupations had their hazards as well. Perhaps the most dramatic occupational injury Binns treated was the case of a young butcher on Saffron Hill who was gored in the left thigh by a bull. Less dramatic were accidents involving horses and horse-drawn vehicles. One groom had his left leg broken 'by a blow of his horse heel'. Others less occupationally qualified were hurt in similar ways. A woman 'had her left leg broke by a coach wheel', 'Mr. Payne broke his left collarbone . . . falling off a horse' and a young man 'fell from a horseback & put his right arm out of joint in the elbow'.[34]

The work of housewives and maid-servants was also dangerous. Mrs Carie, a goldsmith's wife, was treated for a mortified hand and arm after pricking her finger with a needle. Elizabeth Bemis, Mrs Brewer's maid, was 'burned with fire upon the left temple close to the eyelid and under the eye'.[35] The home itself was also full of hazards. Children burned themselves and broke bones tumbling from beds and windows. Adults fell downstairs.[36] Indeed, it is remarkable that the casebook contains so few examples of accidents occurring in the home, considering that in the seventeenth century open fires were the rule, building regulations were non-existent and tools conformed to no standard except the maker's own. To survive, one had to be careful.

Of course, even vigilance could not prevent some accidents. One poor woman, a servant at Gray's Inn, died after receiving a head injury 'being in a boat upon the Thames by a stick thrown from another boat'. Another woman was wounded on the forehead by a tile, which presumably slipped off a roof.[37] Binns did not describe the circumstances which produced many of the injuries he treated. Most of these were simple dislocations, fractures and cuts which he dealt with for very short periods of time. Typical of his commentary on such cases was the following: 'A girl in Shoe Lane put her right elbow out. Put it in. Well.'[38]

He recorded successful treatment of most of the injuries for which he was consulted. What follows is a general description of his therapeutic approach to wounds, fractures, dislocations and bruises. Only brief mention will be made of the preparations he applied to the injured part, the discussion concentrating, rather, on Binns's routines which reveal both the results most important to the surgeon and the procedures patients underwent. In cases of stab wounds Binns first attempted to stop the bleeding with dressings which he called boulsters, pleagetts or rowlers. Sometimes he searched the wound with either a finger or a probe before dressing it, but he usually delayed this procedure for a day or two, presumably to avoid exacerbating the bleeding. He then usually prescribed a laxative or a clyster, to keep the body soluble, and a cordial to support the patient's spirits. He also generally prescribed a light diet, often consisting exclusively of liquids such as broth and posset-ale. After the initial bleeding had stopped, Binns attempted to prevent apostemation by keeping the wound open. This he did by means of a tent (a roll of dressing or other material) inserted into the mouth of the wound to keep open a drainage tract. If the wound was so small a puncture that it could not be easily searched, Binns might dilate it, with an instrument he called a root, before inserting the tent. Binns also occasionally injected medicines into puncture wounds.

Binns's penchant for keeping stab wounds open would almost certainly have elicited criticism from Richard Wiseman, who was strongly in favour of 'bringing the lips of the wound exactly together'. He wrote,

> Nature hath nothing to do here in bring the lips together, that is the sole work of the chirurgeon; who must not lay a pledgit, or crowd a dossil of lint or tent into a little wound; no, that is the way to keep the wound open, and make it painful, whereby defluxions are stirred up, the temperament of the part weakened, and the cure prolonged; contrary to the intention of all who have writ of wounds, and to the practice of our knowing chirurgeons here.[39]

Wiseman used tents, certainly, but only in cases where the wound was suspected or known to contain foreign bodies, or where apostemation was expected or observed.

Wiseman's method of dealing with cuts and lacerations

coincided with Binns's practice. These Binns usually stitched up immediately after stopping the bleeding. The case of a tailor in Postern Lane who cut his own throat provides an excellent example of wound management. Binns sewed up the wound, which did well for twelve days. At this point, it 'began to apostemate', so Binns reopened the wound and changed the ointment in the dressings. The patient recovered.[40]

Gunshot wounds, a favourite subject among military writers, presented special difficulties. Indeed, Wiseman wrote that surgeons of the past assumed that such wounds were poisonous because of 'the deadly colour of these wounds, which in those early days, when the invention of guns was novel, surprised them, by looking not unlike poisoned and burnt wounds'. He went on to say that such beliefs influenced the treatment of gunshot victims in his own time, with disastrous results:

> In these our later times, although they do not call them venomous, yet is it a difficult thing to dissuade many of our chirurgeons from dressing these wounds with tinctures of myrrh and honey of roses, and thrusting in of great tents: by which way of dressing I have seen these wounds undigested the tenth day; one whereof was in the cheek with dry and flaggy lips. These lesser fleshy wounds being undigested, at last gangrene: and in truth it is not to be wondered at.[41]

He advocated less drastic treatment, which, he maintained, was more efficient. However, he did not minimise the danger of such injuries, writing,

> Wounds made by gun-shot are the most complicate sort of wounds that can be inflicted: for they are not only solution of continuity, but have joined with them contusion, attrition, and dilaceration, in a high and vehement kind. To this we may add all sorts of fractures and accidents as *hemorrhagia*, inflammation, erysipelas, gangrene, and *sphacelus*; besides the extraneous bodies which are violently carried into the wound, and multiply indications.[42]

Binns's experience illustrates Wiseman's general statements. Occasionally, the bullet lodged in the body and had to be cut out. Sometimes there were powder burns to contend with. In one case, part of the lining of the injured man's doublet was projected into the wound by the bullet and was removed three days after the man was shot. According to Binns, compared to most puncture wounds and lacerations, gunshot wounds were dirty, yielding 'a dirty black matter' for the first few days of treatment. They could also be foul smelling.[43] Some cases Binns treated similarly to his puncture wounds, keeping the wounds open with flamulae (fabric strips or strings) or tents moistened with medicines. Sometimes he used injections, as with puncture wounds. Other gunshot wounds he simply dressed at the skin surface. Despite their difference from other sorts of wounds, Binns used no special medications for gunshot wounds, and never indicated that he believed them to be poisoned. Once the bleeding had been stopped and foreign bodies removed from the wound, he adhered to his usual routine of frequent dressings, laxatives, clysters and occasional phlebotomy, watching for the signs of apostemation, and trying to prevent that complication if possible. The signs of apostemation included swelling, the build-up of fluid, local heat or fever and sometimes mortification. A moderate discharge from the wound was regarded as normal and healthy.

Binns used numerous preparations, both to bathe and anoint wounds and upon the different parts of his dressings. He expected wounds to heal in a certain fashion, and prescribed different preparations to aid in each stage of the healing process. If a wound were unusually painful, he applied a cataplasm (medicated poultice) to ease the patient's discomfort. He was then most concerned to bring the wound to 'digestion', that is, to cause or facilitate the production of healthy discharge. Wiseman called this discharge 'laudable pus', which was 'a perfect white matter, of good inconsistence, and not foetid or ill scented'.[44] If, in the process, 'proud' or 'spongy' flesh formed in the wound, Binns attacked it with spirit of wine or other preparations designed to remove it. Next Binns wished the wound to 'incarnate', an action signalled by a reduction of discharge from the wound and the generally healthy appearance of it. The final step was to cicatrise or close the wound. Binns was careful not to allow wounds to close until either the threat of apostemation had passed or, in the case of compound fractures and incised bones, splinters of bone had emerged from the wound.

Of course, wounds very often did apostemate. When they did,

they were treated in the same way as other sorts of apostemations and fistulae (see below). Binns dealt with many such wounds – cases so extreme that tendons and bones had become 'corrupt' or 'foul' and extremities threatened to become gangrenous. However, in only one case did he resort to amputation.[45] His caution was not unique. Wiseman advised against this extreme measure, reporting numerous cases similar to Binns's where he used cautery and scarification, along with a suitable regimen, rather than take a risk which was likely to end in the death of the patient. Wiseman indicated that amputation (usually by hot knife) was only the treatment of choice where other measures had failed and 'if the body be youthful, and the habit of body tolerable'. None the less, both Wiseman and the early seventeenth-century surgeon, John Woodall, who preceded Binns on the staff at St Bartholomew's, applied the procedure more often than did Binns.[46] Their relative willingness to amputate almost certainly reflects their experience with battlefield surgery and their greater familiarity with both the techniques and the prognoses involved. Binns's cautious treatment of wounds was quite successful. Out of 79 injuries which involved open wounds, the case-notes report 8 deaths, 21 unknown results, and 50 cures.

Binns treated 58 cases of compound and simple fractures and dislocations, exclusive of head wounds. In his treatment of these patients, his greatest concerns were to prevent or cure apostemation and fever, and to restore the use of the limb. A paramount goal was to get broken bones to knit. In stubborn cases, Binns and his contemporaries resorted to bone surgery to achieve this end. Thus, in one case of a fractured leg where the bones refused to knit, 'the greater fossil being broken obliquely there start up a small corner of the bone towards the inner ankle so as it caused pain so I broke off the sharp point with my nail & applied mixt. ung. after which he had no pain'.[47] Wiseman reported parallel cases, where fractures could not easily be reduced or did not heal, where he either sawed off the end of the bone or reduced 'the prominencies . . . with a chisel-like instrument thrust between the fractured ends of the bone', used 'after the manner of a lever'. In one case, 'the leg remained the shorter, almost as much as had been sawed off of the bone'.[48]

In routine cases, Binns set bones using splints, various sorts of plasters, rollers, laced stockings and pillows to immobilise the injured part. His approach varied from case to case, depending on the patient's general condition and the amount of pain the treatment caused. He regarded broken bones – particularly in the legs – as serious injuries, treating patients for months, applying plaster after plaster, and checking limbs for strength. Mr Fisher, the innkeeper at the Star in Holborn, had his left tibia close to the ankle broken by a coach wheel in March 1640. It was a compound fracture and Binns feared gangrene, so he dressed it twice a day for the first two weeks. Mr Fisher was completely bedridden well into May, being laid on a pallet every two or three days while his bed was being made. Binns was still applying new plasters in August, when the case-note ended, incomplete.[49]

Less serious were broken noses and simple fractures of the arms, wrists, clavicles and ribs. These Binns set; he applied warm dressings to ease pain and reduce swelling, usually delaying application of the long-lasting 'restringent' plaster for a few days until the swelling had gone down. As in other injuries, he occasionally let blood, prescribed clysters or laxatives and recommended a light diet.

Dislocations were usually regarded as less serious than fractures, except when they were accompanied by a wound. Binns reduced the dislocation, then immobilised the limb. His treatment of the following patient is quite typical.

> Jonathan's son the carman fell from a horseback & put his right arm out of joint in the elbow so I put it in myself with little extension by pulling the cubitus & withall bending it inward & thrusting up the eminence of the advitorium all at once & so it slipped in. It slipped out again by putting his arm out at length: it went in again as it did before.

After some twenty days of treatment, during which two plasters were applied, the patient found his joint a little stiff so that he could not straighten it, but 'by carrying it out & motion it came again, all praised be God'.[50]

Head wounds – particularly those involving fractures – were among the most serious disorders Binns treated. Of the thirteen cases for which we have some details, four patients died, five got well and four case-notes were incomplete, so the outcome is unknown. The four patients who died experienced a similar pattern of symptoms. Each seemed reasonably well after the initial dressing of the wound and remained so for at least a week. After between nine and fourteen days each patient developed symptoms – vomiting, fever, or paralysis – which became increasingly severe until the patient's death between thirteen and twenty-five days after injury.[51] In three cases, Binns and the other surgeons consulted followed standard procedure by laying the cranium bare in order to determine whether the skull had been fractured. In two cases the trepan was applied.[52] In Binns's practice this operation was obviously reserved for the most desperate cases, when the patient was expected to die in any event. Both of Binns's patients who underwent trepanning died within 24 hours after the operation.

In contrast, Richard Wiseman performed the procedure more often than did Binns and with greater success. In depressed fractures of the skull, where no wound or fissure existed large enough to give vent to any build-up of fluid under the skull, Wiseman wrote, 'then the trepan ought to be applied, to give vent to the serum, and to make way for the raising the deprest bone'. Even where an obvious fissure existed, the trepan could be applied 'where the fissure lieth untowardly for discharge of matter, or where the depression of the cranium is deep'.[53] Wiseman's observations regarding five trepanations indicated that four patients had survived the operation. One patient died and Wiseman maintained that she might have lived, had she permitted the trepan to be applied earlier.[54]

Not all of Binns's patients suffering skull fractures died. In August 1649,

> Frank the drawer at the Castle Tavern in Paternoster Row . . . received a blow with a pint pot upon the frons near the edge of the left temporal muscle, which made a little depression with a fracture round the depression and a piece of the depressed bone carried away to the side of the wound.

Binns gave Frank the treatment he routinely used for head injuries. He opened a vein and gave a suppository. He dressed the wound, using warm medications and bandages. He then prescribed a suppository every other day, changed the medicines used on the dressings as healing progressed, rolled the bandages loosely and watched Frank's daily progress. Frank recovered quickly.[55]

Binns regarded this treatment routine as necessary. In the case of Will Evims, a patient who died thirteen days after receiving a knife wound on the left side of his forehead, Binns, who merely consulted, criticised the attending surgeon for 'neither [having] given him clyster nor opened vein nor applied anything to his wound more than pleagetts coplaster'. He was, however, flexible enough to learn from what he perceived as his own mistakes. In the case of a boy who died twenty-five days after having been kicked in the head by a horse, Binns apparently felt he was partly to blame for the patient's death, for he wrote, 'Let it be your care not to roll the head too hard'.[56]

In addition to the serious injuries described above, Binns treated a number of patients for sprains, bruises and relatively minor burns. One sprained ankle yielded quickly to several days of hot ointments and soaking, combined with a stiff plaster. In a more stubborn case, a repeatedly sprained ankle resisted a long and varied course of treatment which included fomentations, purges, plasters, a laced stocking and a trip to Bath. The patient remained uncured.[57] Bruises usually responded after several applications of oils and plasters. However, some bruises apostemated, requiring the more complicated treatment described below.

In the course of his career, Binns recorded treating only five patients for burns. In each case the patient recovered. In only one instance was he called immediately after the injury occurred. In this case, that of a maid-servant who scalded her arms in June 1651, Binns produced a cure within three weeks by the use of warm unguent, applied with a feather, and a dressing of lawn (fine linen or cotton) rags kept wet with another ointment and laid over the burn.[58] In two other cases Binns began treating burn victims only when other efforts had failed. When he 'began cure of Elizabeth Bemis Mrs Brewer's maid', the burn on her left temple near her eyelid had caused an ulcer so deep it was 'almost to the cranium'. During his first visit, Binns opened a vein, applied cupping glasses, ordered a clyster and fomented the ulcer with whey. After several of these fomentations, he applied an unguent until the burn had healed. However, after healing had taken place, 'her eyelid began to draw up within a month . . . so that the inside was turned out, it became very painful and swelled like a bladder'. At this point, the patient resorted to a traditional magical treatment, stroking her eyelid 'with a dead hand' (probably belonging to a recently hanged criminal), thereupon finding relief (Binns did not comment upon this therapy). However, 'she had not perfect ease till she had an issue in her arm on the same side'.[59]

Surgical repairs

A significant part of Joseph Binns's practice was concerned with the treatment of such conditions as ulcers, herniae, apostems, fistulae and tumours, in addition to an assortment of less commonly encountered ills, such as hydrocephaly. Again, difficulties exist with regard to terminology. For instance, an apostemation, or matter-filled swelling, might also be described as a tumour, since Binns used the word 'tumour' to refer to any swelling. Also, apostems frequently developed into fistulae. Equally, after opening, they might become ulcers. Thus, any figures mentioned in connection with these terms must be approximate. However, a rough breakdown of Binns's own references to these conditions indicates that he treated 31 patients for ulcers (excluding those caused by syphilis and its treatment), 68 for apostems, 25 for fistulae, 18 for herniae, 35 for tumours and 19 for other disorders requiring repair.

These patients came to Binns hoping to obtain relief from pain and disability. Many also hoped to have their appearances improved. For instance, Mrs Storye, a coachman's wife, had a 'tumour varicosus in the right cheek & coming out at her mouth, in her neck to her shoulder, no bigger than a cherry when she was born but increased as she did grow'. The tumour was only occasionally painful; from time to time it apostemated and required surgical intervention. However, Mrs Storye must also have been concerned about the disfigurement it caused. When Binns saw her, the tumour 'was apostemated from behind her ear to the temple very big'. He was able to cure the apostem and leave 'the tumour less than it used to be, praised be God'.[60]

Surgical repairs were also required by people who were in pain and who, no doubt, feared the possibly fatal consequences of allowing a condition to continue. Many such patients sought a return to their previously stable state, rather than a complete cure. For instance, Mr Arthur Rudle had worn a steel truss to control his rupture for many years. When, after having taken cold, he found he could not replace the rupture in the truss, he first called for the truss-maker, Mr Bostocke, and later for Binns to help him. The surgeon, by means of a series of clysters and warm applications to the rupture, was finally able to replace it in the truss twenty-six days after he was first consulted. Mr Rudle was satisfied. He was also fortunate. Mr Sadler bruised his old rupture, and all the efforts to replace it in his truss made by Binns and the patient's friends were useless. Sadler died five days after he was injured.[61]

Some patients and their families decided to alter a reasonably stable condition in the hope of obtaining a permanent cure. When Mrs Wilson's baby was born,

> it had a little knot or tumour soft in the nape of the neck upon the skull. This grew bigger every month so that in September 1648 it was as big as one's fist, I was satisfied that it was water, the child's head was larger much than children of that age usually are (it was then some 8 months old) I perceived there was a perforation in the skull. I was fearful to open it because of the accidents which might follow[,] but being earnestly desired of the mother of the child, she being well resolved concerning the child, the 15th of September, 1648, I opened this tumour by incision.

There followed a month during which Binns repeatedly opened the baby's head. The child was feverish and sick most of the time. On 16 October it died.[62]

Not all surgical repairs of congenital disorders presented such problems. Binns reported that 'Mr. Webster of Chesterfield his son was cut of a wry neck the 19 June 1640. It was skinned in 5 days. (Mr. Harris his way of cutting)'.[63] Binns made no suggestion that such an operation was either dangerous or unusual. However, Mr Webster was concerned enough to travel a long way in search of expert surgical help. He was not alone. London was used as a medical centre for the whole of England, and Binns's patients had often travelled long distances to consult him.

Apostems

The repair jobs which Binns most frequently undertook were the treatment of apostems and fistulae (the term he used for hollowness left by earlier apostemation). As indicated above, these ailments resulted from various causes. Wounds apostemated. Patients developed apostems and fistulae as complications of conditions such as haemorrhoids, tooth-decay, childbirth, breast-feeding and ague.[64] Whatever the cause or location, Binns's approach was either to open and drain the swelling, making certain that all matter had issued before he allowed the orifice to close, or to open the fistula, cleanse the area, and make sure the flesh as it grew again was sound. His usual method of opening both apostems and fistulae was to apply 'the caustic stone' for several hours, which either opened the affected place on its own or made it easier for Binns to open it by incision. Binns also used 'suppurative cataplasms' which occasionally opened apostems on their own. Very rarely he opened apostems by incision. And sometimes apostems obligingly opened spontaneously.[65]

Like other surgeons, Binns assisted drainage by inserting a tent into the orifice of an apostem. If the opening was not large enough, Binns dilated it with a root. He then encouraged drainage by the use of various medicines, either applying them to dressings, bathing the affected area, or injecting them into the orifice. In cases of fistulae where Binns could find two orifices, he sometimes drew a 'frenum' or string through both openings and tied the string progressively tighter. After several days he was usually able to open the fistula quite easily by incision. In other cases, where such a procedure was not possible, he used caustic.

Wiseman's method of dealing with fistulae was identical to Binns's. In one of his 'observations',

> An officer of the King's Army laboured long of a fistula, occasioned by a gun-shot wound in the upper part of the os tibiae near the knee . . . After general evacuation, I applied a caustic the whole length of the sinus, whereby I took off that callus, gave vent to the discharge of that foetid ichor made in the ulcer, and took out several pieces of the rotten bone which were shut in there. That done I scraped away the remaining rottenness, and drest the bone with catagmatick powders, etc. by which means after some time a callus thrust forth, and united with the neighbouring flesh, which incarned with the lips, and was afterwards cicatrised.[66]

The treatment of apostems and fistulae was often a long frustrating business. Just when it seemed that healing was about to occur, a new swelling would develop, or a new hollowness be found, and the whole process would begin all over again. In May 1645, after suffering from an ague, John the carman's son developed an apostem in his right calf. Binns opened and treated it in his usual manner, but John developed a fistula which became 'full of matter' at least four times before it finally healed in April 1646.[67] Such patients required frequent visits for dressing changes, assessment of the healing process (often requiring alterations in prescriptions), and monitoring of the general physical state, including pain, sleep, appetite, and bowel movements. Many of the working hours of Binns and his servants or apprentices must have been occupied by visits to patients suffering from apostems and fistulae.

Ulcers

Binns treated many sorts of ulcers. Some, as indicated above, came about in the course of treating apostems and fistulae. Many resulted from syphilis (discussed below). Some were cancerous, some were symptoms of scurvy, some were complications of other disorders, such as tumours and corns, and still others appeared spontaneously. Binns kept a number of medications which he used mainly for the treatment of ulcers. He had his own 'ulcer water' and 'unguent mixt'. He also touched ulcers with strong preparations composed of such substances as mercury, antimony and vitriol. His aim was first to cleanse the ulcer of 'escars', discharge and unhealthy spongy flesh, then to promote healing.

His success in healing ulcers was variable. Although he tried a number of different preparations on Mrs Lightfool's facial ulcers between May and July 1633, each new ointment caused much pain, but did no good. Some ulcers, such as the apthous type which Mr Hutchinson's girl Sarah had on her gums and tongue, might possibly have disappeared on their own (Sarah was well in ten days). Others of Binns's cures seem almost miraculous. On 4 April 1655, a 14-day-old infant developed an ulcer on the navel after the umbilical cord had fallen off. Despite the efforts of Binns and the physician Dr Bathurst, the ulcer grew until 'it spread as broad as a xx piece'. At this point Binns used his unguent with an antimony preparation, and reported 'good digestion'. The ulcer healed by 20 April, 'Laus soli deo'.[68]

Although Binns treated a number of ulcers which he described as cancerous, he never approached them with much hope of success. Indeed, he reported a cure in only one case of cancer. This was that of Goodwife White of St Giles in the Fields. Binns removed her cancerous breast in St Bartholomew's Hospital on 3 February 1648. She was alive and well in 1653. Binns attempted breast removal in another patient seven months later, using the ligature method also recommended by Wiseman. Binns

> used a double ligature upon the woman's breast the 9 August at morn 1648. Tied it harder the 11th at morn & the 12, & the 14th it had gained much – the 16th & the 18 – the 22nd the lower string was through the bigness of a finger, the upper one near to an inch . . . so with string cut it off in the ligature. It bled pretty freely. Died a week after.[69]

Thereafter, Binns treated breast cancers more cautiously, dealing with cancerous tumours and ulcers in the same way as those regarded as non-cancerous. In addition to breast cancers, he treated cancerous mouth and tongue ulcers. Regardless of the therapy applied, these patients died.[70]

Binns treated several leg ulcers which, according to the casebook, had been caused by scurvy. These began with swelling and spots in the affected leg. The spots turned to pustules or blisters, and these eventually ulcerated. Binns treated such patients with juice of scurvy grass, purges, and a variety of ointments.[71] Binns successfully treated three cases of ulcers in the eye. In one case, he described the affected eye in detail:

> I found her eye much inflamed [,] upon the pupilla a little whitish dint in the outward coat of cornea like the pressure of a pin's head with little towes from it as if it had been a little piece of flock of wool, which seemed to be an ulcer. Her pain was great pricking & burning.

Binns characteristically treated the woman's whole system, blistering her neck, purging her with pills, applying plasters to her temples, and dropping medicines into her eye. The ulcers got worse at first, so Binns changed the eye medications (including woman's milk in the second preparation) and cupped and scarified the patient's shoulders. After this the eye improved. The woman was relieved of her pain and retained 'some weak sight' in her eye.[72]

Tumours

Binns's practice included the treatment of many tumours. As indicated above, he used the word 'tumour' to describe any swelling. However, he also used the term more specifically, referring to growths which were not apostemated swellings or oedema. He also used other terms, such as 'wen', 'polyp', 'ficus' and 'ascites' to refer to tumours. Some tumours were easier to treat than others. Polyps in the nose, for instance, were not difficult to remove, but tended to recur. Binns wrote in 1650,

> I extracted a pollipus out of Mrs. Cooper's daughter's nostril & made her an issue in her left arm. I had extracted it out of both nostrils 2 years afore this . . . (I expected it again in 1654). They are in both nostrils like a bunch of grapes, injected after a restringent medicine.[73]

Likewise, he had no difficulty treating a 'ficus' in the anus of one Mr Lucas. On 2 February he 'made ligature' upon the tumour. He reported that 'it looked deadish the next day and flacid, it came off going to stool the 6 February at morn'.[74]

However, some tumours were harder to deal with, and Binns approached them with caution. Indeed, his casebook reveals nothing more clearly than this surgeon's reluctance to use the knife. Even when opening the flesh was necessary, Binns preferred gradual (and if possible bloodless) means, such as the caustic stone and ligature. The following case illustrates his caution. On 16 March 1661, he and the surgeon Mr Arris were called to see a Mr Chilsonne who had

> a great tumour on the inside of his right thigh very large in length from the middle of the thigh to the knee in thickness from the forepart of the thigh so to the underside of the thigh to the outside.

They judged that 'it was a schirrus cancerosus' and ordered a cataplasm to be applied. Their prescriptions were used for some two weeks. At this point, a Dr Williams was called in. He was in favour of opening the tumour by means of a 'sympathetic specific medicine' of his own composition. This was first applied on 8 April. On 10 April, incision was tried, but 'there came blood trickling out pretty fast, so clapt on a dosell [dressing] . . . and bound it up till the 11 April, cut a little deeper till blood came', dressed it again, and continued this pattern of treatment until Dr Williams could insert a probe two inches into the incision. On 16 April the patient died. The next day, the tumour was opened. Binns reported 'there was nothing in it but coagulated blood & a substance like rotten liver, & but little thin blood, & a hollowness from it up to the groin full of black grumous blood'.[75] Binns apparently felt that the patient would have been better off without Dr Williams's radical help.

Binns attempted to remove only certain sorts of tumours. These were not always small. In one case, he successfully removed a wen from a woman's shoulder-blade which was 'hanging down as big as a child's head'. On 12 February 1652 he 'incised' a cancerous tumour on a man's thigh. He then treated the resulting ulcer and a new tumour which developed on the patient's ribs until 29 August, when the man died. Despite this outcome, Binns reported 'his thigh is even cicatrised'.[76]

Other tumours he dealt with by using surface applications and internal medicines. In a case of scrofulous tumours of the neck, for instance, Binns prescribed a course of vomits, purges, salves and plasters. This patient was under his care on and off for four years. Her condition did not heal permanently, so she left Binns and looked elsewhere for a cure. Binns noted laconically, 'She was after touched by the King'.[77] Most of the tumours Binns treated were easily visible, occurring on the extremities or the neck and head. He dealt with few tumours occurring in the abdomen and chest, although he did undertake treatment of an 'ascites' or tumour of the belly. He opened this swelling on 24 June 1655, releasing a gallon of fluid the first day and a similar amount on the two following days. The fourth day he released three quarts and the patient felt better, but was very restless. He died that evening. As in the case of hydrocephaly discussed above, and one of another infant who was born with an 'aqueous tumour on the small of the back', Binns was able to drain the swelling, but could not stop production of the fluid.[78]

Hernia

The last major type of repair Binns undertook was the treatment of hernia. He treated eighteen male patients for herniae. Twelve of these had 'hernia aquosa' (also known as hydrocoele), a condition in which one side of the scrotum filled with a watery fluid. Binns's treatment of hernia aquosa followed a routine which was usually successful. The day before surgery, the patient was prescribed a vomit. The next day the swelling was opened by incision. The following case was typical:

> 1652. Dr. Bennet hath had a hernia aquosa 12 months in his testicle [.] I opened it the 8th April in the afternoon the stone lay to the seam in the middle of the scrotum, & I made incision on the outside towards the thigh an inch from the stone, and toward the bottom of the tumour. There came out of clear water three parts of a pint, I used a restringent & warm fomentation for 5 or six days, morn & night, with a hot stupe.

The patient recovered.[79]

Binns treated other sorts of hernia with surface applications and trusses. Mrs Benfield's son developed an intestinal hernia which Binns treated with purges and the application of hot ointments and dressings. The patient was cured in two weeks. Mr Robinson's old intestinal hernia fell down so that it filled the scrotum. Binns and two surgical colleagues, Mr King and Mr Heath, tried to reduce it without success. They treated the patient with clysters, fomentations and cataplasms, but the patient died seven days after he became ill.[80]

In Binns's treatment of hernia, as in his therapeutic approach generally, one can see both his dependence upon medical theory and his empiricism.[81] On the one hand, he prescribed purges, clysters, issues and phlebotomy in order to keep or produce a humoral balance in the body. On the other, he altered the treatments he applied according to his perception of their efficacy. His apparent aim was not to attack the primary causes of disease, about which the casebook does not speculate, but to get rid of an unwelcome symptom or to return the patient to a bearable and stable condition. In this he appears to have frequently succeeded. Of the approximately 194 repairs he undertook, 92 left the patient well, 22 resulted in improvement of the condition, and only seven left the sufferer no better than before. In 31 cases the patients died, and in 44 the outcome is unknown.

Venereal disease

Binns treated many ailments which were produced by acknowledged internal diseases. Some conditions, like the spots, ulcers and swellings which appeared on the legs of scurvy sufferers, fell properly within the surgeon's sphere of operation. Others, such as diarrhoea, sore throat, agues and coughs, might more appropriately have been taken to a physician, as indicated above. Binns treated internal problems with purges and vomits, sometimes adding a typically surgical remedy, such as an issue, to the course of treatment. His general approach to illness has been discussed above, and need not concern us here. What we will investigate at length is his handling of venereal disease, particularly syphilis, which called upon all of his medical and surgical abilities at once.

Binns adapted the remedies he prescribed to the severity and types of symptoms presented, the sufferer's previous experience of 'cures' and the patient's reactions to the means tried. The first manifestation of disease which Binns saw most frequently was 'gonorrhoea', which involved discharge from the penis, 'smarting' during urination, and uncontrollable erection or 'standing'. Binns routinely began treatment with a dose of 'pill Barbarosa', which purged the patient, and an injection into the urethra of his 'green water'. To this he often added a diet drink which contained the purging herb senna. If the condition continued, he moved on to one or both of the two courses of treatment favoured at the time – a month's prescription of either guaiacum or mercury. The guaiacum cure was considerably more pleasant for the patient. Sometimes it apparently succeeded.[82] However, Binns used mercury far more often.

The mercury treatment involved taking mercury internally, applying it in ointments to rashes, scabs and ulcers, and in 'waters' injected into apostems, noses and genitalia. Side effects of treatment were a sore mouth and throat, sometimes involving ulceration, spitting great quantities, occasional nausea and frequent bowel movements. In the hands of an unskilled or unscrupulous practitioner, the cure could be worse than the disease. Thus, Binns treated both the illness and the 'cure'. On 8 May 1639, he first saw Joan Carter,

> who hath the lower mandible corrupt (& the teeth fallen forth) all the chin from the one cheek to the other, the

> cheeks & chin much swollen & hard, she was fluxed by Kixton the Quack 3 years ago, & she continued spitting at times ever since, & at that time where her cheeks were ulcerated for want of looking to they grew so hard cicatrised that she could not well open her jaws so he cut them & after that she had a contraction of some branches of sinews down her neck, that she could neither open well her mouth nor lift up her head much.

By October he could report that 'she [was] very well praised by God, & no great blemish, only her chin a little shrunk in'.[83]

Binns himself was very careful about mercury doses and patients' reactions to them. If the patient had too extreme a reaction, he either reduced the dose or withdrew the mercury for a time. By the same token, if doses did not seem to be working, he increased them. He apparently experimented with different mercury doses and preparations, trying them out on patients in St Bartholomew's Hospital. During one February, he gave three men the same number of 'precipitate pills' on three successive days and compared their reactions. On the first day, five grains gave one man four stools and the others two stools apiece. Eight grains on the second day produced two, five and four stools respectively. On the third day, sixteen grains gave the patients two stools, four stools and two vomits, and six stools respectively. One man had begun to spit at this point.[84]

Even in the hands of a skilled practitioner, mercury cures produced symptoms which themselves required treatment. Mr Thomas Mazeine had first consulted Binns in May 1635, at which time 'the diet' removed all his pains. In March 1637, he had nodes in both shins. Binns prescribed a mercury course which relieved the pain in his legs, but caused ulceration of his tongue and cheeks 'with white sloughs'. Binns treated this problem with 'lotion of barley, althea roots, licorice and violet leaves which cleansed the ulcers in the 7th or 8th day'.[85]

Of course, Binns combined a mercury flux with other prescriptions designed to improve the patient's general health. He almost always prescribed a diet drink, and recommended healthy eating habits. He blamed a repeat patient, Mr John Malett or Merett, for the fact that his ulcerated forehead was slow to heal, writing 'but sometimes it would be all cicatrised, & he keeping no good diet, but disordered, so it would ulcerate by places & some little pieces of bones cast out'. Several months later the patient 'took pills, & became temperate so, he grew fat & in very good health & all his forehead healed save a little moisture came out above his nose, very well in April 1655'.[86] Binns also prescribed sweating for syphilis patients, as did other practitioners.

The nature of the pox required the healers who treated it to apply their skills to particular immediate problems as well as to the disease as a whole. Of particular concern to both sufferer and practitioner were the ulcers on the foreskin which rapidly became gangrenous and caused patients to lose all or part of the penis. In one case, Binns applied 'a strong cataplasm to revocate the spirits and hinder putrifaction', and twice scarified the foreskin. When these measures did not work, Binns cut away the mortified flesh.[87]

Another manifestation of syphilis which was particularly difficult to treat was its invasion of bones which caused tumours and the eventual rotting away of the bone itself. In 1645, Mr Fotiley was cured 'of a pain in his left leg nocturnal a little tumour upon the bone' by a Mr Sase. 'In 1651 he had pain again. The bone foul which Quince [another surgeon] took off with a mallett and chisel & the diet. Took away his pains.' Binns first saw the patient in April 1659, when the bone was 'like a rotten post'. Binns applied dressings to the bone itself and gave mercury internally. In August, Mr Fotiley went downstairs 'and coming up again he turned a little awry & broke the rotten part of the maior tibia in sunder so keeps his bed wholly'. By October, he was feeling a bit better, but still had to return home to Berkshire in a horse litter.[88]

Other symptoms of syphilis which Binns treated separately were ulcerated throats, palates, noses and lips, bubos in the groin, obstructions in the urethra, nodes in the shins and the skull and various pains in the joints and the head. His treatment was apparently successful. In the cases for which the information exists, he recorded 60 as having recovered and 15 as improved. Ten patients remained uncured and two died. These figures do not tell the whole story. No doubt some patients, disheartened by long and inconclusive courses of treatment, consulted other healers. Some who had apparently been cured became ill again years later. Binns's casebook contains references to quite a few patients who repeatedly consulted him along with other practitioners in their interminable efforts to rid themselves of the pox. The most faithful of these sufferers was one Mr Brooks, who underwent some seven courses of treatment in four years.[89] Thus the number of 'cures' indicated above is certainly an overestimate of the patients who were permanently healed, and the small number of deaths recorded is probably an underestimate.

Binns and his patients clearly held that syphilis was sexually transmitted. Mr Baker, a bookseller's man, developed pustules upon the glans 'by dealing with a pocky woman'. Mr Henry Richards 'the 20 July in the night suffered much pain bet. glans & praepution having lain with a wench some 5 or 6 days afore'.[90] Because of its associations with unclean sexuality, syphilis affected people's attitudes and behaviour concerning marriage. Mr Baker was aghast when his syphilis re-emerged shortly after his marriage in the summer of 1655. He had thought he had been cured five years earlier. Mr Egas apparently felt he had been unfairly treated by the pox when it returned after four years' dormancy. He protested 'that he had not dealt with any but his wife who was then very well & had been for long time'.[91]

Syphilis was acknowledged to be loathsome disease which disfigured its victims and lasted a dreadfully long time. A severe case could impoverish the sufferer. In one year of treatment, Mr John Merett or Malett ran up a £35 bill at the apothecary's. Further, owing to its associations with sexual vice, it was also a shameful disease. While a person suffering from scrofula (also a disfiguring ailment) could be an object of pity, a pox-ridden sufferer was likely to be ridiculed. Therefore it is not surprising that many of the people Binns treated for syphilis complained of more innocent sounding individual symptoms, such as chronic headache or sore throat. 'My cousin Spooner's sister' consulted Binns for 'extreme pain in her head . . . it being all her head over & as much by day as night but somewhat worse in the night'. Several days later she developed nodes on her forehead and pains in her shoulders. Binns prescribed a mercury flux.[92] Considering such attempts at concealment, it is probable that more of Binns's patients were syphilitic than the diagnoses indicated in the case-notes reveal. For instance, some of the women who consulted Binns for amenorrhoea, too small an amount of menstruation and the whites may have had the pox. Mrs Elin Barker, who complained of amenorrhoea, 'sloughs & stench', falls within this category. The unfortunate 5-year-old girl who had the whites in very great quantity was another possible victim. Binns wrote 'it was feared [that] one that had the gonorrhoea spent his sperm betwixt the child's legs upon her pudenda, but this was not certainly proved'.[93]

There was, of course, another possible explanation for amenorrhoea. One 20 July Binns treated 'Mary at Mr. Barham's' who 'wants her menses', with laxatives and emetics. He also let blood from the saphenous vein – the classically endorsed treatment for this complaint. Nine days later her menses 'came down very well'. This sounds very like induced abortion.[94] Binns also treated other specifically female problems, such as inordinate menses, fits of the mother and swelling in the hand and arm occurring after childbirth. For all of these conditions he prescribed laxatives or emetics, or both which usually produced the desired result.[95]

Binns's treatment of syphilis and other genito-urinary disorders was conventional. His concentration on this area of practice was also conventional. Surgeons had been undertaking the cure of venereal diseases since the early sixteenth century at least. Binns's therapeutic methods did not change over the entire thirty years covered by the casebook. Venereal disease provided him with an arena where his own special talents – patience, caution, conscientiousness and persistence – could be well employed.

Conclusions

There is much that Joseph Binns's casebook does not tell us, both about his own practice and about the ordinary practice of surgery in seventeenth-century England. Only tantalising hints are given about his 'man' – the servant, apprentice or assistant who is occasionally mentioned in a case-note. Since surgical training was invariably by apprenticeship, and since Binns was an active member of London's surgical community, it is more than likely that he kept a series of apprentices in the course of his career. It is equally likely that, as a well-to-do man, he employed one or more servants. In addition, the casebook provides little information about the prices Binns charged for his services. Money due or received is mentioned only under unusual circumstances. Thus we know nothing about this surgeon's ordinary rates, or whether he charged on a sliding scale, according to the patient's ability to pay. The casebook is not even a particularly good source for the volume of patients Binns dealt with over either the long or the short term. His hospital patients are certainly under-represented in his notes. Indeed, it is quite possible that Binns was erratic in his record-keeping, sometimes noting every patient he saw, at other times recording details only of cases which held some special interest for him.

Nonetheless, Binns's casebook is one of the best sources of information available to us about everyday surgical practice in seventeenth-century England, providing enough material to justify generalisations about his therapeutic routines and his general approach to healing. It clearly demonstrates that, for the most part, Binns's practice did deal with what was designated as the surgeon's domain: external disorders. But, like other surgeons and apothecaries of the day, he was prepared to treat internal diseases. Likewise, the casebook shows that Binns depended upon both theory and empiricism in his approach to treatment. His therapeutic regimes were governed by humoral theory. However, long experience of remedies and surgical procedures, combined with trial and error, influenced the courses of treatment he conducted.

The question remains of how typical Binns was of seventeenth-century surgeons. This paper can offer only speculative comparisons between Binns and better-known published surgical contemporaries and predecessors. In most respects, Binns was apparently quite conventional in his therapeutic routines. Compared to Wiseman and Clowes, he was relatively sparing in his use of phlebotomy. Unlike Woodall and Wiseman, he performed few amputations. And, unlike Wiseman, astrology had no apparent influence on the courses of treatment he pursued.[96] Unfortunately, until other surgical casebooks are found, too little basis for comparison exists to establish just how typical Binns was.

Yet Binns's records provide evidence for a wider range of surgical care than one would expect on the basis of the records left by military surgeons. Both minor and life-threatening disorders were described; both successes and failures were reported. The casebook thus indicates the possibilities of seventeenth-century surgery. According to his own account, Binns's track record was impressive. In those cases for which information is available, 265 patients emerged well from the surgeon's treatment and 62 got better. Twenty-two patients failed to improve and 53 died. Too often historians of medicine dismiss the surgeons of the past because of what they could not do, ignoring what they actually did.

Notes and references

1. J. Binns, 'Surgical casebook, 1633–1663', British Library, Sloane MS. 153, hereafter referred to as Binns. Numbers refer to my own transcription of the casebook.

2. M. Pelling, 'Appearances and reality: barber-surgeons, the body and disease', in A. L. Beier and R. Finlay (eds), *London 1500–1700: the Making of the Metropolis* (Longman, London, 1986), p. 87.

3. Guildhall Library, MS. 5625/1 fo. 89. V. C. Medvei and J. L. Thornton, *The Royal Hospital of St. Bartholomew 1123–1973* (no publisher stated, London, 1974), p. 388.

4. Public Record Office, PCC 1664, 47.

5. S. Young, *The Annals of the Barber-Surgeons of London* (Blades, East & Blades, London, 1890).

6. Ibid., p. 345. See also L. McCray Beier, *Sufferers and Healers: the Experience of Illness in Seventeenth-Century England* (Routledge & Kegan Paul, London, 1987), for discussion of Binns's relationships with and attitudes toward other healers.

7. Binns 199/393, 191/372.

8. Young, *Annals*, pp. 77, 119, 182.

9. Beier, *Sufferers and Healers*.

10. The numbers given here represent a change (due to recounting) from those given in Beier, *Sufferers and Healers*, pp. 55–6. This change does not affect any observations made or conclusions reached.

11. M. MacDonald, *Mystical Bedlam: Madness, Anxiety and Healing in Seventeenth-Century England* (Cambridge University Press, Cambridge, 1981), pp. 20, 26.

12. The casebook refers to only 41 hospital patients.

13. See, for example, W. Clowes, *A Profitable and Necessary Book of Observations, for all those that are Burned with the Flame of Gunpowder, etc. and also for Curing of Wounds Made with Musket and Caliver Shot, and other Weapons of War Commonly Used at this Day both by Sea and Land . . . Last of all is Adjoined a Short Treatise, for the Cure of Lues Venerea* (M. Dawson, London, 1596); J. Woodall, *The Surgeon's Mate* (Laurence Lisle, London, 1617); R. Wiseman, *Several Chirurgical Treatises* (R. Royston, London, 1676).

14. T. Gale, *An Institution of a Chirurgian* (R. Hall, London, 1563), fol. 3.

15. Sir George Clark, *A History of the Royal College of Physicians of London*, 3 vols (Clarendon Press, Oxford, 1964), vol. 1; R. S. Roberts, 'The London apothecaries and medical practice in Tudor and Stuart England', unpublished PhD thesis, University of London, 1964.

16. R. Wiseman, *Several Chirurgical Treatises*, 2nd edn (London, 1686), pp. 355–6, 457. All citations of this work below refer to the second edition.

17. Binns 152/288–91.

18. Binns 241/473.

19. Binns 217/437–8.

20. Binns 8/22. Wiseman, *Chirurgical Treatises*, p. 377.
21. Binns 12/31.
22. Binns 6/17, 10/25, 192/379, 24/55.
23. Binns 123/217, 19/45. Clowes, *Morbus Gallicus* (London, 1597), ch. 3 (no pagination).
24. Binns 96/142.
25. Binns 205/411.
26. Binns 123/215. See also Wiseman, *Chirurgical Treatises*, p. 416.
27. Binns 105/171, 197/388.
28. Binns 213/427, 190/370, 23/53, 198/391, 176/343, 190/371, 34/67.
29. Binns 125/219. See also 139/249.
30. Binns 190/371.
31. Binns 213/427, 96/142.
32. Binns 155/297, 155/298, 155/299.
33. Binns 12/31, 72/102, 201/396, 86/129, 134/231.
34. Binns 32/64, 66/93, 78/115, 140/251, 163/317.
35. Binns 85/128, 105/171.
36. Binns 29/61, 202/402, 67/96.
37. Binns 8/21, 213/425.
38. Binns 141/253.
39. Wiseman, *Chirurgical Treatises*, pp. 341–2.
40. Binns 89/134.
41. Wiseman, *Chirurgical Treatises*, p. 407.
42. Ibid., p. 409.
43. Binns 157/301, 101/145.
44. Wiseman, *Chirurgical Treatises*, p. 415.
45. Binns 214/429.
46. Wiseman, *Chirurgical Treatises*, pp. 443–56. J. Woodall, *Surgeon's Mate.*
47. Binns 163/317.
48. Wiseman, *Chirurgical Treatises*, pp. 475–7.
49. Binns 147/269.
50. Binns 140/251.
51. Binns 8/21, 8/22, 9/24, 167/323.
52. Binns 8/21, 9/24, 167/323.
53. Wiseman, *Chirurgical Treatises*, pp. 380–1.
54. Ibid., pp. 392–9.
55. Binns 198/391.
56. Binns 8/22, 167/323.
57. Binns 32/13, 219/441.
58. Binns 202/401.
59. Binns 105/171. The practice of treating certain ailments in this way is discussed in C. Gittings, *Death, Burial and the Individual in Early Modern England* (Croom Helm, London, 1984), pp. 67–8.
60. Binns 112/191.
61. Binns 369/526, 169/330.
62. Binns 27/60. For a similar case, see 43/81. In both cases, autopsies were performed.
63. Binns 140/250.

64. Binns 46/83, 80/121, 81/122, 82/123, 94/140, 105/166, 137/244, 139/248.

65. Binns 159/310, 95/141, 220/442, 236/460.

66. Wiseman, *Chirurgical Treatises*, p. 459.

67. Binns 181/352.

68. Binns 104/164, 271/530, 259/507.

69. Binns 311/623. Wiseman, *Chirurgical Treatises*, p. 104.

70. E.g., Binns 227/449, 229/450, 198/390, 199/393.

71. E.g., Binns 71/101, 297/573.

72. Binns 111/190.

73. Binns 197/387. See also 310/618.

74. Binns 265/520.

75. Binns 267/525.

76. Binns 16/42, 288/556.

77. Binns 259/506.

78. Binns 277/541, 43/81, 27/60.

79. Binns 53/85.

80. Binns 212/424, 213/428.

81. The word 'empiric' had such a derogatory connotation in the seventeenth century that I hesitated to use it. However, Wiseman himself divided surgery between 'empirical' and 'rational' faculties. See Wiseman, *Chirurgical Treatises*, 'The epistle to the reader'.

82. E.g., Binns 30/60, 162/316.

83. Binns 129/226.

84. Binns 209/420–2.

85. Binns 114/200.

86. Binns 54/87.

87. Binns 18/44, 131/228.

88. Binns 97/143.

89. Binns 14/36, 33/65–6, 36/69, 57/39, 158/304, 317/657, 274/534.

90. Binns 56/88, 131/228. On the wider cultural significance of syphilis in this and the Tudor period, see Pelling, 'Appearance and reality'.

91. Binns 92/138, 122/214.

92. Binns 121/210.

93. Binns 102/154–5, 136/242.

94. Binns 192/379.

95. E.g., Binns 216/435, 191/373, 275/536.

96. See Wiseman, *Chirurgical Treatises*, pp. 391–3.

3
Surgery and scrophula

Roger French

Introduction

This paper explores seventeenth- and eighteenth-century perceptions of scrophula. It is not an attempt to write about the history of tuberculosis, with which scrophula was later identified, which would be a search in the past for signs of a modern disease entity. It investigates what doctors and surgeons saw and meant when they used the term 'scrophula', and how their picture of it was constructed. A large part of what follows is concerned with a particular arena – the Aberdeen Infirmary – in which perceptions of scrophula changed radically during the eighteenth century. At one time the disease seems to have been of pressing urgency to medical men, while later the name vanished from the medical vocabulary. In order to illustrate the pressures acting on the Infirmary's physicians and surgeons in their diagnosis and treatment of the disease a number of case histories are employed. Finally, an explanation is offered for the origins of the different perceptions of the disease.

The King's Evil

Scrophula was not a classical name for a disease and opinion was divided in the seventeenth and eighteenth centuries on the extent to which the condition had been described by the old writers. Some argued that one of the symptoms of scrophula, membranous swellings of the glands of the neck, was to be identified with the ancient term struma. Others argued that struma and scrophula were identical, on the grounds that struma was the essential symptom of the disease. All agreed that scrophula in the more recent past was also known as the 'King's Evil', having been thought for several centuries to be curable at the touch of a king. During the Middle Ages the ceremony of touching was regarded as a miracle performed through the agency of the king.[1] The ceremony survived the Reformation, although the Protestant objection to miracles led the Calvinists to deny the efficacy of the touch. The putatively miraculous nature of the touch, however, was useful for the king and the party that supported him, because it could be taken as a sign that God was acting through his chosen representative on earth. It was, supporters of the touch argued, only the true line of kings, established on their thrones by God's will, that had the divine power to cure the King's Evil. James I of England and VI of Scotland, despite his Calvinist background, saw the advantages of his proclamation of the divine right of kings being supported by the appealing ceremony of touching. During the English Civil War and up to the time of his execution, Charles I continued to touch for the Evil. The popularity of the action and its political message led the Puritans to deny its power and in turn encouraged the Royalists in their association of it with kingship.

The royal touch therefore was open to much political and religious loading. It remained part of the French kings' justification of their position until the Revolution of 1789. Conversely, where the political and religious climate was very different there was no royal touch. In the various countries of Europe there were by the sixteenth and seventeenth centuries different perceptions of scrophula, struma and the value of the royal touch, according to the differing political and religious context. The United Provinces in the seventeenth century, having escaped from a Catholic monarch, being dominated by a Calvinist religion and having a non-monarchical government, was no place where claims for a king-curable disease could be respectable. The seventeenth-century Dutchman Steven Blankaart (Blancardus) identified scrophula with the struma of the ancients and discounted all other symptoms.[2] Blancardus published his medical dictionary in Leyden, where we should not expect recognition of scrophula. The same can be said of publications in German-speaking countries, although, for example, an eighteenth-century edition of the sixteenth-century author Castellus published in Leipzig at least acknowledged that some medical authors believed in the royal touch.[3] The seventeenth-century author Poterius, without mentioning scrophula, discussed the geographical distribution of struma, announcing that it occurred most extensively in Italy.[4]

In England the reign of Charles II, after the the Restoration of 1660, saw the reappearance of the touch, as well as a study of it by the king's surgeon, Richard Wiseman, whose work was the largest single authority on scrophula used by British medical men in the late seventeenth and early eighteenth centuries. Wiseman had been surgeon to both Charles I and II and was responsible for selecting the cases of scrophula to go forward for touching. Wiseman was a devoted Royalist; he had been captured by the Parliamentarians at the Battle of Worcester, had twice been arrested as a civilian for his Royalist sympathies and had been involved in a plot to free another Royalist prisoner. His surgical practice was mostly among the London Royalists. Wiseman had followed the exiled Charles II in his continental wanderings, in which Charles had continued to demonstrate the justice of his claim to the throne by touching for the Evil. This claim was vindicated at the Restoration and the ceremony of touching was triumphantly reinstituted. To supporters of the king it seemed that God had indicated his will in religious and political affairs by putting Charles back on the thrones of England and Scotland. These matters, coming after the conflicts of the Civil War, were more important to Wiseman than his routine surgery (his surgical works were written only during his periods of enforced inactivity) and it was they which determined his views on scrophula. It is no surprise that his medical opinions coincide with his religious and political views, and we need not see, as did his Victorian biographer, a conflict between Wiseman's belief in a 'royal miracle' and his 'scientific' description of surgical procedures.[5] For Wiseman to invoke the royal touch was to invoke the nature of kingship. In scrophula and its cure can be discovered the interaction of his religious, political and medical convictions.

Wiseman and the British consensus

For many ordinary people scrophula existed as a disease for which the touch was effective. What the disease was, that is, what was in the scrophula 'package' of symptoms, must have been defined by something very like a national consensus. No one would begin seeking the royal touch unless, for instance, he or she had been said by neighbours to be suffering from the King's Evil. Nor could they gain support, funds or shelter for their journey if men of some standing did not agree on the nature of the disease. At the top of the selection process in seventeenth-century England was Wiseman. It was he who chose the individuals to go forward to the king. The criteria Wiseman used to define scrophula may well have been known to the individuals who were making application, the more so after Wiseman published his description of the disease in 1676. The consensus about what was in the package therefore was partly dictated by him.

Wiseman's scrophula package was a complex one. In fact he sent to the king only the cases that would benefit least from surgery. In that it was good to show that the king could, uniquely, cure by touch alone, it was better that the disease so cured was seen to be otherwise intractable. Wiseman's *A Treatise of the King's Evil* appeared in his *Severall Chirurgicall Treatises* of 1676. In it he aimed to instruct young surgeons on 'whatever is requisite to the Cure' of scrophula, but noted 'when upon triall he shall find the contumaciousness of the Disease . . . he will find reason of acknowledging the goodness of God' who had given kings 'an extraordinary power in the miraculous Cure thereof'. Wiseman observed that the 'Latines' called the disease *Struma.* But struma, he noted, was only a tumour contained in a cyst. Wiseman added,

> none of these definitions seem to describe sufficiently the Disease which we in England call the Kings-Evil . . . for I appeal to the practitioners of this Nation, Physicians and Chirurgeons, desiring them to say whether there may not be many tumours and ulcers commonly judged to be the Evil, which are contained in no cysts, neither do they concrete into a glandule.[6]

Wiseman thus resisted simple identification of scrophula with struma or tumours-in-their-own-membranes. He drew attention particularly to the bifurcated swelling of the upper lip and the non-encysted tumours of the muscles and bone which were also present in cases of the Evil as it was perceived in England. He concluded, 'either we must exclude all these from the King's

Touch, or alter our Definition'. Wiseman preferred to include them, and insisted on his expanded definition: 'in my History of the Disease I have enlarged the bounds of it further, so as to take in several Tumours and Ulcers upon Muscles, Tendons, Ligaments and Bones: also *Opthalmia, Aegylops, Fistula Lachrymalis, Tonsilae* etc'.[7] In addition to possessing any of these features those cases that went to the king had a characteristic tumour close to the mastoid muscle and a *lipitudo* or protrusion of the eyes. Even after Wiseman's time the scale of the ceremony of the royal touch – James II touched heroically – must have had the effect of displaying and confirming the consensus or 'package'.

Scrophula in Aberdeen

After the revolution of 1688, William III, who had a Calvinist background, made no attempt to restore the practice of touching. The last monarch to touch was Queen Anne, who was persuaded by her Tory supporters to demonstrate visually once more the true line of monarchs. Naturally the Hanoverians, as kings of convenience, made no attempt to touch, and their Whig supporters expressed horror at the old notions of kingship and royal cure. But James and the Stuart line practised touching in exile in France, much as Charles II had done, as a token of their just claim on the throne. As in the case of Charles, there were those who hoped that the true line of kings would return.

Aberdeen had more than its share of Jacobites, and when the Old Pretender arrived there in 1715 there was ill-disguised jubilation.[8] It is said that he touched for scrophula during this period, perhaps indeed in Aberdeen itself. The Jacobites kept up a propaganda war from exile about the efficacy of the royal touch, and when Prince Charles Edward arrived in Edinburgh in 1745 he too touched for the Evil. These were significant political events for the managers of Aberdeen's newly founded Infirmary; in December 1745 the Infirmary was taken over by the rebels, who used it to house their wounded and prisoners. By March 1746 the Duke of Cumberland had arrived and taken over the Infirmary for his own sick and wounded. Until the middle of August 1746 the Infirmary remained a military hospital.

The records of the Aberdeen infirmary are particularly useful for a study of scrophula.[9] To understand why, we must look at the special circumstances of its foundation, circumstances that made its records of patients and their diseases remarkably complete. The Aberdeen Infirmary was first proposed by the town council at a public meeting in 1739. The Infirmary was to be a small-scale emulation of the foundations in Edinburgh and Glasgow. It was part of the town council's wider proposals for social support in which the destitute but healthy poor were to be placed in a workhouse, the mad in a bedlam, and the chronic and infectious sick poor supported by home visits from a physician. Aberdeen was an impoverished city in comparison with Edinburgh and Glasgow. To promote the Infirmary the town council intended that a gift of £5 from a group of donors would secure for them the right to nominate a director for a year. Any individual giving £5 could act as a director for a year. The sum £25 confirmed that privilege for life and £100 for eternity – that is, a heritable privilege. The current Town Provost was to be the President of the directors. Being a director conferred an important right, that of recommending a patient for admission. The scheme was supported by the wealthy families of the area; Lord Pitsligo had the right of being a Director, having paid six guineas, the Dowager Duchess of Gordon paid £15 and Lady Durris's gift of five guineas was recorded shortly after the Infirmary opened. Dr George Cheyne, doing well in London, sent home a donation, as did many other Scots, mostly in the colonies. Most of the contributors, however, were the prosperous townsfolk of Aberdeen, the baillies and, indeed, the medical men. The amount raised for building the Infirmary, although only about one fortieth of that secured by Thomas Guy in London, encouraged the town council to contract with a local builder, by the name of Chrystal, for £480 at the end of November 1739. The foun- dation stone was laid on the first day of the next year and work was completed in a little over five months.

Not all the philanthropic directors of the Infirmary had an interest in its day-to-day management, and in October 1742 the town council appointed a board of managers from among the directors. The board represented those institutions and individuals with an ongoing interest in the Infirmary. The first board comprised William Chalmers and Alexander Robertson, previous provosts, Charles Maitland and Alexander Rose, Aberdeen physicians, the merchant John Burnet, James Ogilvie, Collector of Customs, John Osborn, Principal of Marischal

College, John Gordon, Minister of St Paul's Chapel and John Rickart, a gentleman of apparently independent means. Some of the medical men on the board of managers also served in the Infirmary. Alexander Rose was a practising physician-surgeon, a director with a right of recommendation and an expert in the operation of couching for cataract which he performed at the Infirmary. After the appointment of managers, non-managing directors still seem to have had the right to recommend patients for admission. Admission was a complex business, requiring the consent of the Managers. In practice the physician-surgeon took day-to-day decisions about admission, particularly of urgent cases. Such decisions were, generally, approved retrospectively at the managers' weekly meeting. If the Infirmary's physician-surgeon agreed to admit recommended patients, the recommender had to indemnify the Infirmary against the costs of transport, and burial if the patient died.

The running expenses of the new Infirmary were to be met by the interest on capital of £737, controlled by the town council and ultimately derived from monastic sources. Kirk collections were also held to add to these resources. Such collections were most welcome during the Infirmary's first few years, as it struggled with ever-present poverty. The Infirmary expenses included not only the food and medicine of the patients and the heating of the rooms but also the salary of the physician-surgeon and the matron. The first medical man employed in the Infirmary was Dr James Gordon, appointed in August 1742 at ten guineas a year to act as both physician and surgeon.[10] Gordon was also Professor of Medicine at Marischal College, the New Town's university. The son of an Aberdeen physician, he was thoroughly familiar with the surgical and medical traditions of the city. Gordon's contract stipulated that he was to secure his own medicines and visit the Infirmary every day, prescribing medicine and diet for each patient, notifying the 'Mistress of the House' who accompanied him on his rounds. Gordon and his successors were responsible to the managers, who met once a week. Their minute, or *sederunt*, book provides most of the surviving records.

It was poverty that determined the early character of the Aberdeen Infirmary. Its purpose was to take in the acutely ill poor as part of the town council's wider scheme of social relief. In the early years lack of resources limited the number of beds to six (and one for emergency cases). To be cost-effective and to reach as many acute cases as possible, there was considerable pressure on the Infirmary for a quick turnover of patients. Pressure for efficiency of treatment produced a rigorous admission policy intended to ensure that the Infirmary took only those it was established to take: the acutely ill poor suffering from non-infectious diseases. In this respect the Infirmary was run something like a trading company where the 'profits' – the discharge of patients – were related to the input of charitable funds. Moneywise and penny-sharp Aberdonian merchants, represented by the town council, did not want their coppers wasted; a rapid turnover of patients made good advertising in the Infirmary's frequent appeals for money. On admission the physician-surgeon had to write down a diagnosis and prognosis in his book. In a straightforward case the patient stayed about five weeks, which was regarded as the ideal use of funds. Patients with cancer of the lip, for example, fell into this category. In cases where the physician-surgeon was sure of this diagnosis he could admit the patient as an emergency without waiting for the weekly *sederunts*. Gordon seems have been fairly confident of a good outcome in these instances. Cataract cases stayed about the same length of time. Alexander Rose couched cataracts in the Infirmary some fifty times in the period up to 1753. Often patients for this operation travelled considerable distances. In contrast to Edinburgh, however, no one in Aberdeen was prepared to cut for stone of the bladder and patients were sent south to the capital.

In most other cases the records show that the outcome and the length of stay were much less easily predicted. Since the hospital had only six beds, the case descriptions are unusually extensive for an eighteenth-century infirmary. Besides writing down his prognosis at the time of admission, the physician-surgeon reported each week to the managers the progress his patients had made and if and when they had been cured and discharged. Further, he also had to explain any deaths or why patients had become chronically ill and not discharged. In these two instances the Infirmary was no longer fulfilling its proclaimed role. Indeed, it had been specifically enacted when Gordon was appointed in August 1742, that patients would be admitted, even when recommended, only upon his statement that they were curable.

Scrophula in the Infirmary

The case histories show that in the early years of the Infirmary scrophula and scrophulous were entertained as diagnostic categories by the admitting medical men. The term 'scrophula' occurs rarely but there are a number of references to scrophulous ulcers, tumours and related conditions. Like Wiseman, the Infirmary's medical men employed a wide definition of what could be considered scrophulous. They did not, it is important to note, limit the term to struma. Like Wiseman they allowed that a variety of pathological features could be signs of the disease. The records also show that advanced scrophula was considered incurable and that early scrophulous (or scrophula-like) symptoms were worthy of treatment. Thus patients designated as having advanced scrophula were regularly refused admission. Alexander Middleton, a boy from the workhouse, was thus turned away in April 1744 as 'all over scrophulous and not a fit object'. He was directed to keep his clothes wet with cold water in order to prevent the infection spreading to other boys in the workhouse. Altogether seven scrophulous patients were rejected between 1742 and 1745, more than any other category (the next being inoperable cancers). The Infirmary, however, did take in and treat patients who were designated as possibly scrophulous or having definite scrophula at an early stage. This may, in part, have been the case because the town council could put pressure on the Infirmary to accept patients from the workhouse. In May 1743 the physicians and surgeons of Aberdeen visited the workhouse and recommended that four scrophulous boys should go to the Infirmary. Their symptoms were principally the scrophulous itch, and they were treated by 'frictions' and internal medicines. A considerable improvement was noted and they seemed to have stayed little more than a week.

Suspicion of scrophula in a patient admitted with another disorder did not mean immediate expulsion. One of the early troublesome patients was William Thomson, found to be scrophulous after admission with sore feet in November 1742. Gordon did not suspect scrophula until the end of the year, and then allowed himself two weeks to assess the case. During that period, his notes say, he hit on a method of treatment that seemed to bring benefit. He hoped that Thomson would soon be fit enough to take the waters at Moffat Wells, apparently a recognised treatment for scrophula. Conversely another patient was admitted with a favourable diagnosis but the outcome proved very different. In this instance Gordon went back and modified the earlier entry in the records. Helen Touch, admitted as 'scorbutic', was subsequently designated as incurable, and 'scrophulous' was added to the record of admission.

Gordon, in his surgical capacity, would have been faced with many tumours and ulcers among the patients. There were many kinds of these described in the medical literature of the time, but his notes and those of his immediate successors show that in practice surgeons and physicians did not make fine distinctions. Gordon, as the medical professor at Marischal College, certainly knew of and may have taught students the differences which medical texts made between kinds of ulcer, such as the cancerous, gangrenous, scrophulous, scorbutic, sphacelous, oedematous, schirrhous and phagodenic, as well as spina ventosa, noli-me-tangere, and ulcus depascens. His notes in the Infirmary, however, largely contain non-committal descriptions of ulcers as being, for instance, 'open' or 'fungoid'. In making these notes he was acting under unusual constraints. Unlike the authors of *Consilia*, or collections like the 'centuries' (100 cases) and other sources in which 'practical' medicine appeared in the university classroom, Gordon could not retrospectively select cases that illustrated the superiority of some medicine or technique or some point of medical theory. No *post hoc* rationalising was possible. Every case was admitted on the basis of its being curable, preferably quickly, and every admitted case collected notes as it progressed. A small number of cases were admitted with the express acknowledgement that response to therapy was the criterion determining of their length of stay. Gordon thus often left the diagnosis relatively open until subsequent therapeutic experience allowed a definition of the nature of the case. That this is so is confirmed by the admission of patients designated as 'on trial' (slightly less than one-tenth). One example of the difficulties met with in these circumstances is that in cases without a diagnostic label and with an equivocal response to therapy the medical man had no grounds for prognosis. The long and difficult case of George Anderson's ulcer in 1742 and 1743 illustrates this. After treatment Gordon could not decide what kind of ulcer Anderson had, and could not give a prognosis. All the physicians in Aberdeen were invited to discuss the case; those who appeared included Rose, Alexander

Donaldson, Forbes, Gordon himself and the surgeon Andrew Skene.[11] All they could decide, however, was that the case was dangerous but not without hope.

Gordon finished his year's contract in August 1743 and left, donating his salary to the Infirmary. The managers now contracted with a surgeon rather than with a physician; in practice, about three-quarters of all the cases admitted to the Infirmary were surgical rather than medical. The managers chose Andrew Skene, who practised in Aberdeen and who had already been consulted over doubtful cases in the Infirmary. In 1745 the Infirmary was occupied by the rebel forces and it was not returned to civil managers until September 1746. The new managers took stock of the situation and made some changes. First they wanted to ensure that a patient recommended by a director could only be refused admission by the Infirmary's surgeon if one or two other 'physicians' agreed. The 'physicians' referred to were probably from among the directors, since one of these was to be 'Dr Gordon', no doubt the Infirmary's first physician-surgeon, whose waived salary would have made him a director. Second there was to be more consultation between the Infirmary's surgeon and the town's physicians in cases of diagnostic difficulty. The third change made by the managers was that, in making appointments to the Infirmary, there was to be consultation between the managers and the physicians of the town. Indeed, the agreement of the latter was sought when a new surgeon to the Infirmary was appointed, for Skene resigned a few days after the first *sederunt* meeting after the rebellion, 27 September 1746. The new surgeon, however, was – like Gordon – also a physician, Dr Andrew Burnet, a practitioner in the Old Town.

The new regime arrived at a consensus on the nature of scrophula which was much like the old. Chronic scrophula was incurable and not a category of disease admissible to the Infirmary. Likewise the attending medical man – now in consultation with the town's physicians – could still change his diagnosis after admission. For instance at the end of September 1747, after Burnet had consulted either with Rose or another physician of the town, Alexander Chapman was admitted with 'a sore foot'. A week later, however, Burnet, Rose and Gordon inspected Chapman again and decided he had a spreading scrophula. He was ejected. In June of the same year John Calder of Towie, recommended by his minister, had been admitted on trial. In early September it was agreed that the symptoms were scrophulous and that Calder was also to be ejected. Early cases were still considered curable. Helen Thomas was admitted from the workhouse in March 1748; she had 'scrophulous humours' and was taken in 'on trial' in the hope that a course of medicines and the 'freer air of this Hospital' might prove to be of some help. By early May the medical men had decided that, although they had worked a considerable improvement in her condition, what remained was stubbornly scrophulous; she too was ejected.

We are now in a position to summarise how scrophula was perceived and managed in the Aberdeen Infirmary by what amounted to a small medical community: Rose, Burnet, Skene, Gordon and occasionally others. First, a pre-surgical stage was recognised, in which the symptoms appear to have been largely cutaneous: the 'scrophulous itch'. Medical men considered that they could offer considerable benefit here, with frictions, washing in cold water, and internal medicines. Opinion seems to have been divided on the question of whether this stage was infectious; some patients thus diagnosed were directed to wear wet clothing to prevent cross-infection when returned to the workhouse while others were taken into the Infirmary without mention of any danger of infection. Second, when physicians were faced with severe but non-specific conditions such as ulcers and tumours, scrophula was an important category to be excluded. In some instances of this sort, patients were taken in on trial with no firm diagnosis. When, however, patients failed to respond to treatment scrophula might be invoked. Besides using therapeutic responses as a means to identify scrophulous symptoms the medical men looked for tumours in glands, joints and other places. In confirmed scrophula they expected these tumours to ulcerate. If a condition was truly scrophulous, deep exploration of any ulcers was expected to reveal caries in the bones. Patients with ulcers were sometimes admitted on trial in order to perform this exploration. If the surgeon found 'spoiled bones' then the case was generally regarded as hopeless, and the patient was removed as soon as his strength allowed. Over 40 per cent of the patients on trial were ultimately ejected as incurable.

The medical men also experimented with treatments for doubtful or early scrophula. In particular, patients taken in on trial were given a variety of internal medicines. This was not the case with the large number of patients with definitive surgical conditions. As the first symptoms of scrophula included swollen glands, it was accepted that some sort of blockage had occurred and drugs were administered to relieve the obstruction. The Infirmary records list mercury as being used for this purpose. This was administered in the form of 'sweet mercury' in milk (the Infirmary maintained its own cow for the purpose). The mercury promoted copious salivation and sweating, and this was taken as evidence that the small vessels were clearing. But sweating was much reduced by the cold of an Aberdeen January and, almost from its inception, the managers of the Infirmary were anxious to equip the hospital with specially heated rooms. Coal was bought and appeals were launched for funds to build more warm rooms. By 1749 the managers were negotiating with tradesmen for the modification of existing rooms to increase their warmth. In 1750 the Infirmary had twenty beds, but space was still very short for those on mercury treatment. One scrophulous patient was turned away in the February of that year because the weather was too cold for the 'mercury sweats'.[12] By this time there was a waiting list of scrophulous patients and some were taken in for a rapid course of treatment that would leave them 'as well as can be expected'. They were then sent home with directions for their regimen, which included a spare diet, limewater to drink and lots of air. The physicians and surgeons associated with the Infirmary were now so confident of being able to effect some improvement in scrophulous conditions that they themselves, in their position as directors, recommended patients with these disorders, agreeing to indemnify the Infirmary against the costs of possible burial if the patient died.

Perceptions of scrophula in the Aberdeen Infimary altered radically in 1752 when a new physician-surgeon, Thomas Livingstone, took up his post. After his appointment in August 1751 it was arranged that, before taking up his duties, Livingstone was to travel for a year 'for his further improvement', that is, he was to take medical courses. When he returned to Aberdeen he took the degree of MD at Marischal College. In the interval before Livingstone's arrival some cases of 'scrophulous runnings' were admitted by Rose and the others among the medical managers. But after August 1752, when Livingstone took up his duties, scrophula vanishes from the records. This may in part be because Livingstone's case-notes were much more technical than those of his predecessors. For instance William Swap was admitted with a paranychia of his hand, Marjorie Shirres with a spina ventosa, Agnes Morgan with a marasmus, Alan Anderson with a gutta serena, Joseph Lawris with anasarcous swellings and so on; none of these terms had been used by Skene, Burnet or Gordon. Interestingly too Livingstone seems not to have consulted with the managers as much as his predecessors did.

There was possibly another reason why scrophula was not used as a category by physicians like Livingstone. We need to recall the religious and political 'loading' of the King's Evil and the various perceptions of struma and scrophula which existed in the medical communities of Europe. What was surgically celebrated by Wiseman in Restoration England was probably acceptable in crypto-Jacobite Aberdeen. Unfortunately it is impossible to trace at present the political and theological connections of the physicians associated with the Infirmary. King's College was undoubtedly tainted with Jacobitism well into the century, although Marischal College was staunchly Hanoverian.[13] Nevertheless the defeat of the rebels must have changed the political climate in Aberdeen, and Livingstone can perhaps be seen as a 'new man' fitting more appropriately into a Hanoverian, Calvinist, prosperous, Enlightened Scotland. More relevant no doubt is Livingstone's training, part of which had been at the Edinburgh medical school, which was self-consciously pro-Hanoverian and pro-Union. The medical texts employed there were those of Boerhaave. Scrophula did not exist in Boerhaave's texts. His *Institutes* did not name it.[14] The *Aphorisms* run through eighteen kinds of tumour without mentioning the scrophulous.[15] The disease is not to be found in the large index to the enormous *Commentary on the Aphorisms* by van Swieten, and as far as can be ascertained the word is not mentioned in the text.[16] Yet at the time that these texts were circulating in Edinburgh the Aberdonians were scraping together their shillings to build new rooms containing closets with chimneys to sweat the scrophula out of the patients.

By the mid-eighteenth century there was a variety of views about scrophula in different European countries. Many Scottish, English and French texts acknowledged the existence of the disease, but in most British sources, Enlightenment values and Whig politics no longer encouraged the statement that it was king-curable. While James's medical dictionary deals extensively with scrophula, that of Quincy talks of the 'strange Conceit' of the royal touch.[17] As we have seen in other northern European countries, even before the eighteenth century, it was common either not to mention scrophula or simply to identify it with struma. To discuss simple struma in place of scrophula was to break down the complex package of symptoms that practitioners like Wiseman and the Aberdeen doctors took as constituting scrophula. Boerhaave, for instance, discussed quite separately the ulcers, tumours, caries and so on that were once part of scrophula. Presumably the origins of Boerhaave's avoidance of scrophula lay in the prevailing religious and political sentiment of his homeland. The United Provinces in the seventeenth century had not long since freed themselves of Spanish domination and were no friends of absolute monarchy of a Catholic kind. The Dutch saw themselves as republican or democratic and Protestant. Boerhaave also saw himself as rationalist, mechanist and Enlightened. For Boerhaave scrophula had associations with superstition and its cure by the touch had no possible mechanical explanation. Besides it was a 'cure' that had been used for centuries as a religious sign and political tool by absolutist and Catholic monarchs (in France) or monarchs who would like to be (in Britain).

To return finally to Aberdeen in the 1740s, we can see that the surgeons and physicians at the Infirmary were not practising Boerhaavian medicine. Like many students in the eighteenth century, they had probably studied in a number of places. Gordon and Rose had even spent some postgraduate time with Boerhaave but they had taken their medical degrees at Rheims, as had a third of all the physicians entering the Edinburgh College of Physicians between 1700 and 1737. It was no doubt cheap and convenient to do so, and such a graduation need not imply any extended length of study at Rheims. But it might well be that Gordon and Rose were at least aware that Rheims was a place very different from Leyden. It was here that French kings were crowned and anointed with the unction that gave them their powers of healing. Here were the bones of the saint through whose intercession the healing power had been bestowed. The French royal touch was indeed mentioned in the bull of foundation of the university. Whatever perspective they had adopted from their medical education, it is clear that Gordon, Rose and other physicians had no doubt about the existence of scrophula.

Notes and references

1. M. Bloch, *The Royal Touch* (Routledge & Kegan Paul, London, 1973).

2. Stephanus Blancardus, *Lexicon Medicum Renovatum* (S. Lutchmans, Leyden, 1735).

3. Bartholomaeus Castellus, *Lexicon Medicum Graeco-Latinum* (Leipzig, 1713).

4. Petrus Poterius, *Insignium Curationum et Singularium Observationum Centuria Secunda*, cap. xxviii, in Friederich Hoffmann, *Operum Omnium Physico-Medicorum Supplementum . . . Pars Prima* (de Tournes, Geneva, 1749).

5. Richard Wiseman, *Severall Chirugicall Treatises* (R. Royston, London, 1676).

6. Wiseman, *Chirugicall Treatises*, pp. 245, 248, 236.

7. Ibid., p. 261.

8. P. J. Anderson, *Records of the Aberdeen Universities Commission, 1716–1717* (Aberdeen, 1900), p. 9. The professor of medicine in King's College, Aberdeen, had been Patrick Urquhart, who had 'Illuminations in his windows on the Thanksgiving observed for the arrival of the Pretender', at which there was 'drinking, waveing of Hats and Shooting'. Urquhart's windows were those of the Mediciner's Manse, in Old Aberdeen, next to King's College.

9. The source for patient records of the Infirmary are the *sederunt* books of the Infirmary's managers' weekly meetings, now in the charge of the Aberdeen Medico-Chirurgical Society. The recorded detail per patient is perhaps unique in Britain. The *sederunt* books have been microfilmed. They are the primary sources for all that follows pertaining to the Infirmary.

10. Only the term 'surgeon' is used in the records.

11. Forbes's Christian name does not appear in the minutes.

12. The 'some dozes of Sweet Mercury' given to such patients would be the *mecurial dulcis* of the pharmacopeias. E. Nicolai, *Methodus Concinnandi Formulas Medicamentorum* (Magdeburg, 1747) recommends a course beginning with six grains daily, increasing to half a drachm, when saliva begins to flow.

13. Roger Emerson, 'Aberdeen professors 1690–1800: two structures, two professoriates, two careers', in Jennifer J. Carter and Joan H. Pittock (eds.), *Aberdeen and the Enlightenment* (Aberdeen University Press, Aberdeen, 1987), pp. 155–67.

14. I have used the fourth Leyden edition: Hermann Boerhaave, *Institutiones Medicae in usus annuae Exercitationis Domesticos* (Boutestein, Leyden, 1727).

15. Boerhaave, *Aphorismi de Cognoscendis et Curandis Morbis in usum Doctrinae Domesticae* (Paris, 1728).

16. Gerhard van Swieten, *Commentaria in Hermanni Boerhaave Aphorismos de Cognoscendis et Curandis Morbis* (Wurzburg, 1787–92).

17. Robert James, *A Medical Dictionary*, 3 vols. (T. Osborne & J. Roberts, London, 1743–1745); John Quincy, *Lexicon Physico Medicum: or a New Medicinal Dictionary* (London, 1736).

4

Giovanni Battista Morgagni and eighteenth-century physical examination

Malcolm Nicolson

INTRODUCTION

In recent years knowledge of the medicine of the eighteenth century has greatly improved. Biography and several aspects of medical theory have been extensively investigated.[1] Research into institutional and professional contexts and into education proceeds apace.[2] Lay medical knowledge and activity have at last begun to receive the attention they deserve.[3] But at least one topic remains something of a blank on our map of eighteenth-century medicine. Historians have said relatively little about practical diagnostics and therapeutics.[4] It is clear, however, that we must have some understanding of bedside practice before we can claim a full acquaintance with eighteenth-century medicine. Furthermore, as N. D. Jewson has pointed out, what the doctor does at the bedside of the patient tells us a great deal about the status and power of the practitioner and about the social context within which medical knowledge is produced.[5] Diagnostics and therapeutics are therefore important aspects not only of eighteenth-century medicine but also of the wider history of patient–practitioner relationships.

As Guenter Risse has shown, extant hospital records, case-notes and clinical lectures provide a potentially rich source of information on diagnostic and therapeutic practices.6 Patients' diaries or similar lay testimonies are other obvious resources on which to base a reconstruction of the eighteenth-century consultative encounter.7 However it is an indication of the lack of development in this area of medical historiography that the more readily available printed sources have not yet been fully exploited for the information they contain about eighteenth-century practice.

It must be admitted that, to the twentieth-century reader, medical texts of the eighteenth century often appear to pay little attention to practical therapeutics and diagnostics. When these subjects are treated, the discussion is often abstract or theoretical. Precise descriptions of clinical procedures tend to occur, if at all, only incidentally to accounts of other matters. Furthermore, such descriptions of clinical practice as do occur in the texts cannot always, as we shall see, be taken at face value. These routine matters at the business end of medicine, as it most directly and perhaps most importantly impinged upon the patient's experience, seem not to have been readily incorporated into the written record.

This essay attempts to demonstrate that there are, however, texts which, even in the present limited state of our knowledge of how to read them, shed valuable light on clinical behaviour. Despite many difficulties of interpretation, professorial texts, on occasion, provide opportunities for investigation of practical diagnostics that are too good to ignore. This is certainly true of one of the major medical texts of the eighteenth century: *De Sedibus et Causis Morborum per Anatomen Indagatis* (the seats and causes of diseases as revealed by anatomy), by Giovanni Battista Morgagni.[8]

Giovanni Morgagni, born in 1682, took his medical degree in Bologna in 1701 and remained there after graduation, practising physic in three of the city's hospitals. He also practised in his home town of Forli before moving to Padua in 1711. He was Primary Professor of Anatomy at the University of Padua from 1715 until the year of his death in 1771. His great book, commonly referred to as *De Sedibus,* was published in 1761.[9]

Historians have tended to regard *De Sedibus* as a pioneering work of pathological anatomy. However, as Saul Jarcho has pointed out, the author of *De Sedibus* was not primarily a pathologist or an anatomist.[10] He was, first and foremost, a physician and a teacher of would-be physicians. *De Sedibus* is a treatise on clinical medicine rather than one on pathological anatomy, in the narrow nineteenth-century sense of that term.[11] This is evidenced by the fact that many of the cases described in the book had a successful conclusion, and so never came to the dissecting table. Nor did Morgagni regard post-mortem dissection as an end in itself. The autopsy investigations recorded in *De Sedibus* were undertaken in order to improve the understanding of disease at the bedside.[12] It is to this end that Morgagni indexed and correlated the results of his autopsy investigations against clinical symptoms observed in the living patients.

It may immediately be acknowledged that Morgagni's book, while it is more explicit than most on clinical matters, does not free the historian from all the difficulties inherent in using texts as a guide to bedside practice. Texts are always the product of much artifice on the part of their authors.[13] Thus the relation between their accounts and historical events is a problematic one. *De Sedibus* is no exception. The clinical material which it contains was evidently carefully selected, organised and presented so as to convey a thoroughly favourable image of Morgagni, illustrating his clinical acumen, wisdom and high moral character. It is also clear that Morgagni intended *De Sedibus* as a polemical contribution to the contemporary debate as to the clinical utility of anatomical research. Thus there is often an argument implicit in his clinical descriptions. Moreover, the text is thoroughly structured by literary devices. However it will be argued that the problems of interpretation which these implicit agendas create do not entirely negate the value of the text as a source of information on the clinical practice of Morgagni and his colleagues in Bologna and Padua.[14]

De Sedibus possesses a great advantage over many other eighteenth-century texts in that one of the most besetting obstacles to extrapolation from printed text to actual practice is somewhat obviated by Morgagni's style of presentation. Eighteenth-century medical authors often set out to produce fully comprehensive and authoritative treatises. This enterprise entailed assembling material from literary sources as well as from the author's own experience of practice. These two sources were often not explicitly differentiated in the final text. Thus the presence in Boerhaave's *Aphorisms*, for example, of a good description of how to inspect a hydrocele is not sufficient evidence to support the conclusion that Boerhaave carried out this procedure himself, far less that it was part of his routine practice.[15]

Morgagni borrowed from the literature as much as any of his contemporaries but he was careful to cite his sources routinely and explicitly. This was partly to display the extent of his scholarship but it was also because he and his colleagues in Bologna and Padua employed an ideology of direct experience. Much as they valued the collective wisdom to be found in the medical literature they accorded particular importance to their own observations. This is well exemplified by the long passage which Morgagni devoted to denying that the 'worms' or 'snakes' said to be generated in the chambers of the heart under certain pathological circumstances were anything other than 'polypous filaments':

> But you will reply, that the worm which was found by the physicians in the pericardium of a certain Florentine . . . was still 'alive'. Who says so? Petrus Sphererius. But was he himself present? It does not appear that he was. Was he who related it to him? Not even that. I resided at Bologna, at a time when a rumour happen'd to be spread about, that upon dissecting some horses of a nobleman . . . lizards . . . were found in their hearts . . . [S]ome half-learn'd persons were not wanting, who contended . . . that there might have been so . . . To these Valsalva replied, What need have we of dispute? Let us examine these lizards. Another horse . . . having died in the same stable . . . we examin'd the carcase . . . nor did we need any very long examination, in order to perceive very plainly, that they were nothing else than polypous concretions.[16]

In accordance with this emphasis on direct personal observation, Morgagni frequently used the first person when discussing clinical histories, specifying which aspects of the case he had seen for himself, which came from literary sources and which were told him by his colleagues or by the patient. Thus when Morgagni wrote, 'I perceived a tumour of this kind by examining the epigastrium with my hand', we have reasonable grounds for tentatively accepting that he actually did undertake this procedure.[17]

Furthermore, Morgagni was a wonderfully prolix author. He seems to have been anxious not to leave out anything of consequence. We are also fortunate in having available a considerable sample of Morgagni's consultation letters, which complement and substantiate the testimony of *De Sedibus*.[18] For all the above reasons Morgagni's text is a rich source of material for the investigation of eighteenth-century clinical practice and its professional context. I will argue that the evidence which it provides should lead to a modification of the currently accepted view of eighteenth-century clinical practice.

As noted earlier, the elucidation of the clinical procedures used by Morgagni has wider historiographical significance. As well as discussing the implications of my findings for the Jewson thesis, I will pay particular attention to Owsei Temkin's argument that much of the novel character of nineteenth-century medicine followed from the introduction of surgical modes of thought into physic at the end of the eighteenth century.[19] It seems to me that the Temkin thesis might be extended into an earlier time period and thus made more general. I will argue that, in eighteenth-century Padua, close institutional and professional links existed between physic and surgery and, consequently, forms of medical knowledge were developed by physicians in which the perspectives of physic and surgery were, to some extent, combined.

Physical examination in the eighteenth century

Bedside practice has not, of course, been completely neglected by historians. Charles Newman, in a series of publications which appeared in the 1950s, offered quite a detailed account of pre-modern diagnostic practice.[20] In brief, Newman argued that the eighteenth-century physician relied upon four basic techniques. First and primarily, he listened to the patient's own statement of his complaint. Second, he noted the patient's general appearance, especially the facies, and his behaviour: whether he tended to favour one side or the other as he lay in bed, whether he was calm or confused, and so on. Third, the physician inspected the urine, sputum and faeces. Fourth, he took the patient's pulse. Only relatively rarely, according to Newman's account, would the physician examine the patient's body manually or even visually inspect those parts of the body normally covered by clothes or bedclothes. Newman gathered his evidence from a small selection of casebooks of English physicians of the seventeenth and eighteenth centuries and from clinical records remaining in the London hospitals. He showed that it was not until the 1830s that physical examination became common at Guy's and St Bartholomew's hospitals and, perhaps, not until later at the North London.[21] Before this the patient's verbal complaint provided most of the data on which diagnosis was based. Auscultation, percussion, succussion, and even palpation were held by Newman to be virtually unpractised among physicians of the seventeenth, eighteenth or early nineteenth centuries.

Nothing that has been published since Newman's work has substantially contradicted his description of eighteenth-century diagnostic practice. Kenneth Keele, in his survey of the evolution of clinical methods, noted the variety of clinical techniques – inspection, palpation, abdominal percussion and auscultation – employed in classical times and concluded that it was not until the nineteenth century that clinical methods were again the equal of those of AD 200. Keele argued, for instance, that it was Auenbrugger who, 'for the first time since Aretaeus the Cappadocian, opened up the world of the ear as a clinical instrument'.[22] A similar view was taken by Stanley Reiser. While acknowledging that the eighteenth-century physician might occasionally palpate, Reiser argued that the physician would attach far less weight to the information obtained by his sense of touch than to the patient's narrative. Reiser also pointed to the extent to which many eighteenth-century physicians gave advice by letter as evidence that actual examination of the patient's body was not considered an essential precondition for forming a clinical opinion.[23] In 1980 W. F. Bynum summarised received opinion when he wrote 'the patient's own description of his illness was the pivotal point in the diagnostic process'.[24]

Evidence to corroborate Newman's general description can readily be cited. For instance William Cullen's clinical practice in the Edinburgh Royal Infirmary exemplifies admirably Newman's account. Cullen's clinical lectures provide no direct evidence that, in the course of his hospital practice, he ever touched the bodies of his patients. Indeed it seems very likely that he did not. The clinical procedure in the Infirmary in Cullen's time seems to have been that the clinical clerk took down a written account of the patient's complaint, elicited verbally through systematic and standardised questioning. The clerk's account was read to the physician as he came to each patient on his rounds. He observed the patient's general appearance and asked him if the clerk's account was an accurate one. The only occasion on which the patient's body was routinely handled by the physician or the clinical clerk seems to have been at the taking of the pulse.[25]

Cullen's text, *First Lines of the Practice of Physic*, provides further insight into his clinical techniques. In it he described how to identify and treat a wide variety of diseases. All the conditions were characterised in terms of symptoms observable either to the patient himself or to a physician standing or sitting near the bed. The following account of how to assess the seriousness of chronic menorrhagia is very typical:

> When in consequence of the circumstances and the repetition of these, the face becomes pale; the pulse grows weak; an unusual debility is felt in exercise; the breathing is hurried by moderate exercise; when, also, the back becomes pained from any continuance in an erect posture; when the extremities become frequently cold; and when in the evening the feet appear affected with oedematous swelling; we may, from these symptoms, certainly conclude, that the flow of menses has been immoderate, and has already induced a dangerous state of debility.[26]

Cullen's interest in nosology led him to attend very carefully to the distinctions to be made between diseases. Yet he seems to have employed physical signs of any sort very rarely indeed in differential diagnosis. There are only two examples of physical examination in the lengthy *First Lines*. Cullen wrote that tympanites was distinguishable from anasarca partly by the fact that in the former 'the swelling does not readily yield to any pressure' and 'being struck, it gives a sound like a drum'.[27] In the latter condition, on the other hand, the swelling, when pressed with the finger, 'forms a hollow that remains for some little time after the pressure is removed'.[28] In ascites 'the fluctuation of the water within, may be perceived by the practitioner's feeling, and sometimes by his hearing'.[29] Similarly, Cullen held the 'most decisive' symptom in the recognition of hydrothorax to be fluctuation of water in the chest, 'perceived by the patient himself, or by the physician, upon certain movements of the body'.[30]

Useful as Cullen may have felt palpation or abdominal percussion to be in cases of these sorts, he did not eagerly seek to add further manual techniques to his diagnostic repertoire. This is evidenced by his reaction to Auenbrugger's suggestion of thoracic percussion. In the 1778 edition of *First Lines*, Cullen wrote, 'How far the method proposed by Auenbrugger will apply to ascertain the presence of water and quantity of it in the chest, I have not had occasion or opportunity to observe.'[31] Exactly the same statement may be found in the extensively 'corrected and enlarged' edition of 1786.[32] Throughout the period intervening between these two editions, Cullen was engaged in extensive hospital and private practice. It is clear that undertaking a trial of Auenbrugger's method was not one of his priorities. While the above quoted examples of eighteenth-century physical examination imply that Keele somewhat overstated the case when he argued that the ear was never used as a clinical tool by the physician prior to 1800, Cullen's texts support the general conclusion that the employment of any form of physical examination was rare.

Other Edinburgh sources tell a similar story. Physical examination is virtually absent from John Rutherford's clinical lectures, although he frequently impressed upon students the value of inspecting the facies and noting the colour of the inner canthus of the eyes.[33] There is some evidence of palpation in Andrew Duncan's record of consultations which took place in his charitable dispensary.[34] However Duncan made it quite clear that any direct examination of the patients was done by his clinical clerks and not by himself.[35]

To take an example from another major centre of eighteenth-century medicine, it appears that Boerhaave in Leyden employed palpation only rarely, in particularly interesting cases.[36] When advising a fellow physician on how to distinguish ascites from tympanites, Boerhaave suggested neither palpation nor percussion, but weighing the patient.[37] If the patient was abnormally heavy, this would indicate the presence of water rather than gas in the abdomen. A similar approach to physical diagnosis seems also to have been prevalent in late-eighteenth-century Italy. Loris Premuda has documented the virtual absence of physical examination in Padua from 1770 until 1830.[38]

It must be emphasised that several techniques of physical examination were well known to the medical men of the eighteenth century. The techniques were known because, as Keele has pointed out, they are described in the medical works of antiquity. Greek medical texts were, in the early eighteenth century, still part of the living literature of medicine. They were read for their practical medical value rather than merely for historical or literary interest. Several Greek authors, including Galen and Hippocrates, described palpation and other diagnostic techniques such as succussion, auscultation and abdominal percussion. The absence or rarity of physical examination cannot therefore be explained by the relevant procedures not having been invented.

Why was this part of the Greek legacy ignored? As both Jewson and Foucault have pointed out, diagnostic techniques are not independent variables.[39] They are part of the totality of medical discourse in any historical period. For Jewson, eighteenth-century medical cosmology did not have a place for physical diagnosis because disease was understood in terms of unique qualitative differences between individuals, in terms of subjective experiences, in terms of the sufferer as a psychosomatic totality. This phenomenological conceptualisation of disease accorded both the study of physical signs and the study of pathological anatomy only limited meaning. In Charles Newman's more down-to-earth vocabulary, 'the doctors in those days lived in a different world' – a world in which disease did not have to follow the localised laws laid down by the anatomy of organs and tissues as it did in the nineteenth century.[40] In the eighteenth century, the seat of a disease need not be an essential part of its nature. Diseases could move from site to site, according to their own natural history or the effects of medical management.[41]

Jewson has argued that the most important feature of the eighteenth-century physician's social context was the power of the patient.[42] The dominant mode of eighteenth-century medicine was private practice for a negotiated fee. In this situation the patient was the patron and he was able to judge each practitioner on his individual merits. This meant that both the treatment and the rationale behind the treatment had to be acceptable to the patient as patron. Otherwise the patient could simply summon another practitioner. The patient was therefore autonomous and authoritative. The reliance of diagnosis on the patient's verbal account of his disease reflected this autonomy. The patient's own experience of his illness constituted the primary reality of the medical encounter, the reality with which the physician had to deal. Furthermore the patient was able to insist that, unless he or she specifically decreed otherwise, the physician should abide by the normal social conventions governing physical intimacy. Thus even in his professional capacity, the elite physician was bound by the rules of genteel etiquette maintained by polite society.

The lack of epistemological significance granted to physical examination neatly harmonised with a widely prevalent prejudice against manual work. The eighteenth-century elite physician was deeply concerned with questions of professional dignity and status. His preferred clientele were from the upper strata of society and he aspired to be accepted as a gentleman. Part of the rationale behind this claim to exalted status was scholarship. A scholar worked with his mind, not with his hands. His skills were verbal and rational. Physicians deemed manual procedures appropriate to surgeons, apothecaries and barber-surgeons.

These conventions whereby physicians did not routinely handle or examine too closely the bodies of their patients appear to have been an important aspect of their professional *mores*. They seem to have been defended as such. We can see this from the reception given to Leopold Auenbrugger's diagnostic innovation, thoracic percussion. Auenbrugger's colleagues in the Vienna hospitals responded with indifference to this novel technique. At least part of the explanation for this attitude seems to lie in the antipathy of the Viennese physicians toward handling the bodies of their patients directly.[43] Indeed such a reluctance seems to characterise certain features of Auenbrugger's own work. He recommended that the percussing physician should don a glove of fine leather or that the patient should wear a thin shirt.[44] It is also well documented that, in the first decades of the nineteenth century, many older practitioners in England vigorously opposed the introduction of more physical and intrusive methods of diagnosis such as stethoscopy, apparently because they were unwilling to compromise their professional dignity.[45]

It is interesting to note that Newman's description of changes in diagnostic practice and technique reinforces the view advanced, albeit in rather different ways, by Erwin Ackerknecht and Michel Foucault, that a truly radical change came upon medicine during the period of dominance of the Paris School – from the very end of the eighteenth century until the fifth decade of the nineteenth.[46] This was the period in which hospital medicine became the dominant means of production of medical knowledge and in which pathological anatomy flourished. Within the new institutional environment of the Paris hospitals, relations between doctor and patient changed. Physicians now confidently examined the bodies of their patients with their hands, their eyes and their ears.

Percussion and auscultation were now feasible. The stethoscope was invented. The nineteenth-century pattern of clinical diagnosis was laid down. It was not therefore until the 'birth of the clinic' that physicians actively searched the body for physical evidence on which to base a diagnosis and no longer simply passively listened to the patient's account of his illness. Only then could morbid structure be used as the principal diagnostic indicator.

Morgagni's techniques of physical examination

As noted above, one of the most striking and exciting features of *De Sedibus* is that it contains many passages in which Morgagni clearly and explicitly described his diagnostic procedures. The overall picture of his bedside practice which emerges, however, is not quite what the received account of eighteenth-century clinical procedures would lead one to expect. For instance Morgagni frequently recorded laying his hands upon the living bodies of his patients:

> And so great and so constant a pulsation was there at the region of the heart, and from thence quite to the navel, that I scarcely remember ever to have felt or to have seen a larger. For the whole of it was perceiv'd by the eye; and although it was the most considerable in the breast yet that part of the belly, also, which I have mention'd, struck the hand, when laid upon it, in such a manner, that there seem'd to every one to be an aneurism, not only in the thorax, but in the belly also.[47]

There are literally dozens of similar statements in *De Sedibus* which suggest that Morgagni practised palpation frequently. On occasion Morgagni's palpation seems to have been a very active form of manipulation:

> If you handled it, you perceived it to be an unequally tuberous tumour in its whole surface, and even in the very circumference of it, just as if it has been made up of granular bodies; which seem'd also to be confirmed by the resistance it gave when you press'd it. When it was press'd upon . . . a sense of pain, but not very violent arose in the

tumour . . . by laying hold of the tumour with both hands, I easily drew it to one side or other.[48]

By his own account Morgagni was regarded by his colleagues as having particular acumen in the practice of palpation. He was occasionally asked to give his opinion in cases where the evidence gained by palpation seemed to his colleagues problematic or equivocal.[49] However palpation in early eighteenth-century Padua should not be thought of as something peculiar to Morgagni. There are many references in *De Sedibus* to the technique being used by his contemporaries. For example, Morgagni mentioned having been given tuition in particular aspects of the diagnostic value of the technique by one of his professors in Bologna, Ippolito Francesco Albertini.[50] It seems likely, therefore, that palpation was an unremarkable element of the clinical procedures employed by elite physicians in Padua and Bologna at this time. It may be noted that Morgagni's position as a skilled practitioner of palpation in Padua appears to have been quite different from that of Antoine Portal in Paris later in the century. Portal was also, by his own account, accomplished in the diagnostic use of palpation. However he lamented that only four other physicians in the whole of Paris could apply the technique.[51] He had therefore actively to proselytise for it. To Morgagni, by contrast, palpation was routine practice, collectively accepted and endorsed by his colleagues, as is evidenced by the following passage:

> From this blood-letting the respiration was made somewhat less difficult, but the pulse at most, only a little better . . . I applied my hand to the heart, and found that it beat with equal frequency, but with moderate force. And this pulsation was produc'd even far below the region of the heart, as one of the senior physicians thought, though I could not very well perceive it myself: I so far perceiv'd it, however, that besides the polypous concretions, and the quantity of water in the pericardium, which we had suspected before, I added the suspicion of the increas'd magnitude of the heart.[52]

Palpation was a frequent enough practice among Morgagni's colleagues for him to be able to make a habit of correcting their mistakes in its application:

> pray call to mind, how far the surface of the vertebra is distant from the extremities of their posterior processes, and how much it is curv'd and protuberates forwards into the cavity of the belly: so that I have seen the hardness of it more than once impose, not only upon patients themselves, but even upon the physicians who were but little skill'd in anatomy. And this has happen'd particularly in lean and thin people, where they sometimes ... would fain have convinced me of there being a very remarkable hardness in the mesentery, which I found by laying my hand upon it, to be nothing more than this anterior surface of the spine whereof we speak. And I remember that, once having call'd aside a formerly celebrated physician (as my custom is on such occasions) to admonish him of his mistake, in this affair.[53]

Another noteworthy feature of the practice of palpation in Bologna and Padua at this time is that it was not used only to determine the site and the extent of abnormal structure, but was also used as a means of deciding what the precise prognostic significance of the abnormal structure might be. Whether a tumour was painful to touch or whether or not it adhered to underlying tissue could be of crucial importance, as in the following example:

> When we had withdrawn from the patient, one of the physicians, under whose care he had been, gave us a long dissertation upon the nature and seat of the tumour, the sum of which was this; that he believed the tumour to be scirrhous; but a spurious one, because it was painful when compress'd: and that it had its seat in the omentum, because it was movable and external.[54]

Furthermore Morgagni appears to have palpated robustly and confidently in bodily areas not normally exposed to non-intimates, 'And although it is very difficult in very fat and full-breasted women of that kind: to distinguish this disorder; unless, perhaps, by pressing your fingers very strongly against the chest, at the sides of the breasts.'[55]

As well as describing the practice of palpation, Morgagni discussed the feasibility of the Hippocratic technique of succussion: laying hold of the patient by the shoulders and shaking, and listening to the fluctuation of fluids in the thorax or abdomen. Morgagni regarded this procedure as not practical for most patients.[56] He did value auscultation, however. He pointed out that attending to noises made by water fluctuating in the abdomen or thorax was useful in the identification of dropsy. The precise location of the noises sometimes enabled differentiation between the various forms of dropsy. For instance, the difficult diagnosis of what he called dropsy of the pericardium was made confidently in a case where the physician 'could very distinctly hear the agitation of the water itself in the pericardium, when the heart was pulsating'.[57]

Morgagni was not sure whether this test was truly pathognomic, or even whether it would always be feasible. However his willingness to consider the utility of such a form of examination may be contrasted with the advice other eighteenth-century physicians gave on how to discriminate between dropsy of the thorax and dropsy of the pericardium. Their techniques depended solely upon the patient's testimony and behaviour. Although Cullen knew that fluctuation noises could be used in the diagnosis of hydrothorax he denied that the sounds in the chest could allow the physician to distinguish where exactly the fluid was situated.[58] Greatzius, a student of Hoffmann, held that the best distinguishing criteria were the following:

> the faintings were more frequent in the dropsy of the pericardium, than that of the thorax, and the difficulty of breathing more mild; and besides, that the patient affected with a dropsy of the pericardium, does not feel that the fluctuation of the water so distinctly, in turning himself from side to side, as . . . they are acustom'd to do, who labour under a dropsy of the thorax.[59]

Morgagni attended to a variety of other bodily noises such as the crepitation of fractured limbs. In one case, by listening to such sounds, Morgagni was able to decide that the bones of a child's arms had not been fractured or dislocated, but rather the epiphyses had become separated from the main shaft of the bone, owing, he conjectured, to some internal disease.[60] He also employed the percussive technique for distinguishing whether there was water or gas in a swollen abdomen. For instance, he diagnosed a case of ascites, which another physician had confused with tympany, by using the following procedure:

> In the first place if you placed your left hand on the side of the abdomen, you struck the opposite side with small but repeated strokes of the right hand, you perceived the fluctuation of the water striking against the left hand.[61]

This is by no means the only reference Morgagni made to his use of abdominal percussion. There are also several accounts in *De Sedibus* of this technique being used by his Paduan colleagues.

Morgagni's palpation and percussion were accompanied by a visual inspection which scrutinised the whole surface of the body and extended into its orifices. Many eighteenth-century physicians routinely examined their patients' lips, gums and tongue. As we have already noted, John Rutherford told his students of the value of noting the colour of the lachryma caruncle of the eyelids.[62] But Morgagni's visual inspection extended into other orifices as well. For instance he examined the nasal passages at least as far as the opening of the nasolacrimal duct.[63] Nor was Morgagni's visual inspection confined to those surfaces not normally covered by clothes. Clothing might be removed in order that Morgagni could observe better: 'A child was brought to me for advice, on account of a tumour being prominent about the lumbar vertebrae. While they were taking off the clothes, for me to look at it....'[64] Inspection of the naked surface of the body does not seem to have been confined to children. Morgagni reported the following observation of a man of 32:

> The conformation of the thorax shew'd nothing from whence I could conjecture that he was dispos'd to a consumption; for the shape of it was such, that it lay quite contiguous to the broad bones of the scapulae, and did not, by receding therefrom, render them prominent like wings.[65]

There is evidence that the clinical inspection and examination undertaken by Morgagni were often very intimate indeed. Morgagni recalled that his mentor, Antonio Maria Valsalva, did rectal examinations of both men and women. On one occasion Morgagni noted that Valsalva confidently diagnosed an incurable rectal tumour 'having only ask'd questions of this woman, without so much as introducing his finger, to examine the rectum'.[66] We may surmise, from Morgagni's evident surprise, that this was a departure from Valsalva's normal practice in such cases. Morgagni also recorded an instance of Valsalva differentiating between piles and a rectal ulcer by direct digital examination:

> For in one of them, having introduc'd his finger, pretty high up in the rectum, he point'd out to the others, the certain situation of the ulcer as the apex of his finger being receiv'd into the orifice of it, seem'd to be embrac'd around, with a kind of ring as it were; for in this manner he assur'd them, that the ulcers of the rectum, or vagina, were frequently found, so that a narrow mouth is dilated into a more capacious sinus.[67]

On another occasion, however, Valsalva's diagnosis of a rectal ulcer was made wholly on the basis of the patient's testimony. He concluded that an ulcer was present because the patient complained of a purulent discharge, and that it was situated below the sphincter because the flow of the discharge was continuous.[68]

There is no unequivocal evidence in *De Sedibus* that Morgagni did rectal examinations himself. On one occasion he was consulted by a young priest who complained of a discharge of urine *per anum*. Morgagni questioned the patient and examined the fluid expelled but, in his account of the case, he mentioned neither a digital nor a visual examination.[69] However Morgagni did give detailed accounts of pathological and congenital abnormalities, observed in life, of both male and female genitalia.[70] *De Sedibus* also provides evidence that Morgagni and his colleagues at Padua not only inspected but also palpated in the groins of both male and female patients. A woman with a tumour in the groin was examined by several physicians including Santorini, a close friend of Morgagni. Morgagni recorded that 'All signs of a hernia were absent; except that immediately upon applying their hand to that part, the woman discharged wind.'[71] However before inspection or palpation in this region of the body could take place, the physician had first to gain the permission of the patient. For example, Morgagni recommended the following procedure if a pulse could not be felt at the wrists: 'other arteries are to be examined; as, for instance, the temporal arteries and the carotids; and finally also, *when it is permitted*, the crural arteries, which have a pulsation in the groins'.[72]

As several of the above quotations indicate, Morgagni did not have absolute authority and license during physical examination. His diagnostic practice was finely modulated and controlled by social convention and by the authority of the patient. Certain parts of patients' bodies were, thus, more easily touchable than others. For example, he exercised some circumspection when called to consult with the physicians treating the Bishop of Brescia:

> When I examin'd accurately with my hand what was above, below, and at the sides of, the tumour, except that I did not go on to examine below the navel, (the physicians and the patient, asserting that nothing preternatural was there or nothing hard or resisting was perceiv'd).[73]

We may assume that Morgagni saw no need to ask for special permission to conduct a fuller investigation in this case. The patient might allow certain procedures and not others. Vaginal examination, for example, was often prohibited. Morgagni gave a detailed description of how to diagnose pregnancy by digital examination of the os uteri. He regarded compression of the os uteri as the least equivocal sign of pregnancy in the early months, 'Wherefore I have made use of this sign when it was in my power; but I have it in my power very seldom; the women of our country being for the most part repugnant to an examination of that kind.'[74]

However it was not only the patient that was able to exercise authority within the consultative encounter. We have already seen one example in which Morgagni used the evidence obtained from physical examination to contradict a patient's opinion as to the state of his health. Palpable lumps in the abdomen were not, despite their owner's anxiety, tumours. They were, according to Morgagni, part of a perfectly normal vertebral column. In the following example the contradiction of the sufferer's testimony was more subtle. Morgagni agreed with the patient that a pathological swelling existed in the abdomen but did not accept his opinion as to its having diminished in size. The passage is worth quoting at length because of the vivid picture it provides of Morgagni in action at the bedside:

> In the meantime this extravasation increas'd so that when I happen'd to have occasion to go up to the hospital . . . and being asked to feel the man's belly, I scarcely perceiv'd any particular tumour elsewhere than in the scrobiculus cordis, the abdominal cavity being so greatly distended with water. The tumour was very hard and very unequal, but free from pain, even when you press'd upon it. I inquir'd whether it was troublesome by its weight? whether there was any pain which was produc'd quite to the throat? and whether he was ever troubled with a cough? To all which queries the patient answer'd in the negative. But when I asked him whether the tumour increas'd at that time? he not only answer'd negatively, but even asserted that it had subsided, and was grown much less: I suppose because it was in great measure obscur'd by the increasing water: and indeed, those who had felt it at other times could not perceive it to be diminish'd. The face of the man was somewhat pale but not yellow, nor of a cinereous colour; and even the white parts of the eyes, though I examin'd them very attentively, did not appear to me to have the least yellowness.[75]

Morgagni and the eighteenth-century consultative encounter

The contents of *De Sedibus* seem to allow little doubt that Morgagni's bedside practice constitutes an important exception to Charles Newman's general account of eighteenth-century clinical behaviour. Morgagni inspected and palpated confidently and purposefully almost every part of his patients' bodies. It seems equally clear that Morgagni's use of physical examination was not idiosyncratic. Its employment was common practice among many of his contemporaries in Padua and Bologna. They, like Morgagni, inspected and palpated extensively. They employed the ear clinically, attending to abnormal noises made in the thorax, abdomen and limbs of their patients. They valued internal digital examinations and frequently, if not quite routinely, undertook such investigations.

According to Jewson, the patient's experience of his own illness, or written or verbal accounts derived from it, embodied the real meaning of the disease for the eighteenth-century physician. It is noteworthy that, for Morgagni, the patient's testimony, or a written account derived from it, did not always provide an adequate basis on which to form a clinical opinion. Like most eighteenth-century physicians Morgagni conducted a considerable consultation correspondence. In the majority of cases he felt able to rely on the information provided for him by the patient or the attending physician. Sometimes however he wrote back that he was unable to form a full opinion without having examined the case:

> I would not dare to assert that such was the case at the beginning of this lady's sickness without having first made an exact inspection of the injured place, in order to ascertain whether the sign mentioned by Bassio was encountered.[76]

On occasion it was necessary for the physician to see for himself.

We have also noted that *De Sedibus* provides examples of Morgagni contradicting the patient's opinion on the basis of his own examination of the seat of the disease. On one occasion he denied that a pathological structure existed; on another he held that a tumour was increasing in size despite the patient maintaining that it was getting smaller. There must of course have been many occasions on which the eighteenth-century physician and his patient disagreed over the presence, nature or progress of a disease. We may presume that the physician would frequently have opposed his authority and learning against the opinion of the patient.[77] However the significant point here is that Morgagni was, on occasion, prepared to take the very basis of the understanding of disease away from the patient. The patient was, in these instances, no longer the wholly competent interpreter of his own physical condition. Acceptance of the evidence presented here must entail some revision of Jewson's portrayal of eighteenth-century modes of production of medical knowledge.

There are, on the other hand, many systematic distinctions to be made between Morgagni's approach to physical examination and that of an elite nineteenth-century physician. First, Morgagni only occasionally used the evidence gained by examination to contradict the patient's account. In general the two sources of information complemented each other. In the nineteenth and twentieth centuries, by contrast, the information which the doctor gathered in the process of direct physical examination could make the patient's testimony redundant. Complaints by the patient not supported by clinical signs might be dismissed. The doctor's expertise might thus *routinely* negate the patient's understanding of his own disease.[78] Second, direct examination was a frequent but not a constant feature of Morgagni's consultative procedure. As we have seen, both he and Valsalva were sometimes content to diagnose on the basis of the patient's account even in circumstances where a more direct technique might be simple to apply. Valsalva sometimes did rectal examination, sometimes not. In the nineteenth century, however, once physical examination was established it became routine and obligatory. No doctor would diagnose a rectal tumour without as direct an examination as was possible. Third, the patient's consent regulated and modulated the extent of Morgagni's physical examination. Here again a systematic difference may be noted between the form of physical examination undertaken in early eighteenth-century Padua and that which became common in the following century. In the nineteenth century the intensity of physical examination which was accepted as routine and normal by the patient greatly increased. The nineteenth-century physician became a licensed examiner of the bodies of his patients.[79] Being examined by the doctor became identified as a special form of social interaction – no longer constrained by the normal conventions governing touch between non-intimates, but controlled by ethical standards and modes of conduct established and maintained by the medical profession itself. Physical examination still involved the patient's consent, of course, but effective departure from the normal procedure depended, not upon the patient granting additional consent, as in the examples quoted above, but upon the patient withdrawing consent. Morgagni was able to expand the extent of his physical examination when additional permission was forthcoming; a nineteenth- or twentieth-century hospital doctor would contract his normal diagnostic procedure when permission for certain forms of examination was withdrawn.

It is worth emphasising that Morgagni's theory and practice was overall very typical of an eighteenth-century, indeed an early eighteenth-century, physician. His diagnostic procedures were modulated in a characteristic manner. The patient's account generally had a central place within Morgagni's understanding of disease. His materia medica and the means whereby it was applied were likewise quite typical. One would not, for instance, find shavings of human skull or renderings of human fat in a nineteenth-century pharmacopoeia.[80] In fact these preparations were already old-fashioned in Morgagni's time, yet he placed great store upon them, choosing the sources of the fat he used with great care.[81] Morgagni also extracted items of practical value from the classical texts. His disease theory was humoral, modified along the lines of eighteenth-century iatromechanism.[82] Many of the passages of *De Sedibus*, even the anatomical ones, fit very well within Foucault's description of the eighteenth-century medical gaze.[83] For all these reasons Morgagni must be regarded as lying unequivocally on the far side of the transformation that separates eighteenth-century from nineteenth-century clinical medicine. This realisation prohibits one possible explanation for the character of his diagnostics and for his being exceptional to Newman's accounts. That is the explanation which is frequently advanced to explain the apparently progressive nature of Morgagni's pathological anatomy – namely that he somehow anticipated the nineteenth century and its anatomico-clinical preoccupations.[84] The clearer we see Morgagni as a creation of the eighteenth century, the more apparent it becomes that the character of his diagnostic practice must be understood wholly in eighteenth-century terms.

Real as the effect of the patients' authority was in modulating and constraining the behaviour of the eighteenth-century physician, the importance within the medical context of the normal social conventions governing physical contact between non-intimates can be exaggerated. It is obvious that patients frequently consented to be examined very intimately indeed by surgeons, if not by physicians. Otherwise no operations for hernia, bladder stone or anal fistula would ever have been done. Yet these operations were common enough in the eighteenth century.[85] Bladder catheterisation was also quite frequent.[86] If social constraints did control physicians' diagnostic behaviour, the explanation for the efficacy of such constraints must lie, at least partly, in physicians choosing to be bound by particular social conventions and patients coming to expect physicians to behave in a particular way. In other words, physicians' utilisation of physical examination was circumscribed by their cultivation of a social role distinct from that of other medical practitioners.

What the Morgagni example shows us is that the exact configuration of physicians' choices and patients' expectations was a cultural variable. The fact that the professional boundaries between physician and surgeon were often not clear-cut reinforces and exemplifies this conclusion. We have therefore to abandon the idea that a single monolithic form of diagnostic practice existed as standard wherever and whenever diagnosis was practised by physicians in the eighteenth century. While perhaps provisionally accepting Newman's description in its broadest outlines, we ought to be alert to the possible existence of a much more finely-textured pattern of variation in practice, corresponding to the wide range of different cultural and professional contexts within which the eighteenth-century physician worked. Likewise Jewson's account of the social constraints upon the production of medical knowledge in the eighteenth century will not develop its full value until the precise social circumstances under which it may be said to apply, fully or partly, are elucidated.

Surgery and internal medicine

Why was Morgagni, a typical eighteenth-century professor and physician, apparently untypical in that he employed auscultation, abdominal percussion, and external and internal physical examination? Why were the diagnostic techniques employed in early eighteenth-century Padua and Bologna different from those employed in Paris, London or Edinburgh? Owsei Temkin has argued that much of the novel character of nineteenth-century medicine was the result of a process of cross-fertilisation between surgery and internal physic.[87] This cross-fertilisation started in the latter half of the eighteenth century and was intensified in the work of the Paris school. In France reforms consequent upon the Revolution abolished the professional and educational distinctions between surgery and physic and created a unified medical profession. The cognitive consequence of this union of the two disciplines was a body of medical knowledge in which internal disease was newly conceived of in localised, structural, anatomic terms as opposed to the whole-body, humoral pathology of eighteenth-century physic. Physicians began to think, in a word, surgically. Their new structural outlook was expressed in their interest in pathological anatomy and in their development of techniques of physical examination. The aim of the new diagnostic procedures was to anatomise the living, to see the structural effects of disease at the bedside. The new conception of pathology thus gave physical examination primary significance.

It has not been pointed out how similar Temkin's conclusions are to those of recent studies in the sociology of science. Sociologists of science have given careful attention to the movement of personnel from one scientific speciality to another.[88] Such migrations have been identified as major sources of cognitive change and innovation. The skills learned in the original field are applied to the problems presented by the new one. In this way the character of the receiving speciality may be altered. Likewise Temkin explained much of the character of medicine at the Paris school in terms of an influx of personnel from surgery. Thus Temkin's explanation for the difference between the form of internal medicine dominant in the early nineteenth century and the form of internal medicine dominant in the eighteenth would seem, on both empirical and theoretical grounds, to be a very promising one.

The corollary of the Temkin thesis is that where physic and surgery were close together, socially and educationally, or where surgeons were exceptionally powerful one might expect to find, in the eighteenth century, forms of practice more like those which were to become dominant in the nineteenth. Toby Gelfand has shown this to be the case in his careful study of the Paris school of surgery in the late eighteenth century.[89] He has demonstrated that the anatomico-clinical approach of nineteenth-century medicine was prefigured in certain aspects of late eighteenth-century French surgery. This was due, he argues, to the relatively greater professional power of surgeons in Paris compared to other European centres.

It is interesting to note that, in Padua and indeed in Italy generally, throughout the first half of the eighteenth century, physicians and surgeons were not so rigidly separated from one another as they were elsewhere.[90] Trainee surgeons attended classes at the Italian medical faculties. Surgery was taught by professors who were also professional surgeons. Furthermore, in Italy men who had the right to call themselves physicians and who actively practised physic, also practised surgery. For instance Morgagni remarked that his colleague Antonio Gallio was a 'very skilful physician and surgeon, in which last capacity he was particularly famous'.[91] A total of eight eminent physicians were described by Morgagni in *De Sedibus* as being also fine surgeons; pre-eminent among these was Morgagni's teacher and mentor, Valsalva, who according to Morgagni 'loved and cultivated' the profession of surgery.[92] One could find no such distinguished coterie of dual practitioners in contemporary Edinburgh, Paris or London.[93]

No doubt the cultivation of surgery was made easier by the fact that, in Morgagni's professional circle at least, there seems not to have been a serious stigma attached to what one might call scholarly manual work. Morgagni was the sort of person who would have been sensitive to such a prejudice if one existed. He seems to have been very jealous of his dignity as a university professor and upper-class physician. For instance, he quite disdained to inquire after the names of his plebeian patients in the hospitals.[94] But he was apparently quite unselfconscious of the work he did with his hands. He boasted of his skill in experimentation and in anatomical dissection.

As Temkin has pointed out, Morgagni did not perform operative surgery himself.[95] However he should not be regarded as neglecting surgery solely on this account. Operations were a relatively small part of eighteenth-century surgical practice. Morgagni undertook many other procedures which would have been regarded as falling within the normal repertoire of the eighteenth-century surgeon. For instance he used a magnet to remove iron splinters from the eye.[96] He investigated the position of foreign bodies in the ear.[97] He employed the techniques developed by the French surgeon, Dominique Anel, for the treatment of lachrymal abscesses and fistulae.[98] These involved the use of very fine sounds and tubes to clear obstructions from the lachrymal passages and to effuse the cavities with medicinal injections. Morgagni wrote an important defence of Anel's controversial methods.[99] Furthermore, while he did not operate on humans, Morgagni did do something very similar in the course of his experiments on live animals. His investigations of the cervical arteries of the dog were virtually experimental surgery.[100]

It is also clear that physicians in Bologna and Padua often undertook the overall supervision of surgical cases, even though the cutting and mending were done by a specialist operator. Several of Morgagni's surviving consultation letters record him providing detailed advice on surgical matters. As well as giving comprehensive instructions on how to apply Anel's techniques, he made specific suggestions on the use of the cautery and the urethral bougie.[101] Morgagni was also consulted on the treatment of wounds and on the pre- and post-operative care of surgical patients. In the course of his normal practice, Morgagni had many surgical cases presented to him in the first instance. He did not confine himself to advising whether or not an operation was required.[102] Using his great knowledge of human anatomy he made detailed suggestions as to how the operation should be carried out, what especial precautions the operator should take, and so on.[103] This co-operative relationship between physic and surgery may be contrasted with the situation in the Edinburgh Infirmary, later in the century, where the physician might never see the surgical cases at all. They were segregated in surgical wards and attended only by surgeons.[104]

Morgagni regarded it as part of his duty as a physician to exercise quality control over the work of surgeons. On one occasion a child died after an operation to remove a tumour. Morgagni had seen the child beforehand and regarded the surgical intervention as misconceived. He was curious to inspect the body and asked the parents' permission:

> There . . . having met with the surgeon . . . I did not omit to blame, as indeed my duty was, his late supreme confidence and destructive boldness . . . yet that he might be more cautious and considerate for the future, as he was now very docible, and entreated it of me, I immediately consented, and promised him that I would be present, while the tumour was dissected, and explain the contents of it to him.[105]

Morgagni's professional role also required him to provide expert arbitration should disputes arise between surgeons and their clients. *De Sedibus* describes several occasions on which his opinion was sought under such circumstances.[106] In the exercise of these duties anatomical knowledge and skill in physical examination would have been invaluable.

It seems that the right to supervise which the physician traditionally claimed over the surgeon did have, in early eighteenth-century Padua and Bologna, a significant effect in shaping the character of patient care. It is understandable therefore that Morgagni argued vigorously and frequently that a detailed knowledge of surgery was part of the essential equipment of a physician. Morgagni's professional situation allowed and required him to be capable of surgical modes of thought. As is well known, Morgagni championed a view of pathology which entailed considerable structural localisation. This too may be seen as a link with surgery since all surgeons have perforce a structural understanding of disease. The abnormalities which Morgagni's dissection knife exposed constituted an anatomical explanation of the patient's clinical symptoms. Moreover, the abscesses, tumours and gangrenes which Morgagni found on the internal surface of the body were precisely the same kind of phenomena as those seen by surgeons on the external surface of the body.[107] For all the above reasons, it is not far-fetched to say that Morgagni, great physician as he was, employed, on appropriate occasions, a surgical view of disease.

Post-mortem enquiry was quite commonly practised throughout the seventeenth and eighteenth centuries. It was, however, generally undertaken in isolation both from physical examination and a structural perspective on disease. Temkin and Gelfand have both argued that what linked all three together in the work of the Paris school was the surgical outlook of its leading physicians.[108] A surgical perspective on internal disease, being necessarily structural and manipulative, is likely to accord primary relevance to both pathological anatomy and physical examination. In this cognitive framework, pathological anatomy and physical examination may be seen as the joint expressions of a single tenet of pathology: that the disease process is somehow associated with perceivable structural change.

Despite the great differences between early eighteenth-century Padua and early nineteenth-century Paris, there are certain obvious similarities. In both cases physic and surgery were intimately linked. Pathological anatomy and physical examination were routinely practised and were taken to what were, in contemporary terms, very high levels of technical excellence. Clinical manifestations were explained in terms of structural changes. Thus, the quasi-surgical nature of Morgagni's theory and practice of physic provides a fresh display of the explanatory value of the Temkin thesis. The contents of *De Sedibus* suggest that the triangular fructification between surgery, pathology and physical methods of diagnosis which Temkin describes also occurred, albeit to a lesser extent than in Paris, in the major medical schools of northern Italy, in the early eighteenth century.[109] It was, thus, the existence of a close social and professional association between physic and surgery which gave the diagnostic practice of Giovanni Morgagni its distinctive character.[110]

Acknowledgements

I am grateful to Michael Barfoot, Catherine Crawford, Mary Fissel, Christopher Lawrence, Andrew Pickering and Virginia Smith for their careful scrutiny of several of the earlier versions of this paper. It was also presented to History of Medicine seminar groups in Manchester and Edinburgh, and to a Wellcome Institute symposium. I owe a considerable debt to the many comments and questions I received on these occasions. Throughout the period of preparation of this paper I have been supported by the Wellcome Trust, to whom I wish to record my gratitude.

Notes and references

1. For example, C. Rosenberg, 'Medical text and medical context: explaining William Buchan's *Domestic Medicine*', *Bulletin of the History of Medicine*, vol. 57 (1983), pp. 22–42; R. Porter, 'William Hunter: a surgeon and a gentleman', in W. F. Bynum and R. Porter (eds), *William Hunter and the Eighteenth-Century Medical World* (Cambridge University Press, Cambridge, 1985), pp. 7–35.

2. For example, W. F. Bynum, 'Physicians, hospitals and career structures in eighteenth-century London', in Bynum and Porter, *William Hunter*, pp. 105–28; T. Gelfand, *Professionalising Modern Medicine: Paris Surgeons and Medical Science and Institutions in the Eighteenth Century* (Greenwood Press, Westport, 1980); R. Stott, 'The incorporation of surgeons and medical education and practice in Edinburgh, 1696–1755', unpublished PhD thesis, University of Edinburgh, 1984.

3. For example, see Roy Porter, 'Lay medical knowledge in the eighteenth century: the evidence of the *Gentleman's Magazine*', *Medical History*, vol. 29 (1985), pp. 138–68; 'The patient's view: doing medical history from below', *Theory and Society*, vol. 14 (1985), pp. 175–98.

4. This is despite the fact that it is more than twenty years since E. H. Ackerknecht pointed out the advantages of such subject matter. Ackerknecht, 'A plea for a "Behaviourist" approach in writing the history of medicine', *Journal of the History of Medicine*, vol. 22 (1967), pp. 211–14.

5. N. D. Jewson, 'Medical knowledge and the patronage system in eighteenth-century England', *Sociology*, vol. 8 (1974), pp. 369–85; 'The disappearance of the sick man from medical cosmology 1770–1870', *Sociology*, vol. 10 (1976), pp. 225–40.

6. G. Risse, *Hospital Life in Enlightenment Scotland: Care and Teaching at the Royal Infirmary of Edinburgh* (Cambridge University Press, Cambridge, 1985).

7. For example, J. Lane, '"The doctor scolds me": the diaries and correspondence of patients in eighteenth-century England', in Roy Porter (ed.), *Patients and Practitioners: Lay Perceptions of Medicine in Pre-Industrial Society* (Cambridge University Press, Cambridge, 1985), pp. 205–48.

8. G. B. Morgagni, *De Sedibus et Causis Morborum per Anatomen Indagatis* (Remondini, Venice, 1761); translated by B. Alexander as *The Seats and Causes of Diseases Investigated by Anatomy*, 3 vols (A. Millar & T. Cadell, London, 1769); reprinted, with some new material by P. Klemperer (Hafner, New York, 1960).

9. For more information on Morgagni see S. Jarcho, 'Giovanni Battista Morgagni; his interests, ideas and achievement', *Bulletin of the History of Medicine*, vol. 22 (1948), pp. 503–24.

10. Ibid., also P. Klemperer, 'Morbid anatomy before and after Morgagni', *Bulletin of the New York Academy of Medicine*, vol. 37 (1966), pp. 741–60.

11. Another way of expressing this would be that the eighteenth-century phrase 'morbid anatomy' encompassed clinical implications. Pathological anatomy was not, in the eighteenth century, an autonomous discipline.

12. Morgagni also opened bodies in the course of forensic and public health investigations.

13. A similar point was eloquently made by T. S. Kuhn, *The Structure of Scientific Revolutions*, 2nd edn (University of Chicago Press, Chicago, 1970), pp. 137–43.

14. A further problem of interpretation is imposed by the fact that I have largely used Morgagni's text in translation. However, Alexander's translation is universally acknowledged to be a very literal one. It certainly seems so to me. Furthermore I have checked each quotation in the original, and not used any in which Alexander's translation did not seem accurately to convey Morgagni's sense. Misinterpretations may still remain, however, and I would be very grateful if scholars more skilled in classics would bring any such to my attention. I have used Alexander's translation on the authority of Jarcho, 'Morgagni', p. 503.

15. Hermann Boerhaave, *Aphorisms*, translated by J. Delacoste (B. Cowse & W. Innys, London, 1715), p. 339.

16. Morgagni, *The Seats*, vol. 1, p. 737.

17. Ibid., vol. 2, p. 340.

18. Enrico Benassi's Italian edition of Morgagni's consultation letters has recently been translated and revised by S. Jarcho, *The Clinical Consultations of Giambattista Morgagni* (University Press of Virginia, Charlottesville, 1984).

19. O. Temkin, 'The role of surgery in the rise of modern medical thought', *Bulletin of the History of Medicine*, vol. 25 (1951), pp. 248–59.

20. C. Newman, *Evolution of Medical Education in the Nineteenth Century* (Oxford University Press, London, 1957), pp. 86–104; 'Physical signs at King's', *King's College Hospital Gazette*, vol. 27 (1958), p. 77; 'Physical signs in the London hospitals', *Medical History*, vol. 2 (1958), pp. 195–201; 'Diagnostic investigation before Laennec', *Medical History*, vol. 4 (1960), pp. 322–9. But see also S. C. Lawrence, 'Science and medicine at the London hospitals: the development of teaching and research, 1750–1815', unpublished PhD thesis, University of Toronto, 1985, vol. 2, chs. 10 and 12.

21. The North London Hospital later became University College Hospital.

22. K. D. Keele, *The Evolution of Clinical Methods in Medicine* (Pitman, London, 1963), p. 44.

23. S. J. Reiser, *Medicine and the Reign of Technology* (Cambridge University Press, Cambridge, 1978), pp. 5–6.

24. W. F. Bynum, 'Health, disease and medical care', in G. Rousseau and R. Porter (eds.), *The Ferment of Knowledge: Studies in the Historiography of Eighteenth-Century Science* (Cambridge University Press, Cambridge, 1980), pp. 211–53.

25. My picture of the clinical practice at the Edinburgh Royal Infirmary is a composite one, drawn from Risse, *Hospital Life*; G. Stewart, 'Sketch of the history of the Royal Infirmary and the development of clinical teaching', *Edinburgh Hospital Records* (Pentland, Edinburgh, 1893), pp. 1–17; and M. Barfoot, personal communication.

26. W. Cullen, *First Lines of the Practice of Physic*, 4 vols (C. Elliott, Edinburgh, 1786), vol. 3, pp. 13–14.

27. Ibid., vol. 4, p. 228.

28. Ibid., p. 277.

29. Ibid., p. 323.

30. Ibid., p. 314. The interpretive difficulty noted above with regard to Boerhaave's description of how to inspect a hydrocele must also be borne in mind when considering all these examples from *First Lines*.

31. Quoted in S. Jarcho, 'The introduction of percussion in the United States', *Journal of the History of Medicine*, vol. 13 (1985), pp. 259–60; see also his 'Auenbrugger, Laennec and John Keats: some notes on the early history of percussion and auscultation', *Medical History*, vol. 5 (1961), pp. 167–72.

32. Cullen, *First Lines*, vol. 4, p. 314. Interestingly Cullen's colleague, the physician Alexander Monro *secundus*, had apparently experimented with percussion on corpses. See Christopher Lawrence, 'Ornate physicians and learned artisans: Edinburgh medical men, 1726–1776', in Bynum and Porter, *William Hunter*, pp. 153–76.

33. J. Rutherford, 'Clinical lectures', student's manuscript notes, Edinburgh University Library, Dc.10.28, p. 20.

34. A. Duncan, *Medical Cases, Selected from the Records of the Public Dispensary at Edinburgh*, 2nd edn (C. Elliot, Edinburgh, 1781), p. 108, for example.

35. Ibid., p. 4.

36. See L. S. King, 'Description of another dreadful and unusual disease drawn up by Herman Boerhaave', *Journal of the History of Medicine*, vol. 23 (1968), pp. 331–48; W. J. Derbes and R. E. Mitchell, 'Herman Boerhaave's "*Atroci, nec Descripti Morbi Historia*" the first translation of the classic case report of rupture of the esophagus, with annotations', *Bulletin of the Medical Libraries Association*, vol. 43 (1955), pp. 217–40.

37. G. A. Lindeboom, *Boerhaave's Correspondence* (Brill, Leiden, 1962–79), vol. 2, p. 79. There is only one letter, vol. 3, p. 195, in this collection in which Boerhaave sends the details of a case to a colleague for his opinion. This contains no reference to Boerhaave having undertaken either palpation or inspection, despite the fact that disorders of the gall-bladder and the hypochondrium are under discussion.

38. L. Premuda. 'The revival of the anatomico-clinical method in Padua: the fundamental contribution of F. S. Verson (1805–1849) from Trieste, a disciple of the Vienna School of Medicine', *Janus*, vol. 67 (1980), pp. 30–9; also 'Die Anatomisch–Klinische Methode: Padua–Paris–Wien–Padua', *Gesnerus*, vol. 44 (1987) pp. 15–32; and 'Die Klinische Forschung in Padua im Zeitraum vom Tode Morgagnis bis zur Einführung der Physikalischen Diagnostik', *Acta Congressus Internationalis XXIV Historia Artis Medicinae* (Budapest, 1976), pp. 815–24. As will be seen from the remainder of this paper, it would seem that the situation in Padua as regards the use of physical diagnosis differed between Morgagni's time and the end of the century.

39. Jewson, 'Sick man'; M. Foucault, *The Birth of the Clinic* (Tavistock, London, 1973).

40. Newman, 'Diagnostic investigation', p. 328.

41. For the use of theories as to the movement of disease around the body see Malcolm Nicolson, 'The metastatic theory of pathogenesis and the professional interests of the eighteenth-century physician', *Medical History*, vol. 32 (1988), pp. 277–301.

42. Jewson, 'Medical knowledge'.

43. For background see J. B. Herrick, 'A note concerning the long neglect of Auenbrugger's *Inventum Novum*', *Archives of Internal Medicine*, vol. 71 (1943), pp. 741–8.

44. L. Auenbrugger, *On Percussion of the Chest*, translated by John Forbes in *Bulletin of the Institute of the History of Medicine*, vol. 4 (1936), pp. 373–403. The passage referred to is on p. 382.

45. See S. J. Reiser, 'Aspects of the role of the stethoscope in the introduction of auscultation to Great Britain and the United States', *Proceedings, Twenty-Third International Congress for the History of Medicine* (London, 1974), vol. 1, pp. 832–40; E. J. Bluth, 'James Hope and the acceptance of auscultation', *Journal of the History of Medicine*, vol. 25 (1970), pp. 202–10; see also Reiser, *Reign of Technology*, pp. 37–8; M. Nicolson, 'Percussion and stethoscopy in early nineteenth-century Edinburgh', in W. F. Bynum and R. Porter (eds), *The Five Senses in Medicine* (Cambridge University Press, Cambridge, forthcoming).

46. E. Ackerknecht, *Medicine at the Paris Hospital 1794–1848* (Johns Hopkins University Press, Baltimore, 1967); Foucault, *Birth of the Clinic.*
47. Morgagni, *The Seats*, vol. 1, p. 762.
48. Ibid., vol. 2, p. 382.
49. Ibid., p. 206.
50. Ibid., pp. 178–9. For further information about Albertini's use of physical diagnosis, see S. Jarcho, 'The *Animadversiones* of Ippolito Francesco Albertini (1748) on cardiac and precordial diseases which cause dyspnoea', *Proceedings of the American Philosophical Society*, vol. 116 (1972), pp. 163–81.
51. Ackerknecht, *Paris Hospital*, p. 26.
52. Morgagni, *The Seats*, vol. 1, p. 723.
53. Ibid., p. 220.
54. Ibid., vol. 2, p. 382.
55. Ibid., pp. 638–9.
56. Ibid., vol. 1, pp. 407–8.
57. Ibid., pp. 394–7.
58. W. Cullen, 'Clinical lectures', notes taken by Sir Charles Blagden, Wellcome Institute Library, MS 1948, p. 40.
59. Quoted in Morgagni, *The Seats*, vol. 1, p. 391.
60. Ibid., vol. 3, pp. 312–13.
61. Ibid., vol. 2, p. 304.
62. Rutherford, 'Clinical lectures', p. 20.
63. Jarcho, *Clinical Consultations*, p. 212. See also G. B. Morgagni, *Adversaria Anatomica Omnia* (Cominus, Padua, 1719), part 1, tabula IV, fig. 1.
64. Morgagni, *The Seats*, vol. 1, p. 271.
65. Ibid., p. 673.
66. Ibid., vol. 2, p. 102.
67. Ibid., p. 109.
68. Ibid.
69. Ibid., p. 544.
70. For example, ibid., pp. 618–22, 647–53. In the last case Morgagni advised a woman that an 'obstructing membrane' in her vagina was not merely an abnormally thick hymen but a major congenital deformity. She was urged not to submit to surgical intervention but to allow her marriage, 'which was improperly contracted', to be dissolved.
71. Ibid., p. 556.
72. Ibid., vol. 1, p. 718, emphasis added.
73. Ibid., vol. 2, p. 382.
74. Ibid., p. 696.
75. Ibid., p. 206.
76. Jarcho, *Clinical Consultations*, p. 4; see also Morgagni, *The Seats*, vol. 1, p. 337.
77. I have discussed this aspect of eighteenth-century doctor–patient interaction in Nicolson, 'Metastatic theory'.
78. S. J. Reiser, 'The decline of the clinical dialogue', *Journal of Philosophy and Medicine*, vol. 3 (1978), pp. 305–15; also Reiser, *Reign of Technology*; W. R. Arnery and B. J. Bergen, *Medicine and the Management*

of Living: Taming the Last Great Beast (University of Chicago Press, Chicago, 1984).

79. Jewson, 'Sick man'; also D. Armstrong, *Political Anatomy of the Body: Medical Knowledge in Britain in the Twentieth Century* (Cambridge University Press, Cambridge, 1983).

80. For example, Morgagni, *The Seats*, vol. 1, pp. 191–2.

81. See D. L. Cowen, 'The Edinburgh Pharmacopoeia', in R. G. W. Anderson and A. D. C. Simpson (eds), *The Early Years of the Edinburgh Medical School* (Royal Scottish Museum, Edinburgh, 1976), pp. 25–45.

82. For an account of Morgagni's disease theory, see Jarcho, *Clinical Consultations*, pp. xxxvi–xc.

83. Compare, for example, Morgagni's description of vomited 'membranes', *The Seats*, vol. 2, p. 55 with the passage from Pomme quoted by Foucault, *Birth of the Clinic*, p. ix.

84. See, for example, G. Lazorthes and L. Campan, 'Jean-Baptiste Morgagni (1682–1771), initiateur de la méthode anatomo-clinique', *Bulletin de l'académie nationale de médecine*, vol. 166, no. 9 (1982), pp. 1317–21; J. Feroldi, 'À propos d'un tricentenaire: J. B. Morgagni, essor de l'anatomie pathologique et naissance de la méthode anatomo-clinique', *Conférences d'Histoire de la Médecine: Cycle 82–83* (Institut d'Histoire de la Medicine, Lyons, 1983), pp. 55–68.

85. See O. H. Wangensteen and S. D. Wangensteen, *The Rise of Surgery: from Empiric Craft to Scientific Discipline* (Dawson, Folkestone, 1978).

86. This may be gauged from the frequency with which the procedure is mentioned in the major texts of the period, not only *De Sedibus* but also, for example, G. Van Swieten, *Commentaries on the Aphorisms of Herman Boerhaave* (Horsfield & Longman, London, 1771).

87. Temkin, 'Role of surgery'. See also note 110 below.

88. J. Ben-David, 'Roles and innovations in medicine', *American Journal of Sociology*, vol. 65 (1960), pp. 557–68; J. Ben-David and R. Collins, 'Social factors in the origin of a new science: the case of psychology', *American Sociological Review*, vol. 31 (1966), pp. 451–65; N. Mullins, 'The development of a scientific specialty: the phage group and the origins of molecular biology', *Minerva*, vol. 10 (1972), pp. 51–82.

89. Gelfand, *Modern Medicine*, esp. pp. 149–92.

90. For information about medical education in Italy, see L. Belloni, 'Italian medical education after 1600', in C. D. O'Malley (ed.), *History of Medical Education* (University of California Press, Berkeley, 1970), pp. 111–12; and J. J. Bylebyl, 'Commentary: early clinical teaching at Padua', in L. G. Stevenson (ed.), *A Celebration of Medical History* (Johns Hopkins University Press, Baltimore, 1982), pp. 200–11.

91. Morgagni, *The Seats*, vol. 2, p. 477.

92. Ibid., vol. 3, p. 34.

93. See Stott, 'Incorporation of Surgeons'; Gelfand, *Modern Medicine*; Lawrence, 'Ornate physicians'.

94. 'A woman of Padua, by the name Jacoba, the wife of Angelo Zanardi (for by reason of finding thirteen ribs of each side of her, I enquir'd out her name and noted it down, which I am not us'd to do among the common people)', Morgagni, *The Seats*, vol. 1, p. 98.

95. Temkin, 'Role of surgery', p. 493.
96. Morgagni, *The Seats*, vol. 1, p. 304.
97. Ibid., p. 325.
98. See Jarcho, *Clinical Consultations*, p. 96.
99. See ibid., p. 402.
100. Morgagni, *The Seats*, vol. 1, pp. 519–20, see also vol. 2, p. 103.
101. Jarcho, *Clinical Consultations*, pp. 214–22.
102. For an example see note 70 above.
103. See Morgagni, *The Seats*, vol. 3, p. 48 for Valsalva's technique for avoiding major blood-vessels when operating upon tumours.
104. See note 25 above and Stott, 'Incorporation of surgeons'. Risse remarks how Cullen's consultation letters 'reflect the perennial diversity of approaches between surgeons and internists': G. Risse, '"Doctor William Cullen, Physician, Edinburgh": a consultation practice in the eighteenth century', *Bulletin of the History of Medicine*, vol. 48 (1974), pp. 338–51.
105. Morgagni, *The Seats*, vol. 1, p. 273.
106. For example ibid., vol. 2, p. 477.
107. A similar point, relating to the French anatomists of the late eighteenth century, is made by Temkin, 'Role of surgery', p. 492.
108. Ibid. and Gelfand, *Modern Medicine*, pp. 173–92.
109. It should also be noted that by Morgagni's time there had been a long history of clinical instruction in Padua; see Bylebyl, 'Commentary'. It is probable that the concerns I have described as characterising the clinical behaviour of Morgagni and his colleagues, in the first half of the eighteenth century, had their roots in a tradition of clinical practice and pedagogy which stretched back at least as far as the 1540s.
110. The character of late eighteenth- and early nineteenth-century medicine was shaped by the increasing importance of the hospital as a locus of clinical investigation as well as by the coming together of physic and surgery; see, for example, O. Keel, 'The politics of health and the institutionalisation of clinical practices in Europe in the second half of the eighteenth century', in Bynum and Porter, *William Hunter*, pp. 207–56. Morgagni worked in hospitals in Bologna and Padua and was well aware of their utility for the advancement of medicine:

> The more opportunities hospitals are offering to us to observe unusual diseases and even more the usual ones the oftener I feel sorry for the physicians of antiquity who were deprived of this advantage . . . What progress medical knowledge would have attained in the subsequent ten centuries after the foundation of the hospitals if it would have been permitted to investigate diseases not only in the living but also in cadavers after every malady, can easily be surmised from the advances which have been made after both opportunities began to be offered since around the early 16th century. (Morgagni, *De Sedibus*, vol. 2, p. 255.)

This material was not translated by Alexander, but is in the Klemperer reprint, *The Seats*, p. xxxi.

However the mere fact that Morgagni enjoyed the advantages of hospital practice cannot fully explain his expertise in localisation and physical examination since most eighteenth-century hospital physicians did not develop such interest. In other words we need to answer a further question: why did the Paduan tradition of hospital medicine develop distinctive anatomico-clinical characteristics? It is in the elucidation of this matter that I invoke the Temkin thesis.

5

Physiological principles in the surgical writings of John Hunter

Stephen Jacyna

Introduction

Since the turn of the nineteenth century John Hunter has been presented as the father of scientific surgery. An influential and persistent historiographic tradition has maintained that Hunter was the first to grasp that surgical practice did not rest upon clinical experience alone, but that it must also be informed by a knowledge of physiological and pathological principles if it were to attain its full potential.[1] Hunter himself said as much in the introduction to his lectures on surgery. At the outset he rejected the usual course of treating particular diseases and operations, 'these being taught by Anatomists and others – The principles are what are the most necessary and these shall be the object of our inquiry.'[2] Without a sound knowledge of such principles, Hunter declared, 'a man cannot be a surgeon'.[3] Recent studies of Hunter have tended to consider his physiological theories in the abstract – as one thread in the varied texture of bio-medical thought at the end of the eighteenth century.[4] This is to overlook the instrumental character that Hunter himself ascribed to his physiology: the primary use of such knowledge was the improvement of the art of surgery. It is also to ignore the dominant image of Hunter's significance that has been handed down to succeeding generations of surgeons. In this essay I shall ask whether there are, indeed, discernible areas of interaction between Hunter's theory and his practice. Was he truly a 'scientific surgeon'; or is there a discontinuity between Hunter the physiologist and Hunter the medical practitioner?

Theory and practice in eighteenth-century surgery

It was a common stratagem among Hunter's eulogists to portray pre-Hunterian surgery as (with a few honourable exceptions) purely 'empirical' in character, in contrast to the 'scientific' approach of the post-Hunterian era. It is certainly possible to find bluff assertions of the superiority of knowledge gained by experience over any form of theory in surgical texts of the eighteenth century. In 1765 the Irish surgeon Sylvester O'Halloran denounced previous surgeons who had relied upon their theoretical preconceptions when formulating therapy; 'by admitting a theory, repugnant to experience, in most instances, have conclusions been drawn, highly detrimental to the sick, and to surgery!' The diversity and complexity of the phenomena which daily confronted the surgeon proved 'the futility of attempting to draw general conclusions, from particular experiments', and supplied 'concise and cogent reasons' for rejecting 'general systems, either of physic, or philosophy'.[5] Edward Alanson in 1782 boasted in similar vein that 'Since all speculative reasoning on these [surgical] subjects is very fallacious, when placed in competition with experience, it has been my aim to deduce the doctrine of this work from practice only.'[6] It is worth noting that even a 'post-Hunterian' surgeon could in 1814 consider it 'mortifying to the pride of theory to see how often it is humbled before the conviction of practice'.[7]

Others recognised, however, that *all* surgical practice was to a degree dependent upon some theoretical notions of the working of the animal economy. William Bromfield in his *Chirurgical Observations and Cases* denounced the widespread practice of bleeding and purging patients suffering from concussion '*usque ad deliquium*[.] And is not this repeated, if the symptoms continue, till death convinces us, that this method will not *always* succeed?' This pernicious 'practice is founded on our fixed idea of *inflammation*, viz. that it is owing to obstruction in the vessels from various causes, and kept up by a plethora; therefore emptying the vessels, by every possible means, is supposed to be the only rational method of cure'.[8]

Bromfield suggested opium as an alternative treatment in cases of head injury. It had first come to his attention, indirectly, from the practice of a 'celebrated empiric', who had justified this treatment on grounds of experience alone. Bromfield, however, sought a *physiological* rationale (drawn from the writings of

William Cullen) for this method; he speculated that if 'inflammations are frequently caused by spasm and . . . the nerves sent to the muscular or vascular fibres may be so irritated as to produce spasm, this doctrine may be worthy of attention: for certainly *opium* is the most likely remedy to take off spasm, as many of us, I dare say, have experienced in the most threatening case of that sort, I mean, what is called, the locked jaw'.[9]

While criticising a practice based upon one particular theory, Bromfield did not, therefore, reject theory as such. Rather, he drew upon the common stock of eighteenth-century physiological concepts to provide grounds for understanding why an alternative, at first sight unlikely, therapy might work. William Hunter in his anatomical and surgical lectures developed the same strategy in a much more elaborate form. Referring to the prominence of the lymphatic system in current physiological thought – for which he and his brother were largely responsible – Hunter suggested that 'Besides explaining a considerable Part of the Animal Oeconomy, the use of this system will be found in explaining a variety of appearances in diseases especially in the Scrophula which is a disease in which the Lymphatic glands are first and most principally effected [*sic*].' Hunter thus rejected 'the common opinion that the Scrophula is caused by a bad humour in the Body'. Moreover, if the pathological doctrine of the role of the lymphatics, itself resting on physiological premises, were true,

> we may perhaps at length hit on some method of treating this Disease more Successfully than hitherto has been Done, this will not consist in purging or carrying off bad humours out of the constitution but by correcting the faulty absorption, the remedies that have been found most successful in this Disease serve to confirm this Doctrine they are the [Peruvian] bark and sunbathing the first braces the body and in some measure stops absorption the other appears to act in much the same manner, while the Shock from the frequent plunges in the Sea may probably produce some changes in the system.[10]

Such explicit and elaborate attempts to base therapy upon physiology were rare, but few surgical texts were entirely free of theoretic constructs – although their authors might not have recognised them as such. This was true even of the avowed anti-theorists such as Edward Alanson.

The distinction between John Hunter and his contemporaries was not, therefore, as absolute as has been suggested. Attempts to found surgical practice upon some species of physiological theory were not unknown before Hunter wrote. Hunter's originality lay in the scale upon which he pursued this project and the vast quantity of empirical materials he brought to its realisation. Moreover, while Hunter was undoubtedly an innovative thinker, his physiological and pathological theories had deep roots in traditional doctrines of the workings of the body in health and disease. In order to approach the question of the relation of Hunter's physiology to his surgical practice, it is necessary to grasp the basic tenets of his system.

The principles of Hunter's pathophysiology

Central to Hunter's conception of the operations of the body in health and disease was his notion of the 'wisdom' of the organism; indeed, this can be regarded as the fundamental doctrine of Hunter's physiological system. Hunter's discussion of bodily actions is pervaded by teleology. It is teleological not merely in the sense that he assumes that the parts combine to create a functional whole; but also in the more direct sense that Hunter often ascribes *purposes* to the body and goes on to consider the means by which it endeavours to attain them. The ultimate end to which the organism strives is 'the propagation of the species, for preservation (of the individual) cannot be called the ultimate effect'.[11] In the wording of the Somerville manuscript of Hunter's surgical lectures, 'The great purpose of all animals, seems to be that of propagation, Man does but little more.'[12] But while propagation was the ultimate goal of the body, its proximate end had to be self-preservation. This applied to the part as well as to the whole. Each organ possessed a portion of the *materia visae* [*sic*: presumably a misprint for *vitae*] *diffusa* which Hunter regarded as the true seat of life; and this *materia* acted in the 'interest' of the part. Hunter, in fact, assigned a kind of 'consciousness' to each part of the body, which was comparable to the consciousness that had its seat in the brain; the 'Actions of the body' were, he claimed, 'similar to those of the mind'. This quasi-mental representation of organic processes is well exemplified in Hunter's discussion of the phenomena of lymphatic absorption. He maintained that

> The remote cause of Absorption of parts must arise from one of the following Causes – 1st a consciousness of the part to be absorb'd of an unfitness to remain – that is says Mr. H. the only manner which we can explain what you all readily understand and with this enlarged mode of speech the English language will be sufficient to convey every Idea – this becomes ready to be absorb'd – 2ndly the Absorbents are ready to do it – or seeing work to be done – are ready to set about it – When the part to be absorb'd is intended as nourishment, or as extraneous Substance – then the Absorbents do the whole.[13]

Hunter recognised that by employing such language he was leaving himself open to various objections. In answer to such criticisms he replied:

> I have used the word *consciousness* because we have no language existing answerable to all my views of the animal oeconomy, and to coin words would not answer the purpose, because then I must have a dictionary of my own. I have not a word for expressing the cause of those actions which take place in the body, as if it was conscious that such and such things were going to take place. There are actions in the body which come the nearest to the consciousness of the mind of anything that I can conceive, and therefore I make use of this word; but it is commonly applied by philosophers only to the mind.[14]

From this justification it might appear that the language of consciousness served in Hunter's physiological discourse merely as a useful shorthand for explaining processes that were otherwise unintelligible. There was, however, within his physiology the basis of a more literal understanding of this use of language. The vital properties possessed by the brain were not, in Hunter's view, essentially different from those of other organs. On the contrary, Hunter held that

> something similar to the materials of the brain is diffused through the body, and even contained in the blood; between this and the brain a communication is kept up by the nerves; I have, therefore, adopted terms explanatory of this theory; calling the brain, the materia vitae

> coascervata; the nerves the chordae internunciae; and that diffused through the body, the materia visae [*sic*] diffusa.[15]

Given this common material composition, it was not unreasonable to suppose that all organs possessed, in some degree, properties analogous to those of the brain.

It is only in the light of these assumptions that one of the best known aspects of Hunter's teaching – the doctrine of the vitality of the blood – can be fully understood. Because the blood possessed a portion of the *materia vitae diffusa*, it shared the same vital properties as other organs; however, the blood was motile and communicated with all parts of the body. This ubiquity made it uniquely important; Hunter saw the blood as the instrument by which the growth and nutrition of the other organs was obtained. The blood was 'conscious' of the needs of the various parts through which it passed and sought to supply them from its own substance. This was the case in normal tissue nutrition; but the same mechanism underlay the body's responses to injury.

The pathological, in short, was an altered form of the physiological. Hunter repeatedly asserted that this continuity between the normal and the morbid was the principal reason why the surgeon must also be a physiologist; it was on this basis that he justified the pedagogic strategy he adopted in his lectures on surgery. 'In the present lectures,' he wrote, 'it is my intention to begin with the physiology of the animal economy in its natural or healthy state; and then to come to pathology, or the physiology of disease, which may be called the *perversion of the natural actions of the animal economy*'.[16]

Hunter's conception of a pathological physiology is illustrated by his discussion of the topic of blood coagulation. He refuted current notions that coagulation was merely the result of a drop in temperature or of stasis on the grounds that they were too mechanistic; in other words, they were deficient because they ignored the essentially teleological character of coagulation. Hunter's own view was that the blood coagulated as the result of an 'impression'. That is, 'its fluidity under such circumstances, being improper, or not longer necessary, it coagulates to answer now the necessary purpose of solidity . . . Coagulation I conceive to be an operation of life'.[17]

In the case of injury, coagulation was the process by which

the body sought to repair the dissolution in continuity of its fabric. Blood was thrown out at the site of an injury and there it performed a variant of its physiological office; it coagulated and was gradually transformed into new flesh. If the process succeeded the loss of substance caused by the injury was repaired.[18] If the process failed, then other actions were summoned up to achieve healing. Although these secondary contrivances were often accompanied by evidently pathological phenomena, their ultimate effect was, Hunter, insisted, therapeutic. Indeed, he regarded the whole gamut of 'simple' inflammatory symptoms, not as a disease, but as the side-effects of the body's efforts to rid itself of a harmful impression.[19] Hunter discussed such salutary operations as adhesive inflammation in great detail. Enough has already been said, however, to give an overview of the most salient features of his pathophysiology. It remains to consider how such doctrines might impinge upon Hunter's surgical practice, and whether there is any evidence that they did in fact do so.

Nature's handmaid, Art

Given his concept of the organism as an intelligent entity that responded to injury in a remedial way, it is clear that Hunter did not regard the body as the passive material upon which the surgeon must work according to his own lights. Rather, there had to be some attempt to harmonise the efforts of the healing art with the inherent curative power of nature. In short, Hunter saw the surgeon as acting – ideally – in co-operation with the body's own intelligence. As well as the human surgeon there was the 'natural surgeon', whose opinion needed to be consulted and whose remedies had to be respected in order to maximise the prospects of recovery.[20]

The notion of the wisdom of the body or the curative power of nature was, of course, an ancient one, beginning with Hippocrates. Neuberger has shown that it was widely professed by British medical practitioners of the eighteenth century.[21] Although Neuberger draws his examples almost entirely from among physicians, the doctrine was also canvassed in surgical texts. Thus on successive pages Bromfield remarks first on the 'astonishing effects' that might be observed in the healing of fractures among the young – 'especially where Nature exerts herself'; and then notes that

> The ill effects of suppressing habitual discharges, by the healing of old ulcers, have made me not quite so sanguine for amputating merely for a *caries*, which is the effect of such kind of sores, Nature having fixed on the ulcerated part as the outlet of some noxious humours, which will not without danger, be totally stopped.[22]

As the latter quotation suggests, the notion of certain actions as expressive of nature's own attempts to cure could influence decisions on what therapeutic strategy the surgeon should adopt. In general terms, the greater efficacy and extent the surgeon ascribed to nature's curative power, the more circumscribed would his own role become. In the course of the eighteenth century there is reason to believe that the balance of opinion shifted markedly in favour of nature, with a corresponding diminution in the scope of art. This was most noticeable in the management of wounds.

Richard Wiseman, in his *Treatise of Wounds* of 1672, held that the healing of wounds

> is the work of Nature and Art: both must mutually join their helping hands, and unless both the vital faculties and nourishment of the part do assist the Art of the Chirurgeon, it will be a lost labour, here must be a joynt meeting and agreement of all in one.[23]

Wiseman maintained that

> In small and superficial wounds . . . there Nature of her own accord is wont to effect the cure, without the help of any Medicament; from us only is required that the Lips of the wound be brought close together by bandage, that neither hair, nor dust, nor any other thing fall between them.

In 'great wounds', however, a much more active strategy was necessary; as well as bringing the lips of the wound together the surgeon was required to sprinkle and spread a variety of powders, pastes and oils over the wound to ensure its healing.[24] If the wound was 'compound', with a loss of substance, then the surgeon 'must assist Nature with his *sarcotics* [i.e. medicines supposed to promote healing], for regaining what is lost'.[25]

It was these attempts to 'assist' the natural processes of healing that called forth the condemnation of a later generation of surgeons. John Bell in 1795 asserted that

> When a modern surgeon allows himself to talk about the 'mundifying, incarning, and cicatrizing of wounds, or directs how to fill the wound up with good and sound flesh', . . . he but proclaims his own ignorance of the properties of the living body.

Bell called upon his colleagues to

> cast behind us a jargon of words, and a farago of useless drugs which belonged to the times of ignorance; and we shall find our duties happily reduced within the narrowest bounds, viz. of saving the patient from immediate bleeding, and of laying the wounded parts so cleanly, so neatly, and so evenly, in contact with each other, that they may adhere. The rest we leave to nature.

Efforts by the surgeon to do more and to effect healing through his own devices,

> will rather interfere with the regular processes of nature. It is an old, but it is a becoming and modest thought, that in our profession, we are but as the ministers of nature: and indeed the surgeon, still more than the physician, atchieves [*sic*] nothing by his own immediate power, but does all his services by observing and managing the properties of the living body.[26]

The 'chief perfection of modern surgery', in Bell's view, lay in the fact that it no longer sought to secure the 'incarning' of wounds by means of useless drugs and applications. Instead, 'we . . . trust all to nature, whose business it is, to make those surfaces adhere which will adhere, or to restore by suppuration and granulation the parts that are lost'.[27] This change in practice was particularly evident in the management of stumps following amputation. Bell held that no one individual could take the credit for this shift in practice, but that Edward Alanson had played an especially prominent role.[28] Alanson had criticised the previous mode of dressing stumps, which had promoted suppuration, on the ground that 'this was going against nature, which is most successful in restoring diseased parts, when the least interrupted by art'.[29]

Hunter's stress upon the natural curative powers of the body was not, therefore, idiosyncratic. To a certain extent, he was merely participating in a general shift in surgical thought. His view of the proper principles for dressing wounds accorded with the ideas of Bell and Alanson; dressings should be 'as simple as possible', and in most cases the efforts of the surgeon should be secondary to those of nature.[30] His notion of the salutary operations of nature was, however, more extended than that of most of his colleagues. Nature operated at the environmental level. Warm and moist climates were peculiarly unhealthy; 'Nature', Hunter held, 'seems to be aware of this, and provides in such Countries abundance of insects, to devour such matters as would be noxious'. Within the body the 'benevolence and wisdom of nature' was apparent in such contrivances as the fact that 'when a circumscribed cavity is wounded, the adhesion [*sic*] inflammation only extends to join the lips of the wound together, but does not extend to unite the other parts', despite the fact that all the parts in the body cavity were in contact.[31]

Hunter did not, however, confine himself to platitudes about the wisdom of nature, nor even to substantive, but elementary, observations on the best means of promoting wound healing. Instead he sought to comprehend the pathophysiological laws according to which nature acted, in order to understand better how the surgeon should, or should not, intervene to aid the processes of healing. Thus Hunter thought it necessary to enquire into the mode in which nature originally laid down the parts of the body because essentially the same processes were employed in regeneration after injury. Restoration, he held,

> seems in general to depend on the same principle as that original principle on which depended the first form^{n} of the parts . . . Nature's adherence to her original principle may be exemplified by observing that in the regeneration of a bone which was originally cartilage, as the long bones, there cartilage is first formed; and where it was originally membranes, as the bones of the skull, there membrane is first formed.[32]

Similarly, mortification was, in Hunter's view, merely a special form of the normal process of lymphatic absorption; it could not be treated rationally, therefore, without a knowledge of how the absorbent vessels acted. He complained that

> Without having my idea of how parts that were mortified are thrown off surgeons have treated all cases of this sort in the same ways and they have been led into error by not knowing how far nature ought to be assisted by art.[33]

Hunter was capable of berating himself for mistaking or ignoring the processes of nature, and, as a result, falling into error. He broke into his lectures on one occasion to show his class a preparation illustrating the following case:

> A man in St. George's Hospital had a hernia, for which I laid the integuments open, and then the Sac; when I found that the intestine had a tendency to mortify, and had formed adhesions to the sac. – These adhesions, which were newly formed, I separated; when the part of the intestine which had adhered to the sack [sic] gave way, and the excrement came out; I therefore returned the [viable] intestine and retained the torn part to the external wound, which became the Anus; but there was still a communication between the upper and lower part of the Gut, so that could the opening in the Groin have been stop'd the faeces would have passed the natural way; to produce this, I dissected off the skin round the opening, and then brought it into contact with ligature, compress, etc. but this would not do, although the granulations by their contractions . . . lessened the size of the opening: I therefore repeated this operation, hoping that at last I might close it; but all my efforts were in vain.

Hunter concluded that

> in the above case I acted like a blockhead, being ignorant of what nature was here doing, for, admire her work, she was forming adhesions all round [the part of the intestine] that mortified, whereby she could not only have preserved the continuity of the Canal, but by the same process would have prevented any escape of faeces; all which I prevented

> by separating those adhesions. If the case was to happen again I should not separate the adhesions, after taking off the stricture.[34]

More generally, Hunter followed the current trend of magnifying the powers of nature and diminishing the role of the surgeon. It was, he held, 'a poor conceit to suppose that Nature needs an ext^{l} Applicat^{n} to be excited to a wise Operation'.[35] When he was himself stricken by angina he swallowed 'a number of hot things according to the usual custom'; but this was, Hunter believed, 'to no purpose' and he attributed his gradual recovery to 'the operations of nature'.[36]

Hunter criticised the usual methods of dealing with the cases of an extravasation of blood on the grounds that they placed too little confidence in the curative power of nature with minimal assistance from art. The common practice was to scoop out the blood and to distend the external surface with warm dressings in order to bring on inflammation, 'and a sore being the consequence of this method it goes on as sores commonly do'. This procedure thwarted the natural process whereby the skin would gradually contract over the coagulated blood, 'as if it were a part to be preserved'; and, ultimately, only so much of the coagulum would remain in the wound as was needed 'to serve as a bond of union to the parts'. The wound would thus heal without suppuration.[37]

Even in dealing with major wounds, Hunter showed a similar tendency to trust to the skills of the 'natural surgeon'. So great was his confidence in 'The Operation of Nature in curing Accidents' that he adopted a passive – even complacent – attitude when confronted with serious injuries. Thus he recounts the case of

> a Man who had three Balls shot thro his Body, and while the adhesive infl^{n} went on (for this was the event) he felt little pain; none of the bowells were materially hurt; he had bloody water, but not bloody stools and had the Intestines been transfixed, the faeces would have passed into the cavity of the Abdomen etc etc – Finding these moderate Symptoms I concluded that adhesions were going on; three tubes were formed by the adhesions so that all communic^{n} between the hurt parts and rest of the abdomen were cut off therefore in ten days I pronounced

> him out of danger, knowing that the adhesions had set bounds to the inf^{n} and mischief.[38]

This optimistic prognosis was in accord with Hunter's conception of the ultimately therapeutic character of inflammatory processes. He concluded that 'whatever cavities the balls had entered, there the surrounding parts had adhered, so that the passage of the ball was by this means become a complete canal'. Nature thus ensured that no foreign bodies entered the abdominal cavity, 'but must be conducted to the external surface of the body, either through the wounds, or from an abscess forming for itself, which would work its own exit somewhere'. Later, he reports, faeces were seen to emerge from the wound; but even this

> new symptom did not alter my opinion, respecting the whole operations of nature to secure the cavity of the abdomen, but it confirmed it, (if a further confirmation had been necessary) and therefore I conceived it could not affect life; but as I saw the possibility of this wound becoming an artificial anus, I was sorry for it.[39]

The sole application of Hunter's physiological principles was not, however, to dissuade surgeons from taking action; they also served as the basis for calls for more effectual intervention. He brought his understanding of bodily operations to bear, for example, on contemporary methods of treating hydrocele. Hunter's discussion of this topic is interesting because it reveals that he was not an unqualified admirer of the curative powers of nature; on occasions he realised that the surgeon's efforts to effect a cure were thwarted by nature's own responses to injury. In such cases it was doubly necessary that he be acquainted with pathophysiological principles if he were to outwit the wisdom of the body.

Hydrocele, Hunter asserted, 'Tho a simple business is not understood by any Surgeon in Europe: All of them say they have seen every mode fail except their own favourite one but none of them thought of enquiring into the cause of the failure.'[40] According to Palmer, Hunter's editor, each of the London hospitals had in the late eighteenth century its favoured manner of extirpating hydrocele.[41] But Hunter held that the success of all these methods was frustrated by an ignorance of nature's responses to injuries – including those inflicted by the surgeon. Hunter maintained that the reason for this failure could be derived 'from a principle, and fixed law in the oeconomy'.[42] More often than not the hydrocele recurred because

> when a breach or waste or loss of substance is produced in the outside of any cavity (and probably in every other part) there immediately takes place an irritation suitable to this cause, and this irritation produces an extravasation of coagulable lymph on the inside, to preserve the cavity or part as entire as possible.

This protective action was, Hunter argued, the common cause for the failure of operations to extirpate hydrocele. It was

> as if Nature was making the same opposition as we should do if a neighbour was endeavouring to make a way through the wall of our house, and, as we could not prevent his endeavours on that side, we should barricade further on this side, by raising up another wall.[43]

As a result, the cavity was preserved despite the surgeon's labours, and could later become once more distended by fluid.

To circumvent these obstacles, Hunter recommended that the surgeon should abandon his usual objective of obtaining union with the fewest possible complications. In this instance the success of the operation could only be assured if nature was prevented from attaining an uneventful cure. Hunter therefore recommended the insertion of a tent or seton into the wound to provoke inflammation and suppuration. But, even then, 'we find Nature taking all the steps she can to frustrate our operations whenever thay are violent upon her'.[44]

Other instances of Hunter presuming to question the wisdom of nature could be adduced. He took her to task quite severely for the false economy of making the male urethra the channel for both semen and urine. This anatomical niggardliness had dire consequences in cases of venereal disease.[45]

Hunter's pathophysiological principles impinged upon his diagnostic practice as well as his therapeutics. On occasion, he drew upon concepts derived from his physiology in making a judgement. Perhaps a more revealing way of regarding this practice is to say that during his physiological and pathological investigations Hunter was confronted by certain appearances to which he attached a significance in terms drawn from his theories. When he encountered comparable phenomena in a clinical setting, he was provided with an explanatory framework in which to accommodate them, and from which the appropriate action could be inferred. For example, an important term in Hunter's pathology and physiology was 'coagulable lymph'. This was the portion of the blood that supplied tissue nutrition; during adhesive inflammation a process of excited nutrition occurred and large quantities of coagulable lymph were thrown out which formed accumulations and led to tumefaction within an organ. As a result a part might appear pathologically altered, giving rise to a misdiagnosis. This occurred in the case of a man labouring under a hydrocele:

> at length the Tumour inflamed, suppurated, and ulcerated as a common abscess and broke, the Surgeon whose Care the Patient was under enlarg'd the opening and taking it for granted that it was Cancerous; he was about to perform the operation and immediately upon seeing it, I thought the suppuration too general for it to be cancerous, and when I got the history of the Case it confirm'd me in the Opinion – The Instruments were all ready and the Patient also and how to settle matters so as to save the Credit of the Surgeon, I was at a loss to know; I could not possibly think of letting the Poor Man loose [sic] his Testicle and therefore took advantage of the fear he express'd on account of the operation, painting it in the most horrid light to him, when he enquired of me what was to be done. This had the desir'd effect; for he declar'd he would not have it performed at any rate. We then told him we wou'd do our utmost endeavour to find out a Medicine that should do him service, and accordingly gave him some trifling [medicine] under which he recovered.[46]

Whether nature was to be followed or frustrated, Hunter's principal contention was that she must be understood by the surgeon. Moreover, there is sufficient evidence to confirm that Hunter did employ his physiological principles when making some clinical decisions. It should not be supposed, however, that such reasoning is evident in *all* his recorded cases; usually he relied upon his experience of previous cases when deciding how to treat the current one. Even so, he was undoubtedly a 'scientific' surgeon on occasion.

While confirming in broad terms the traditional image of Hunter, I hope to have drawn attention to a number of necessary revisions. Firstly, Hunter was not quite the lonely genius that his panegyrists depicted; aspects of his thought are mirrored in the works of his contemporaries. What remains to be done is to define more closely Hunter's relations to the late eighteenth-century medical world in order to determine where his true originality lay. To this end, the *anti*-Hunterians require more attention than they have hitherto received; for example, John Bell who, as we have seen, shared many of Hunter's biases, was frankly bewildered by some aspects of his system.[47] Hunter himself, even quite late in his career, seemed to consider himself as isolated within the surgical community. In his discussion of the proper treatment of gunshot wounds, he noted that although surgeons recognised – as a matter of theory – that balls often emerged from wounds unaided or could remain in the body without occasioning inconvenience, they still persisted in widening the mouths of wounds in an effort to extract the foreign body rather than trusting to nature. Hunter advised his students,

> if you were examined at Surgeon's Hall how you wd treat a gun shot wound, you would do well not to mention my doctrine, but to say according to the old plan, I would open the edges of the wound. They do not ask the reasons of things there.[48]

An eagerness to 'ask the reasons of things' is usually accounted as Hunter's most distinctive characteristic. In this paper I have tried to show that the *answers* to which these enquiries led had con- sequences for Hunter's surgical practice. Whether these patho-physiological principles truly revolutionised the practices of the surgical community as a whole seems more doubtful. However, the full import of the 'Hunterian legacy' for surgery at the turn of the nineteenth century has still to be assessed.

Acknowledgements

The research on which this paper is based was made possible by the generous support of the Wellcome Trust. I would like to thank Edwin Clarke, David Hamilton and Chris Lawrence for their comments on an earlier version.

Notes and references

1. L. S. Jacyna, 'Images of John Hunter in the nineteenth century', *History of Science*, vol. 21 (1983), pp. 85–108.
2. Henry Somerville, 'Mr John Hunter's lectures on surgery', Newcastle University Library, Pybus Collection D. ii. 3, vol. 1, p. 2.
3. J. F. Palmer, *The Works of John Hunter*, 4 vols (Longman, London, 1835), vol. 1, p. 208.
4. S. J. Cross, 'John Hunter, the animal oeconomy, and late eighteenth-century physiological discourse', *Studies in History of Biology*, vol. 5 (1981), pp. 1–110; F. Duchesneau, 'Vitalism and John Hunter', in W. F. Bynum and R. Porter (eds), *William Hunter and the Eighteenth-Century Medical World* (Cambridge University Press, Cambridge, 1985), pp. 279–95.
5. S. O'Halloran, *A Complete Treatise on Gangrene and Sphacelus; With a New Method of Amputation* (Peter Wilson, Dublin, 1765), pp. ii, iv.
6. E. Alanson, *Practical Observations on Amputation, and the After-Treatment* (Joseph Johnson, London, 1782), p. xix.
7. C. Bell, *A Dissertation on Gun-shot Wounds* (Longman, London, 1814), pp. 3–4.
8. W. Bromfield, *Chirurgical Observations and Cases*, 2 vols (T. Cadell, London, 1773), vol. 1, p. 9.
9. Ibid., pp. 10–11.
10. [?] Howison, 'Lectures anatomical and chirurgical by William Hunter', 2 vols, 1775, Newcastle University Library, Pybus Collection H. iii. 5, vol. 1, pp. 75–6.
11. Palmer, *The Works*, vol. 1, p. 225.
12. Somerville, 'Lectures', p. 15.
13. 'Manuscript notes of the lectures of Mr John Hunter', Wellcome Institute Library, Hunterian Society of London, MSS HOOO/32, pp. 17–18.
14. Palmer, *The Works*, vol. 1, p. 236.
15. J. Hunter, *A Treatise on the Blood, Inflammation, and Gun-Shot Wounds* (George Nicol, London, 1794), p. 89.
16. Palmer, *The Works*, p. 211.
17. Hunter, *A Treatise*, pp. 25–6.
18. Ibid., pp. 92–3.
19. Ibid., pp. 201 ff.
20. Ibid., p. 444.

21. M. Neuburger, *Die Lehre von der Heilkraft der Natur in Wandel der Zeiten* (Ferdinand Enke, Stuttgart, 1926), pp. 88–99.

22. Bromfield, *Chirurgical Observations*, pp. 44–5.

23. R. Wiseman, *A Treatise of Wounds* (R. Norton, London, 1672), p. 3.

24. Ibid., pp. 23–4.

25. Ibid., p. 4.

26. J. Bell, *Discourses on the Nature and Cure of Wounds* (Bell & Bradfute, Edinburgh, 1795), pp. 1–2.

27. Ibid., p. 3.

28. Ibid., p. 8.

29. Alanson, *Practical Observations*, pp. 41–2.

30. H. G. Clough, 'Lectures on surgery: by John Hunter', 1779, Wellcome Institute Library, MS 2959, p. 95.

31. J. Hunter, 'Surgical lectures', Royal College of Physicians of Edinburgh, MS M8 47, pp. 169, 229.

32. 'Manuscript notes', p. 120; Hunter, 'Surgical Lectures', (RCPE), p. 300.

33. W. Hamilton, 'Lectures on surgery by Mr John Hunter', Edinburgh University Library, MS Dc 2.441–3, pp. 114–9.

34. J. Parkinson, 'A transcript of copious notes taken from Mr John Hunter's lectures on the principles of surgery . . . ', 1785–6, Royal College of Surgeons of London, MS 49. e 23, pp. 98–100.

35. 'Lectures on surgery by Mr John Hunter', Royal College of Physicians and Surgeons, Glasgow, MS/1/9/57, p. 112.

36. 'Manuscript notes', pp. 12–13.

37. Hunter, *A Treatise*, pp. 195–6.

38. 'Lectures on surgery', (RCPSG), pp. 97–8.

39. Hunter, *A Treatise*, pp. 550–1.

40. Hunter, 'Surgical lectures', p. 273.

41. Palmer, *The Works*, p. 454.

42. Parkinson, 'A transcript', p. 4.

43. Palmer, *The Works*, p. 471.

44. Ibid.

45. J. Hunter, *A Treatise on the Venereal Disease* (J. Hunter, London, 1786), pp. 110–11.

46. 'Lectures on the principles of surgery by John Hunter', 1791, Royal College of Surgeons of London, MS 49. c. 10., pp. 208–9.

47. Bell, *Discourses*, pp. 12, 23–4.

48. Hunter, 'Surgical lectures', pp. 284–5. This MS is post-1781.

6

Practising on principle: Joseph Lister and the germ theories of disease

Christopher Lawrence and Richard Dixey

> Antiseptic surgery is simply a struggle with the causes of putrefaction. I have not mentioned the germ theory of infective disease at all. That has no essential bearing on the *principles* of antiseptic surgery. (William Watson Cheyne, 1882)

Introduction

Joseph Lister's antiseptic system of surgical treatment was developed over a period of about thirty-five years between 1865 and 1900. From a variety of more or less critical perspectives, Lister's theory and practice have been regarded as the foundations on which were built modern aseptic surgery and the conceptual framework deemed inseparable from it, the germ theory of disease. Versions of this story are well known to medical historians and, indeed, to a more general audience, and will be assumed in what follows. Here we argue that a crucial dimension of Listerian surgery has been ignored by historians: the pathological theories employed by Lister and his most important collaborator and publicist, William Watson Cheyne. Investigation of this limited area, we suggest, reveals the history of antiseptic surgery in a new light and demonstrates that many of the practical and theoretical origins of aseptic surgery were not Listerian. That the origins of aseptic surgery lie in non-Listerian traditions has been suggested by other authors.[1] None, however, has explored the means by which the Listerians were so successful in representing their work as the sole legitimate precursor of modern surgery.[2] The correct reconstruction of Lister's pathological theories makes this possible. It also makes it possible to write the history of late Victorian surgery as a malleable cultural form, not as a practice whose details were determined by biological agents.

Recovering Lister's pathological theories is not an exercise in reconstructing an ossified body of ideas employed by Lister throughout his life. Although there are continuities, Lister continually modified his views. He did, however, always maintain that surgery was only practised properly when it was based on true, scientifically ascertained, pathological principles. This view, if not unusual at the time, was by no means universal. In the late 1860s Lister justified his practice by reference to a germ theory of putrefaction. By the mid-1870s this theory had been elaborated into a comprehensive account of the putrefactive origins of epidemic disease. At this time Lister invoked Pasteur's experiments as the inspiration for the theory and practice of antiseptic surgery. In the late 1870s and early 1880s Lister and Cheyne began to remould their views in the light of the new, and quite different, German germ theory of infective disease. At first they subordinated German views to their putrefactive theory then, around 1880, the theory of infection was given equal and independent status. Finally, in the mid-1880s, putrefaction was subordinated to a germ theory of infection. In these years the experiments of German workers, notably Robert Koch, were increasingly cited as the basis of the theory and practice of antiseptic surgery. Theory and practice by now were both very different from their originals. In 1867 Listerian practice was directed to creating local conditions such that severe wounds involving bone damage might heal by granulation or by organisation in a clot. During the late 1870s and 1880s Listerians increasingly absorbed the techniques of their critics, such that, by 1900, most surgical practice was centred on the creation of a general environment in which such wounds might heal by simple apposition of their edges (first intention healing). Lister's early ideas and practice, therefore, were by no means like his later ones, and the change from the one to the other was complex and contingent, not simple and necessary. Nevertheless by the 1890s Listerians could represent the practice of aseptic surgery which was based on the, by now recognisably modern, germ theory of infection, as deriving from a simple elaboration of early Listerian ideas and practice.

It is the 'discovery' of late Listerian ideas in Lister's first formulations which has permitted the construction of a Listerian 'revolution'. This discovery was, as already suggested, begun by the Listerians themselves. It is a reading which has been perpetuated by subsequent historians. For example, Richard Fisher in his biography of Lister coalesces two very different processes: suppuration and fermentation (specifically putrefactive fermentation). Fisher writes, 'Antiseptic surgery emerged when Lister realized that the analogy between suppuration and fermentation which Pasteur had drawn could be applied in practice.'[3] We will argue that suppuration was a process quite different from fermentation or putrefaction and that it did not have the same significance for Lister in the 1870s that it does for the modern surgeon. Although he considered the obviation of suppuration theoretically ideal at this time, it was not a central concern until much later. Until the mid-1880s Lister, along with other surgeons, used a nutritive theory of pus production; the prevention of putrefaction was the central object of Listerian (and indeed all other) surgery. Another related example of the reading of modern views into Lister's early work comes from Fielding Garrison's *History of Medicine*, 'These [the 1860s] were the days of "laudable pus", yet Lister had already begun to think of the old Hippocratic healing by first intention as the surgeon's ideal.'[4] This account represents the goal of modern aseptic surgery, first intention healing, as a Listerian objective. We argue (as did Lister's opponents), that first intention healing was not *and could not be*, the goal of Listerian surgery. Aseptic surgery was created by abandoning the original Listerian objectives not by attempting to achieve them. Suppuration is central to the Listerian story, and by close attention to theories of it we hope to shed some light on what, to modern eyes, is an oxymoron, laudable or normal pus. We do not claim here to reveal what laudable pus actually was, rather the reverse. We attempt to show what it was not. Laudable pus, we will argue, is actually an anomalous object when considered in the light of modern pathological theory, the perspective from which it is usually viewed. The significance of this will be clear when we review the 'pus' produced in Lister's cases and the changing status he attributed to it.

The concept of a Listerian revolution was, to a great extent, created by depicting Lister as being, for twenty years, an embattled champion of a controversial germ theory. The disputes about 'germs', however, have a much more complex history than later narrators suggest, not least because there were *many* germ theories, not just one. Lister's 'germs' were only controversial early on and the view that there was a single 'germ theory' to which he continuously adhered is a historical fiction. In the 1870s 'germs' of putrefactive disease, adopted by the Listerians from Pasteur, were undoubtedly a subject of some suspicion in the medical community. Koch's very different 'germs' of the 1880s were by no means the exclusive property of the Listerians and Lister did not have to engage in dispute over their existence in the way that he had done over Pasteur's germs. German infective theory was, in fact, taken up quite readily by the medical community and, indeed, aspects of the this theory – notably the pus-generating action of micrococci – were contested by the Listerians long after they had been adopted elsewhere in Britain (see below). Listerians, we argue, were obliged to endorse German theory in order to continue representing themselves as being at the forefront of scientific medicine. Thus the tradition which credits Lister with tenacious commitment to a germ theory of disease in the face of opposition disguises the fact that the germ theory which was finally and generally accepted by the medical community was quite unlike Lister's original theory. The controversy over 'germs', made so much of by later authors, was also relatively minor. Much more antagonism was aroused by other issues, for instance, Lister's assertion that what mattered most in the management of wounds was the discovery of a sound method of treating the wound itself. If this could be achieved, Lister argued, hospitals would become more salubrious places. Lister never wavered from this commitment. He regarded the unquestionable decline in hospital fevers in the late nineteenth century as his achievement, based on his wound treatment. His followers also claimed this achievement on his behalf. Thus in his biography of Lister, his nephew, Rickman Godlee, condemning the pavilion system of hospital construction of the late nineteenth century, noted that the buildings built by this movement were,

> as Lister maintained, needlessly extravagant. Time has shown that his opinion was correct. They still stand as an outward and visible sign of the stages by which scientific

> thought advances, but they are no more healthy than many an old hospital that escaped the pick, but set its house in order *by revolutionizing its method of treatment*.[5]

Lister's contemporaries, however, fiercely attacked this position on the grounds that the increasing success of wound management followed from the banishment of fevers from the wards which, in turn, they argued, derived from general sanitary, dietary, nursing and architectural reform.

Another area where Lister provoked controversy was in his claim that he was the sole custodian of the true theory of wound sepsis. Throughout his career Lister repeatedly enunciated pathological 'principles' which, he said, he had discovered and which were the basis of his therapy. As already noted, however, these true theories or principles were continually modified so that scarcely a vestige of the 1867 principles remained in 1900. Contemporaries, such as the Birmingham surgeon, Lawson Tait, pointed this out and criticised Lister on these grounds. Listerians also generated friction by their claim that their techniques (based on their true principles) produced better results than any other practice. Surgeons responded that the technique was both incredibly complicated and undergoing continual modification. More important, they said, simpler methods could bring about the best form of union, first intention healing. Lister's opponents also claimed that their methods were as productive of success as Lister's were. At no time during the years of controversy were *any* statistics set forth, which all could agree, comprehensively showed the greater efficacy of one method of treating wounds over another. Indeed comparison, as many noted, was impossible, since all surgeons were constantly modifying their techniques in an endeavour to achieve better results. By the 1880s the Listerians had effectively acknowledged this.

We argue that in the ten years after 1867 Listerians claimed unrivalled success for their practice, a success which they asserted was based on the truth of their theory. Faced with the relative failure of this approach, since other surgeons claimed equal success, Listerians changed their arguments and began to acknowledge the efficacy of other techniques, claiming that they were effective because, unknowingly, they were based upon Listerian theory – a Listerian theory which was, at this time, being severely modified to incorporate German germ theory (as well as being presented as an anticipation of it). In this way the Listerians were able to present their antiseptic surgery as the forerunner of modern aseptic surgery, although this was in fact created from many of the techniques and assumptions which Listerians had previously disparaged.

Unfortunately Lister's claim to have produced superior results has been accepted, almost unquestioningly, by many historians.[6] Acceptance of this superiority, however, has been contingent on the acceptance of the Listerians' account of their own history. Listerian theories produced in the 1890s are now, more or less, taken as a *true* account of wound sepsis since they approximate closely to modern germ theory. For those who adopt the position that the 1890s account was, more or less, the account given by Lister in the 1870s, it follows that Lister's early results *must* have been superior, because they derived from his use of a modern theory of sepsis. There is a sense in which hardly anything in this paper is new. The whole argument about practice and theory was visible to contemporaries, especially to Lawson Tait, but it has been lost as the Listerian account was eventually endorsed as a true record. As usual the past was the past of the victor.

Surgery and pathological theory at mid-century

In contrast to other accounts we argue here how strikingly similar many of Lister's early ideas and practices were to those of his contemporaries. Lister's work in the 1860s was based on assumptions about pathology which he shared with surgeons and the medical community at large in the mid-Victorian period. Many of these assumptions and the explicit principles underlying mid-century surgery can be found in a 'state-of-the-art' text of 1860, Timothy Holmes's four-volume *System of Surgery*. This was a multi-authored work with contributions from some of the most distinguished surgeons of the day. The section on wounds was written by James Paget. The simplest form of healing, Paget said, was 'immediate union'.[7] If, however, any new material, such as lymph, exuded into a wound, 'adhesive union' might occur.[8] Both of these species of union were forms of healing by first intention. Such healing, Paget noted, should be the surgeon's goal, both after a simple surgical incision and in the contused wounds which followed injury because, he explained, such 'cases very often turn out much better than appeared likely'.[9] Failure of first intention healing led to union by one of the secondary mechanisms. The commonest of these was healing by granulation. Granulations, Paget said, consisted of blood vessels and rapidly proliferating, undifferentiated cells, gradually organising into scar tissues from the depths of a wound. In the early stages of healing granulations appeared as pinkish, friable tissue covered with albuminous liquids. Later, healthy granulations were characterised by 'pus . . . constantly being produced on their free surface'. This 'normal' (or laudable) pus was 'creamy, opaque, uniformly liquid, yellowish white and sufficiently abundant to cover completely the whole surface of the granulating wound'.[10] Pus in small quantities was simply a new tissue element; it was part of normal granulation.

In both first intention healing and in healing by granulation a small amount of inflammation was considered essential to initiate the healing process. In the former, Paget observed, a degree of inflammation was necessary 'for the production of the new reparative material. But it should not go beyond this.' In healing by granulation, inflammation produced 'the first material for granulations'. After this any persistent inflammation retarded the 'organization and continued healthy formation [of granulations]'.[11] Thus normal 'pus' production was *not* the product of ongoing inflammation. Treating wounds which were healing by healthy granulation required leaving them exposed or regularly changing the dressings so that the 'pus' and other fluids did not accumulate.

There was a final form of healing, 'healing by scabbing', which Paget described as 'the most natural and in some cases, the best' of all the healing processes. In this form of healing a dry crust formed over the wound and the healing processes were not visible. No granulations or exudations were produced, indeed if they were, healing by scabbing could not occur. To obtain healing by scabbing he advised,

> if the wound be recent, the blood and exuded fluids, or, if it be granulating, the pus, should be left exposed to the air till it dries on the wound, adhering to the edges and the surface, and completely excluding them from air. Nothing more need be done, unless that the scab thus formed should be lightly covered with dry cotton-wool to protect

> both it and the subjacent surface from whatever may excite inflammation.[12]

Like first intention healing, scabbing was sometimes designated a form of so-called primary union, since no granulations were formed.[13]

Continued inflammation or its reappearance in a wound, Paget explained, was one of the worst impediments to healing. In these circumstances inflammation would be accompanied by its usual signs: redness, swelling, heat, pain and the usual pernicious consequences, that is, ulceration, gangrene, excess and morbid suppuration.[14] This was sepsis. Pus produced in these circumstances was dreaded by the surgeon. It collected in abscesses, buried into sinuses, tracked into fistulas and was absorbed into the circulation giving rise to pyaemia. Its nature (by virtue of its process of production and its effects) was quite different from 'normal' pus.

Inflammation had a chapter to itself in Holmes's work. It was written by John Simon and complemented Paget's account of wounds. Inflammation, Simon noted, was the essential response to tissue injury, it was the beginning of adhesive union and the precursor of granulation in secondary healing. This productive inflammation led to a quantitative change in tissue life, the rapid production of new elements which 'because of their excess . . . tend to be unelaborated and crude'.[15] The pus cells of granulations were 'derivatives of textural overgrowth'.[16] This pus was a sign of the hypernutritive activity that constituted healing.[17] It should be noted that, although Paget and Simon described pus production as integral to granulation, this secondary form of healing was regarded as less desirable than one of the primary forms.

All surgeons recognised that when inflammation persisted or reappeared in a wound, tissue proliferation got out of hand and a mass of dead and dying cells accumulated. Such was the case in abscesses. Abscesses were produced by a stimulus to the tissues which set up inflammation and suppuration. The confined dead elements were, in turn, a continuing irritation to the living tissues and further stimulated inflammation and pus production. Even more serious than this, however, was that the dead cells produced by intense inflammation, whether in wounds or abscesses, could become the seat of one of the most lethal pathological processes of all, decomposition or putrefaction. Putrefaction was the fundamental model around which preventative and curative medicine were organised in the mid-nineteenth century. With a few notable exceptions it has scarcely been noticed by historians, who have continually combed the period for the dawn of modern theories of infection.[18]

Putrefaction was the decay or decomposition of *dead* tissue, the process seen in the post-mortem room, in the rotting of meat or in the decaying of leaves on the forest floor. Decomposition was a necessary part of the cyclical renewal of nature. However, when it occurred in dead tissues *which were still in contact with the living body*, it was productive of dire results. Dead tissue in wounds became dark and foul-smelling. By some means, generally agreed to be ill-understood, a single putrefying wound in a hospital patient was known to be followed by similar changes in the wounds of other patients and with outbreaks of febrile disease. As the *St Bartholomew's Hospital Reports* for 1867 put it,

> Pyaemia commonly supervenes upon foul wounds, or wounds which furnish decomposing matter. Now, such matter may not only be absorbed into the system furnishing it, and thus provoke pyaemia, but, impregnating the atmosphere, it may be carried to adjacent healthy wounds in other persons, and create morbid action in them, whereby foul matter is again formed and then absorbed; for the decomposing matter thus given off is the very matter likely by its presence to excite corresponding changes in healthy wounds.[19]

For this sort of reason, one surgeon noted, 'Healthy men who had wounds, etc, should be separated carefully from those who were unhealthy, as the pus in one case was very different from that in the other.'[20]

Putrefaction was universally regarded as a process of fermentation. As to the circumstances giving rise to it, surgeons agreed that it was associated with such factors as 'the state of the atmosphere . . . inattention to cleanliness . . . the application of morbific matter from sponges'.[21] The immediate agent involved, however, was the subject of debate. Some held putrefaction to be purely a chemical process, others argued living organisms were involved. For example, at the BMA meeting of

1864 decomposition and its relation to multiplying 'spores' and 'sporules' were discussed.[22] In the same year the ovariotamist, Spencer Wells, reported the 'remarkable labours of Pasteur' and noted an association between 'germs' and the decomposition of shed blood.[23] There were various theories too about the exact cause of hospital fevers. Some held that erysipelas, for example, was produced by absorption of toxic chemicals from the wound; others, employing Liebig's zymotic theory, held that fermenting agents themselves could enter the body in the presence of lowered vitality.[24]

Surgeons had various techniques for preventing decomposition, a process which was particularly associated with compound fractures. Some insisted on the cleansing of wounds of all dead matter, apposing the edges and applying simple dressings in the hope of achieving first intention healing. Others used chemical agents, antiseptics, prophylactically. Many of these were also used as disinfectants in situations where non-surgical septic processes occurred, for instance in fever epidemics. When putrefaction did occur, or primary union seemed impossible (in very lacerated wounds), antiseptics were applied and the surgeon endeavoured to bring about healing by granulation. Putrefaction could affect not only new wounds but also old sores, preventing them from healing. A report by James Watson on carbolic acid, a quite widely used antiseptic, in the *Edinburgh Medical Journal* of 1864, noted,

> Several respectable surgeons speak favourably of its use as a lotion – one part of the acid to forty parts of water – in all kinds of fetid ulcers, gangrenous and offensive sores . . . Dr Calvert states that it is the most powerful preventative of putrefaction with which he is acquainted.

Watson observed that 'carbolic acid is a decided antiseptic' and that 'a very small quantity prevents . . . the odour of decomposition'. Dr Calvert had reported it, an 'anti-ferment'.[25]

Lister's theory of inflammation and suppuration

We now examine the assumptions and explicit theory used by Lister in the 1860s and 1870s in order to compare them with those of other surgeons. It will also provide the basis for examining how different were these views of Lister's to those he held in the late 1880s. Joseph Lister published his first papers on antiseptic surgery in 1867 when he was Professor of Surgery at Glasgow University. Most of Lister's opinions at this time were similar to those of other surgeons; nevertheless he also employed one or two unusual ideas, which he had first advanced in 1858, in a paper on the early stages of inflammation. These ideas were refined and used by Lister throughout his working life. This extremely difficult paper admits of various readings. None the less a number of assertions seem possible. First, Lister claimed that he had discovered that the essence of the early stages of inflammation was not, as was commonly held, exalted vitality, but that 'the tissues are for the time being reduced still more towards the condition of ordinary solid matter'.[26] Second, Lister reported that he had distinguished two sorts of inflammation. The first was a direct sort and this was the inflammation which was the necessary precursor of healing. He noted that after a surgical incision direct inflammation follows and the liquor poured into the wound is 'essential to primary union [first intention healing]'. The second sort of inflammation was 'that which is developed indirectly through the medium of the nervous system'. Nervous inflammation was pathological. When provoked 'it interferes with the healing process in a degree proportioned to its intensity'.[27]

This theory of inflammation can be discerned as a structuring element in Lister's famous papers of 1867, which announced his antiseptic surgery. In the first of these papers Lister argued that the inflammation produced immediately after a wound had been inflicted was both necessary and dangerous. On the one hand it was the essential precursor of healing. On the other, because the fluids (lymph, blood, etc.) pouring into a wound were deemed to be nearer the condition of dead tissue, inflammation made putrefaction possible. Lister then described the mechanism of healing by granulation, which like most surgeons he supposed a likely outcome in the contused wounds which were associated with compound fracture. He took the familiar view that granulations were characterised by 'remarkably active cell-development'. Granulations, he noted, *since they were alive*, were immune to putrefaction and, 'being composed of an imperfect form of tissue', were 'insensible', that is, they lacked the sensory nerves which triggered secondary inflammation. Lister then advanced a claim which he was to develop over the next ten years. Airborne putrefaction, he argued, even though long recognised as a cause of mischief by surgeons, had 'probably been underrated' as a source of disaster. That putrefaction was the principal danger, he said, was proven by very small wounds in which a 'scab' protected the wound from decomposing. In these cases healing took place just as in a simple fracture.[28]

Lister then outlined the means by which putrefaction exerted its evil effects. The source of mischief was dead material in wounds; 'access of the atmosphere, decomposition of the blood . . . losing by putrefaction its natural bland character, and assuming the properties of an acrid irritant, occasions both local and general disturbance'. This process could take place on the 'raw surface' of a wound before granulations had formed, or it could attack the fluids on the surface of a healthy granulation. Putrefaction was a rapidly occurring process, often taking place within 24 hours, and signalled by 'the odour of decomposition'.[29]

To explain these effects Lister employed his theory of inflammation. Putrefying fluids were extremely acrid and irritant and thus could excite the 'sensory nerves' on a raw surface and set up the pernicious indirect inflammation and general fever. This promoted rapid cell turnover, with consequent cellular death and the effusion of even more putrescible material into the wound. Lister then noted that, if indirect inflammation did occur, sloughs were produced 'which must be thrown off by a corresponding suppuration'.[30] This sort of suppuration, therefore, was that dreaded by surgeons; it was the heightening of granulation in the presence of inflammation. Suppuration of this sort took two, three or, most commonly, four days to be produced. At this point Lister made an observation that was soon to be central to his claim to be an enunciator of pathological principles: putrefaction, he considered, was the only significant initiator of this pernicious inflammatory process.

Discussing the cause of putrefaction Lister then made what has become the most famous (and most misinterpreted) part of his claim. He noted that the 'decomposition of organic substances' had recently been identified by Pasteur not as owing to any of the 'gaseous constituents' of the atmosphere, but to another 'property' of the air, the 'germs of various low forms of life'. The putrefactive effect of these germs, he added, was produced in the same way 'as the yeast plant converts sugar into alcohol'.[31] It is important to note how indirect was the relation of pus production to germs. Lister's germs were scavengers in dead tissue, they were not parasitic on the living.[32] The pathological process occurring in wounds was analogous to the decomposition of broth in glass bottles or the fermentation of grape juice in vats.

Lister then argued that these findings dictated that the surgeon should aim to find a material capable of killing these germs, or at least of preventing them gaining access to dead tissues in the wound. It is here that he described how his attention was directed to carbolic acid. The acid, he stated, 'proved in various ways well adapted for the purpose'. First, 'It exercises a local sedative influence upon the sensory nerves', an action beneficial when construed in terms of Lister's theory of inflammation. Second, when mixed with blood 'it forms a tenacious mass that hardens into a dense crust', allowing the raw surface beneath to granulate, protecting it from the agents provoking putrescence.[33]

Lister then described eleven cases of compound fracture in which carbolic acid was employed. All were cases in which healing by granulation occurred and only three of them did not suppurate (cases 7, 10 and 11). In two cases the pus was described as 'imperfect' (cases 1 and 9). In none of these instances did Lister regard the pus as significant, *since it was not associated with inflammation* or putrefactive change. This indeed was the basis of his claim in these papers; his 'system' was an important contribution to surgery because, in wounds associated with compound fractures, he had achieved significant success in *attaining healing by granulation without inflammation.* Although theoretically ideal for Lister at this time, the elimination of suppuration was not the goal of therapy. In a paper published shortly afterwards he noted the 'object' of antiseptic treatment was 'not the avoidance of suppuration, but the prevention of putrefaction'.[34] Like any other surgeon, Lister did not regard a small amount of suppuration appearing on a healthy, non-inflamed granulation as a cause for alarm. For example, he reported in case 2 that 'on the fourth day . . . under ordinary circumstances, [inflammatory] suppuration would have made its appearance' but it did not do so. Such a report would have been welcomed by any surgeon. But Lister *did* have in this and other cases what other surgeons might have called laudable pus; he noted that 'the formation of pus [was] . . .

limited to the surface of the granulations'.[35] This was an appearance without grave significance.

Also in this paper Lister described the use of his antiseptic technique to evacuate pus from abscesses. Lister's view of abscess formation was similar to that of other surgeons, although modulated by his theory of inflammation. Lister described how abscesses were set up by some local stimulus, inflaming the tissues by way of the nervous system. Pus was produced by tissue proliferation and its production was sustained by the mechanical pressure of the 'pent up' pus continually irritating and inflaming the lining of the abscess (the 'pyogenic membrane'). Thus, Lister observed, in abscesses 'no septic organisms are present'.[36] The aim of the antiseptic treatment of abscesses was to remove the pus and to prevent agents entering the cavity and decomposing any remaining dead tissue. Lister again stated that these agents were 'germs' and that carbolic prevented their ingress.

The second of Lister's papers on antiseptic surgery also appeared in 1867. Lister claimed that he had, on the basis of his experimental work on inflammation, come to the conclusion that 'the essential cause of suppuration in wounds is decomposition'.[37] This pronouncement needs careful handling. First, it stipulates *wounds*; Lister had other views about pus formation in other sites. Second, as the paper later demonstrates, although he designated decomposition as the 'essential' cause he did not consider it the *only* cause of suppuration in wounds. Third, surgeons would have agreed that decomposition was a cause of pus formation in wounds. The pronouncement, we suggest, is best glossed as follows, '[I have discovered that] the [only important] cause of suppuration in [inflamed] wounds is decomposition.' Lister would have been read as referring to pathological pus formation associated with inflammation, the *sine qua non* of mischief in surgical practice.

That he was referring to the universal dread of pus in an inflamed wound is clear from his appeal to a surgical consensus, 'To prevent the occurrence of suppuration, with all its attendant risks, was an object *manifestly* desirable.' Lister then averred, in a statement that seems wholly inaccurate when measured against other sources, that until recently 'oxygen . . . was universally regarded as the agent by which putrefaction was effected'.[38] Pasteur's work, he claimed, now provided the basis for the belief that 'decomposition in the injured part might be avoided without excluding the air by applying as a dressing some material capable of destroying the life of the floating particles'. He added, 'Upon this principle I have based a practice.' The results of that practice, he pronounced, 'establish conclusively the great principle, that *all the local inflammatory mischief and general febrile disturbance which follow severe injuries are due to the irritating and poisoning influence of decomposing blood or sloughs*'.[39] Lister was repeating his priority claim. He had discovered or at least had established a 'great principle': not that decomposition was *a* cause of mischief, but that it was the *only* cause of mischief in wounds. The strength of this claim had increased since his first paper, where he had merely noted that, in his opinion, other surgeons had not taken enough notice of this effect.[40]

In this second paper Lister also declared that surgeons must persevere with the antiseptic treatment in spite of the appearance of suppuration. Carbolic, Lister argued, prevented decomposition but, in turn, induced suppuration. 'The surgeon', he noted, 'is extremely apt to suppose that any suppuration, is an indication that the antiseptic treatment has failed'.[41] In the face of such an assertion Lister noted, 'I feel it necessary' to defend this view on 'pathological principles'. Then, in what may have been a departure from contemporary opinion, he noted that, 'granulations have no inherent tendency to form pus, but do so only when subjected to a preternatural stimulus'. He pointed out, 'In so far, then, carbolic and decomposing substances are alike – namely, that they induce suppuration by chemical stimulation'. The difference between them was that carbolic acid 'stimulates only the surface . . . [but] decomposition is a self-propagating and self-aggravating poison'.[42] The decomposing tissues provided the nidus for more poison formation and pus, provoked by the decomposition, could itself (because of its high proportion of dead cells) become the seat of putrefaction. Lister was arguing that the pus formation that he said was induced by carbolic, was a simple, non-inflammatory cellular pro- liferation. It was indeed Lister's equivalent of 'normal' pus. Lister, like any other surgeon, could countenance pus in a wound as long as inflammation was not present. Whether the 'pus' was actually caused by the carbolic or not is immaterial here. Pheno- menally speaking, Lister's criteria for normal and abnormal healing by granulation were, at this time, much the same as those used by any other surgeon. Healthy healing was never accompanied by inflammation.

In this paper Lister also began to extend the significance he attributed to putrefaction. Decomposing wounds, he argued, were the source of the surgical diseases of hospitals. Again this was not a novel assertion although it was by no means a general assumption (see below). Lister claimed that after employing his new method, his wards had completely changed their character, 'wounds and abscesses no longer poison the atmosphere with putrid exhalations . . . during the last nine months not a single instance of pyaemia, hospital gangrene, or erysipelas has occurred in them'. The nature of these 'putrid exhalations' Lister did not explain, nor how they produced hospital fevers.[43]

Late in 1867 Lister published again. He iterated the claims made in his earlier papers and added a new observation on the agents of putrefaction which is significant in the light of subsequent developments. He noted that 'the character of the decomposition which occurs in a given fermentable substance is determined by the nature of the organism that develops in it'. On these lines Lister suggested that the agents of vinous fermentation were yeasts and the agents of putrefaction were, possibly, 'vibrios'. At the end of this paper Lister declared that on the basis of his theories he was the creator of a 'trustworthy treatment' for compound fractures and contused wounds.[44]

In 1868 Lister first used, in print, the expression 'the germ theory of putrefaction'.[45] This was a phrase Lister, and later Cheyne, were to employ recurrently. Throughout the 1870s Lister insisted that it was the truth of this theory which had enabled him to achieve greater surgical success than his contemporaries. He recurrently claimed that, by adopting it, he had discovered the true nature of healing, inflammation and sepsis. This paper contained another significant development. Lister affirmed that healing by organisation in a clot, not by first intention, was the ideal to be striven for in the treatment of compound fractures and other complex wounds. Organisation was widely agreed to be an ill-understood process of new tissue formation; it was similar to granulation but involving less proliferation and thus producing less scar tissue.[46] As with all other surgeons, Lister deemed granulation second best both to organisation under a scab and first intention healing. Lister reported a case in which he inflicted a surgical wound (that is, cutting intact skin) to correct a bony deformity. He described how he dressed the wound in exactly the same fashion as he treated wounds in compound fractures and how he anticipated healing by 'scabbing'. Although it is not obvious from published material at this time, Lister, along with all surgeons, endeavoured to achieve first intention healing in simple incised wounds. But in compound fractures, complex bone operations and, later, joint evacuations and excisions Lister explicitly deviated from the normal practice. He did not appose wound edges.

Lister's basic approach to the dressing of wounds of whatever sort was always the same, although he varied the details considerably over time. In the early days he used a dressing of carbolic putty designed to kill or prevent the entry of putrescence-inducing germs. Very shortly after using this he employed a 'protective', an impermeable substance which lay directly on the wound, to prevent what he described as carbolic induced suppuration. Lister eventually settled on oiled silk as the best protective. On top of this were piled eight layers of carbolic-impregnated gauze which overlapped the protective and absorbed the wound's discharges which seeped around the edge of the protective. Below the outermost layer of gauze lay yet another impermeable layer to prevent the discharges running through the dressing and washing out the carbolic.[47]

As he developed his ideas about healing by organisation in a clot, he slowly changed his views on healing by 'granulation and suppuration'.[48] Granulations were now described as a product of abnormal stimulation. Describing tissues in a recent wound he observed,

> It is only when they have been gradually changed under the influence of prolonged abnormal stimulation into that rudimentary form of tissue which, when we see it on the surface of a sore, we term granulations, that they are liable to produce, when still further stimulated, the still more rudimentary pus corpuscle.[49]

Antiseptic treatment, he argued, although initially stimulating the tissues in a wound, subsequently allowed it to heal without granulation. By 1870 he was arguing that if granulations were produced, protection from abnormal stimuli allowed them to develop immediately into 'higher forms'.[50] Refining the practice of healing in a clot, and developing a physiological and pathological theory of how this occurred, or failed to occur, were central to Lister's work over the next fifteen years. Although in the early days Lister called this 'healing by scabbing' it was quite unlike the healing of that name described by Paget. Lister's wounds always had fairly copious discharge. Equally, although like other surgeons Lister regarded healing by granulation as second best, his case reports (like those of other surgeons) make it clear that, not surprisingly, granulations were common.[51]

It is worth reviewing the situation at this point in order that the responses to Lister's publications can be understood. All surgeons, including Lister, regarded some form of primary union as the most desirable object of therapy. All, including Lister, regarded healing by granulation as less desirable. All, including Lister, regarded pus as a nutritive product, the consequence of granulation. Where Lister differed was in his favoured form of primary union in complex wounds. Lister preferred organisation in a clot as opposed to first intention healing. The alternative contemporary practice is exemplified by the work of a Cambridge surgeon, G. M. Humphry. Unlike Lister, Humphry had no qualms about exposure to the atmosphere,

> Cut surfaces seldom fail to adhere together and grow together – that is, to unite by first intention – if they be kept in apposition, however much they may have been exposed to air, as in wounds of the face, scalp and fingers, where this may commonly be done.

Like Lister he saw retained blood in a wound as a problem.

> The obstacle to [first intention] . . . is the accumulation of bloody fluid in the wound keeping the surfaces apart, decomposing, and causing suppuration. No precautions hitherto have assured against this . . . The decomposition may be lessened sometimes, though not commonly prevented, by antiseptics, but fail to provide for escape by drainage.

Where Lister's solution was to cover the clot and hope for organisation, Humphry drained the wound, apposed the edges, left it uncovered and dry and hoped for first intention healing.

> No dressing being used, the pain of removing and reapplying plasters, etc., is avoided. This combined with

some antiseptic or blood-coagulator to the surface of the wound, and a space left for escape of bloody fluid, was, he believed, the mode most likely on the whole, to promote quick union of large deep wounds.[52]

Developing the theory and responses

The responses to Lister's work have been fairly well chronicled and will only be outlined here in so far as they demonstrate the pathological framework employed by Lister and his contemporaries. Initial responses took the form of anecdotal case reporting. Later, surgeons produced statistical series. It should be noted, however, for the first few years at least, Lister's work did not loom large in the medical press. It was perceived as contribution to a shared problem rather than a unique intervention.[53] According to the *Medical Times and Gazette* of November 1867 Lister's publications had led to experimentation with carbolic among the London surgeons. It concluded, 'To sum up our experiences thus taken at second hand . . . the verdict of the Profession in London is in favour of carbolic acid as a disinfectant but that its value as a healing agent is somewhat doubtful'. It reported that surgeons believed that cases might have done as well with any other agent 'which would have thoroughly cleansed the wound from semi-putrid matter'.[54]

Among the responses were priority claims, notably those put forward on behalf of the French surgeon, Lemaire. Lister's replies to these are interesting when read in the light of the germ theory of putrefaction. Lister was perfectly prepared to own that others had toyed with ideas of germs and carbolic. His claim to be a discoverer and expositor of pathological principles, however, was always tenaciously defended.

> I may repeat that I have never claimed to be the first to use carbolic acid in surgery. The success which has attended its employment . . . depends . . . on the wonderful powers of recovery possessed by injured parts when efficiently protected against the pernicious influence of decomposition . . . whether [surgeons] . . . employ this agent or some other of analogous properties, it is only by the light of *sound pathology*, and strict attention to practical details,

> that they can hope to attain in their full measure the magnificent results which the antiseptic treatment is capable of affording.[55]

That the injured parts must be 'efficiently protected against the pernicious influence of decomposition' precisely summarises Lister's theory and practice.

In 1868 the first broadside appeared from Lister's most persistent critic, Lawson Tait. Of carbolic, he wrote,

> I have not been able to discover the slightest benefit from its use . . . [in] twelve cases of compound fracture where there existed a probability of union without suppuration, the only cases in which suppuration did occur were two in which I employed the acid paste exactly as recommended by Mr Lister.[56]

If he did apply the paste as Lister advised, such a result was exactly in keeping with Lister's predictions. Tait made it clear that he regarded first intention healing as quite possible in many compound fractures.

Another attack on Lister's methods was mounted at the BMA meeting of 1869, where Thomas Nunnely of Leeds voiced a conclusion which was to remain central for Lister's detractors: first intention healing occurred in wounds exposed to the air.

> Suppuration, per se, is not an unhealthy action, nor is pus itself always an injurious substance; *but when the process can be prevented by union by the first intention so much the better for the patient*; for, wherever pus or effused blood exist, there is more or less the danger of their becoming decomposed, absorbtion taking place, and the system being poisoned by them. If freely exposed stumps heal up most readily and well, it must be at once apparent that those which do so when most elaborately swathed in carbolised wrappings, do so rather in spite of, than as a consequence of the treatment.

In Lister's system, he complained, surgical science is 'reduced' to 'plentifully imbruing the injured parts with carbolic acid'.[57] As he made clear, this was a deliberate caricature of Lister's approach intended to make the point that surgery was being 'reduced' to the pathology and physiology of wound healing; the general condition of the patient, the state of the hospital etc. were not being given attention. The caricature captured what seemed to many to be Lister's claim and, indeed, was later proclaimed by Godlee to be the core of the achievement. Concentrating on local methods of wound treatment would set surgery, and medicine at large, to rights.

In November 1869 Lister developed his views on the germs which caused putrefaction. He described experiments he had performed on 'a decoction of meat' which was kept free from decay in a flask and he explained that the agents of putrefaction were 'living organisms developed from germs floating in the atmosphere as constituents of its dust'. Lister asserted that these organisms were 'vibrios' sprung from 'pre-existing similar organisms'.[58]

In spite of his proclaimed goal of achieving healing by scabbing, healing by granulation and normal suppuration seems to have been as common for Lister as they were for other surgeons. Indirect evidence for this is the amount of labour Lister invested in the theory of granulation. In 1870 he digressed at great length on the nature of suppuration. He began by referring to his 1858 paper in which, he said, it 'fell to my lot to . . . establish . . . that the . . . essence of *intense* inflammation' was 'a temporary . . . suspension of vital energy' brought about either by 'direct operation of a noxious agent' or by the action of the nervous system. Lister then declared that he had now discovered that the same 'law' operated in the instance of suppuration. Granulation tissue could be provoked into suppuration when stimulated either by the nervous system (inflammatory suppuration) or by chemical agents acting directly (chemical suppuration). Suppuration was only an advanced stage of such granulation, the pus cell 'being the extreme of excess of quantity and impairment of quality in the product of abnormally excited nutrition.'[59] This was virtually identical to Simon's account ten years earlier, employing the nutritional model of pus production.

The nervous type of suppuration, Lister then explained, was typically found in abscesses. That caused by local 'chemical stimuli' was exemplified by antiseptic and putrefactive suppuration. He observed,

> Thus, in their effects upon a granulating sore, an antiseptic and a putrid dressing are alike: both excite superficial suppuration by direct chemical stimulation of the granulations . . . but putrefaction . . . [is a] self-propagating ferment.

Thus, putrefaction set up pus formation and inflammation, and rapid putrefaction could even cause death by 'blood-poisoning before suppuration has had the time to be established'.[60]

When granulations were not stimulated, Lister explained, 'the imperfect tissue of which they consist is ever disposed to develop into higher forms', that is become fully organised. Thus, he observed, by using carbolic 'superficial suppuration is induced without any appearance of inflammation'. And, he concluded, 'Antiseptics, then, though they do produce suppuration when applied continuously to a recent wound, are superficial in their action and utterly trivial compared with the deep and virulent effects of putrefaction.'[61] The gloss here might be as follows. Surgeons frequently saw non-inflamed granulating wounds with a small amount of pus on the surface. These they regarded, *ceteris paribus*, as satisfactory. Lister simply had a different theory of why this phenomenon was satisfactory in his patients.

Also in 1870 Lister detailed his operative results over a five-year period, and described how his methods had, he said, converted 'some of the most unhealthy [hospital wards] in the kingdom into models of healthiness'. Again, he made the claim that wound management had cleared the hospital of fevers. Antiseptic treatment, he said, had reduced the incidence of pyaemia, erysipelas and hospital gangrene because it reduced 'emanations from foul discharges . . . the great source of mischief in a surgical hospital'. Lister considered every other contributory cause as minor. He ridiculed the idea of what was known as 'hospitalism'. Everything, he said, was of 'trifling consequence' compared to 'emanations from sores' and 'putrid exhalations'. What these exhalations were and how they acted Lister did not indicate. That Lister considered revolutionising therapy was central to salvaging the great hospitals as the locus of medical excellence and the seat of medical education is evident in his view that substituting 'cast-iron cottages' for hospitals was expensive, interfered with patient supervision 'and with the teaching of students at the bedside'.[62]

During these years various surgeons took up, selectively used, dropped or modified Listerian techniques. His opponents claimed equal or greater success for their methods and accused Lister of creating an over-complicated system of treatment and abandoning first intention healing. This, as Holmes Coote said, could be achieved by 'simplicity and cleanliness of dressings' and apposition of cut surfaces. It was 'nature and not the surgeon [who] healed the wound'. It is noteworthy that in Coote's case this view was coupled with another anti-Listerian position; hospital fevers were the source of trouble, not the result. He observed,

> that general opinion seems to incline to the belief that [the] . . . origin and propagation [of hospital fevers] are due to general and not to local causes; that the source whence poison is introduced into the system is the air and *not the secretion of the wound*.[63]

Lister's system had certainly had become more complicated by this time. The famous spray had been introduced to provide an atmosphere of carbolic in the operating room to kill the air-borne germs. In the paper in which he described the spray Lister gave an account of the management of a surgical incision. This was not sutured but, after carbolic-soaked sponges and cloths had been applied and removed, the incision was 'enveloped in lac-plaster'. The next day the dressings were changed and the 'gaping wounds' were found 'filled with blood-clot'. The 'oiled silk "protective"' was then applied to the wound, and the limb wrapped in lac-plaster. Two days later the dressing was changed again. Four days later, he reported, the clots were 'extensively converted into vascular tissue'. There was no pus. First intention healing was not attempted; union by organisation in a clot was the goal.[64]

In August 1871 Lister addressed the BMA meeting in Plymouth. He iterated the significance of Pasteur's experiments, arguing that they showed that 'putrefactive changes, are occasioned by particles of dust suspended in the atmosphere'. He then described a series of experiments, inspired by Pasteur's, which, he said, showed that pus, 'a highly putrescible liquid' could be kept 'perfectly sweet' in a flask by use of a carbolised cotton wool plug. Lister then described a further practical innovation: the use of drainage tubes. Lister's wounds, self-admittedly, produced a large amount of discharge. Explaining the use of drains Lister invoked his concept of 'tension' as a cause of suppuration. Carbolic, he said,

> causes an unusually large flow of serum during the first twenty-four hours or more, and you must provide a special exit for the serum, else you will have inconvenience from tension, which will lead to suppuration, though not of the putrefactive kind.[65]

This was another sort of suppuration, also caused by carbolic, this time indirectly. Tension of retained fluids, as in an abscess, set up inflammation and suppuration by the secondary nervous mechanism. Again it indicates how different Lister's model was from the ideal of healing by scabbing, which was described by Paget as occurring only in the absence of any fluid production. It was also another acknowledgement by Lister that he had wounds which produced pus. Again, however, his account of why this was so was differed from other surgeons.

Lister's supporters shared his views on pus formation. Some form of primary union was the most desirable form of healing but granulation with pus in small quantities but without inflammation was an acceptable alternative. Thus W. MacCormac of Belfast found carbolic dressings either prevented pus formation or 'when pus is found it proves quite innocuous not prone to decomposition, and not injuring the wounded surface, with which it is in contact'.[66] The Manchester surgeon Edward Lund also found that antiseptic surgery prevented pus formation or limited its production to 'harmless quantities'. Presumably Lund's 'harmless quantities' would have been much the same as were observed by surgeons (including Lister) practising under any other principle.[67]

At the BMA conference of 1873, John Wood, Professor of Surgery at King's College Hospital, reported a comparison of surgical dressings: dry lint, chloride of zinc and carbolised bandages. All, he said, proved equally effective, so long as the hospital was free from erysipelas and pyaemia. Thus,

> In some cases of psoas abscess treated by Lister's method we had marked success as long as the hospital was healthy. When erysipelas and pyaemias appeared, however, we had others in which the pus in the abscesses became putrid

> and offensive after the first evacuation under the spray and with all the precautions.[68]

Again this was the claim that pyaemia and erysipelas caused sepsis, not the reverse.

Both *The Lancet* and the *BMJ* carried editorials which endorsed Wood's position:

> Wounds heal by *first intention* although exposed to healthy atmospheric influences, and no amount of care will ensure this when the condition of the patient is unhealthy. The disciples of Mr Lister are somewhat difficult to convince, because they have the convenient saving clause, that if the treatment fails some error must have been committed.[69]

The 'saving clause' was invoked when the surgeon George Thompson from Oldham Infirmary visited Lister's wards. Cases looked much the same as elsewhere and in two inflammation with suppuration was present. He commented that the cases were explained away as owing either to the access of germs or to the premature removal of the drainage tube.[70] One of Lister's former house surgeons addressed the failure of the technique in other hands:

> I am at a loss to account for the many failures which those who try the system meet with, unless it be the want of faith in the "Germ Theory" of putrefaction. If this is believed in, the system becomes easy, and the minutiae which seem to trouble so much are mere matters of intuition.[71]

In 1873 Lister delivered two rather more theoretical papers on putrefaction. In the first he referred to a publication of John Burdon-Sanderson's. On the basis of experimental work Sanderson had reached a number of conclusions, including the view that the dust of the air contained no bacteria. Lister doubted this view which, if correct, he said, ought to lead him to jettison the spray. His own work, he reported, showed the inaccuracy of Sanderson's conclusions.[72] These papers are interesting for more than this, however, for, on what he declared was the basis of his own work, Lister revealed a much more detailed and extended germ theory of putrefaction. First Lister developed the view that there was no fixed morphology for bacteria and yeasts. Form was plastic and governed by the local environment. German taxonomic views were, at this time, unacceptable: 'any classification of bacteria hitherto made, from that of Ehrenberg to that of Cohn, based upon absolute morphological characters is entirely untrustworthy'.[73] Indeed it was Lister's opinion that putrefactive bacteria (rod-shaped organisms) were the buds of yeasts. The second development in this paper was the view that, although bacteria might appear similar, they might give rise to quite different fermentative changes, some of which might be non-odiferous. For instance 'an albuminous fluid may be affected with a fermentative change without the occurrence of smell'. Lister gave two clinical examples of this effect.

> I have seen, for example, a psoas abscess furnish merely a slight oozing of serous discharge under antiseptic management, till a single careless application of the dressing admitted, as I believed, some fermentative organism, which, without giving rise to any odour, so altered the character of the discharge, as to stimulate the diseased part to profuse suppuration, leading to death by hectic. I have also observed erysipelas occur in spite of antiseptic treatment, and occasion profuse suppuration without smell.

He concluded, 'from analogy there is reason to suspect that the virus of that disorder is of the nature of an organism, operating as a ferment upon the animal fluids'.[74] The putrid exhalation theory of hospital fevers had been dropped or, at least, had been elaborated into something much more detailed. Highly plastic organisms, which could ferment fluids in wounds, were now cited as a cause of hospital fevers. The central assumption of the earlier theory, however, remained the same. It was the process occurring in decomposing sores which gave rise to hospital fevers. Lister now outlined how his new observations explained how this occurred. Benign organisms, normally present in hospitals, could, he said, become pathogenic. Thus if harmless forms gained access to the decomposing fluids existing in unhealthy wounds they could change both physiologically and morphologically. For example, in the instance of hospital gangrene, in which surgeons had previously assumed that a 'special virus' was at work, Lister observed,

> We now see that it is not essential to assume the existence of a special virus at all, but that organisms common to all the sores in the ward may, for aught we know, assume specific properties in the discharges long putrefying under the dressings.[75]

Lister now elaborated a full-blown germ theory of putrefaction and used it as an explanation of *all* contagious diseases. It is important to note this was *not* a theory of specific organisms causing specific diseases, quite the reverse. Contagious diseases were highly variable because of the great environmentally determined plasticity of organisms.

> Facts of this kind may tend to elucidate points of great importance in the history of contagious diseases, such as the greater virulence of such disorders at some periods than at others. For it seems highly probable from analogy that the *materies morbi* may be of the nature of minute organisms; and if this be the case, we can understand, from what we have seen of the plant under consideration, that differences of energy in the virus may be occasioned by varying circumstances.[76]

Anachronistically it might be possible to call this *a* germ theory of disease, but Lister never did call it that. This seems to be the nearest he came to such a generalisation. It is noteworthy too, that, although cast in the form of a 'germ' theory, how similar Lister's assumptions were to those used by all other physicians and surgeons in the mid-Victorian period. It was changes in the environmental constitution (in this case mediated by germs) which produced febrile diseases which, therefore, necessarily differed in different circumstances. Another feature of this germ theory of putrefaction was that germs do not act on, or invade, the living body. Almost by definition putrefactive germs were confined to dead or dying tissues; 'healthy tissues', Lister declared, 'are capable of preventing the development of these low organisms'. This, he said, claiming priority, was a 'principle I enunciated'.[77] Whether 'germs' could invade less than healthy tissue or whether disease was owing to chemical poisoning was not indicated.

In 1875 a meeting of the Clinical Society was convened specifically to discuss antisepsis. *The Lancet* prefaced its report of the meeting with two long editorials questioning whether all aspects of Lister's increasingly complex scheme were necessary, particularly since Humphry's system of open dressings and Callendar's use of cotton wool and cleanliness were increasingly popular and, it was claimed, equally effective. The success of these systems should, *The Lancet* pointed out, be impossible if Lister's theoretical ideas were absolutely correct. What was evident, *The Lancet* concluded,

> was that few of the speakers either place faith in Lister's theory or carry out his practice in full . . . On the other hand, there were but few who did not express their belief in the utility of some portions of the method, especially in those which relate to the scrupulous care and cleanliness of wounds, and the avoidance of external sources of irritation or putrefaction.[78]

On 20 November 1875 the *Medical Times* ran an editorial on what it now called 'Aseptic Surgery'. One of the best examples of such surgery, it said, 'is certainly the opening of a large abscess on Mr Lister's method'.[79]

In 1875 Lister published again on the salubrious effect on hospitals of his antiseptic treatment. This time he evidenced the experience of continental hospitals as proof of his view that concentrating on the wound cleared hospitals of fevers. Further, he noted,

> it is said that greater cleanliness is involved in the antiseptic treatment. This, again, is an entire mistake. If we take cleanliness in any other sense than antiseptic cleanliness, my patients have the dirtiest wounds and sores in the world. I often keep on the dressings for a week at a time, during which the discharges accumulate . . . and, when the wounds are exposed after such an interval, the altered blood with its various shades of colour conveys often both to the eye and to the nose an idea of anything rather than cleanliness. Aesthetically they are dirty though surgically clean.[80]

This encompasses all that surgeons found objectionable in Lister's method. All his paraphernalia kept wounds open, discharging and filled with clot, when, apposed and covered with a simple dressing, they might heal by first intention. Again it is an indication of how far Lister's method was from producing the simple healing by scabbing described by Paget.

In 1875 and 1876 Lister reported a number of successful cases. Many of these were primary incisions for complex bone and joint conditions. Some Lister left open and draining. In others, however, the wound edges 'were brought together by carbolized silk sutures'.[81] How far Lister attempted to juxtapose wound edges at this time is hard to determine. In one wound which had not been sutured, removal of the dressing after fifteen days revealed a healthy blood clot. This, he said, was a phenomenon impossible without his form of antiseptic dressing. There was, he observed, no pus, 'not even any granulation'. He added,

> How the tissue which is thus formed in an organising blood-clot differs histologically from that of granulations, *I have not had time to investigate.* But that it differs from granulations functionally is certain, and that in two ways. First, it has not nearly the same tendency to contract that granulations have; and, secondly, instead of forming pus under the influence of the very slightest stimulus, as granulations do, this tissue resembles normal textures in requiring protracted stimulation to induce it to granulate and suppurate. Now, cicatrization in an open wound without granulation is something new; it never happened in the world's history without antiseptic means.[82]

In 1876 the controversy over antiseptics was nicely summed up by the military surgeon, Sir Thomas Longmore. Longmore described how the Peninsular War had taught surgeons the value of simplicity, hygiene, atmospheric purity and cleanliness. Today, he noted, there was a 'natural school', who were attempting to achieve first intention healing by manipulating these factors alone. There was, he said, 'Another body of surgeons, at the head of whom is Professor Lister, who assert that there are unavoidable impediments to simple healing, to union by the adhesive process, under this natural method.'[83] It was not until the 1880s that the Listerians responded to the question recurrently posed by the 'natural school'; why do wounds heal when exposed to the air? For, as *The Lancet* put it in 1875, 'Mr Lister tells us that the air is as it were, darkened with disease producing germs.' But his opponents, it noted, 'affirm, and the experience of most persons seems to bear them out, that they have seen cases do perfectly well, notwithstanding the freest admission of ordinary air . . . and where nothing but simple water is used as a dressing'.[84] One important member of the 'natural school' was the Birmingham surgeon Sampson Gamgee who, in a clinical lecture of 1878, claimed that the 'majority of wounds heal rapidly and painlessly under dry and infrequent dressing, uniform gentle pressure, and absolute rest'.[85] It was Lister's view that wound discharges were particularly vulnerable to putrefaction, whence he took care to absorb them in a massive carbolic impregnated dressing. Gamgee and other surgeons, however, dressed wounds with dry, absorbent substances and allowed any discharges to soak into them. In their experience such discharges did not putrefy.[86] Gamgee did acknowledge that Lister's method might prove useful in unhealthy wounds but, under normal circumstances, he held it unnecessary.

In 1877, in a much cited address, the Manchester physician William Roberts discussed the 'doctrine of contagium vivum'. Roberts's paper is interesting since it contains the first statement of a position that the Listerians were soon to adopt, the argument that all successful surgical methods were employing their antiseptic principle. Roberts outlined how putrefaction and fermentation were caused by living creatures, saprophytes. In septicaemia, he argued, a poison, the product of microbial decomposition of wound products, entered the blood. He then noted,

> We should probably differ less about the antiseptic treatment if we took a broader view of its principle. We are apt to confound the principle of the treatment with Lister's method of carrying it out. The essence of the principle, it appears to me, is not exactly to protect the wound from the septic organisms, but *to defend the patient against the septic poison.*[87]

Seen in this light, he said, the open method was simply 'another way . . . of defending the patient against the septic poison'. Roberts's putrefactive model shared many elements with Lister's. He observed, 'You cannot successfully inoculate the healthy tissues with septic bacteria'.[88] His address, however, also included recognition of a new, predominantly German, infective theory of disease, characterised by the idea of morphologically specific organisms *invading living tissues* and always producing the same disorder. Roberts then noted that there were strong analogies between septic (putrefactive) diseases and fermentative activity *in vitro*. These, however, did not extend to species-specific infections where the analogies lay with parasitism. The organisms producing these disorders he observed, unlike septic bacteria, could invade living tissue, as Koch's animal experiments had demonstrated. Roberts was insistent that putrefactive activity and infective pathogenesis (as in diseases such as relapsing fever) were *not pathologically similar processes*.[89] That is, he distinguished a germ theory of putrefaction and a germ theory of infection.

In 1878, the year following Roberts's publication, Lister chose as his introductory address to King's College Hospital, London, the nature of fermentation. He digressed on the 'large class' of diseases which were 'zymotic' or whose 'essential nature is fermentative'. He instanced puerperal fever and wound sepsis as paradigmatic of the group. Once again the truth of Pasteur's experimental findings was iterated. Lister exemplified alcohol formation as a typical fermentation and noted the ferment was 'capable of self-multiplication'. He added that he believed this to be 'the essential property of a true fermentation'. Putrefaction of shed blood was also 'a true fermentation', the cause of which was 'microscopic organisms, termed bacteria from their rod-shape'.[90]

In 1878 Lister described an excision of the knee joint, in a little girl with an atrophied leg, locked in flexion. The hamstrings were divided, the knee joint opened and extension performed. Lister noted, 'Next to the importance of the avoidance of putrefaction in wounds is the prevention of tension by providing a free escape for effused blood and serum'. Lister used a horse-hair drain. The wound drained 'blood and serum'. There was no 'particle of pus'. Lister also observed, 'The skin is still as it has been all along, free from inflammatory blush or puffiness'.[91] Lister was distinguishing several processes here. The carbolic had not stimulated the tissues to granulation and suppuration. There was no inflammation, therefore there were no retained fluids (also produced by carbolic stimulation) irritating the nervous system. There was obviously no putrefaction. Once again a simple wound had been converted into an organising clot.

Lister's opponents continued to publish in these years, claiming equal success for their simpler techniques, insisting that wounds healed when exposed to the air and that first intention healing should be the goal of surgery. At the BMA annual meeting of 1879, what proved to be a controversial address was given by William Savory of St Bartholomew's Hospital. He noted,

> Antiseptic surgery! Unhappily there is much confusion in the current employment of this phrase. This ought to mean – and with some, but a few only, it does mean – the principle which aims to secure healthy wounds and their repair as speedily as possible . . . by the most scrupulous cleanliness – by cleanliness, I repeat not only the common, but in the surgical sense, which means the prevention or removal or destruction of all matter which may prove poisonous. This, I take it, is the only adequate conception of antiseptic surgery: and, as thus understood, the term antiseptic ought in fact to become superfluous, being simply equivalent to good surgery.[92]

Having detailed how the wards in his hospital were run with cleanliness and overall care of the patient in mind, Savory criticised the use of drainage tubes and carbolised dressings which could convert wounds into germ traps and hotbeds for the cultivation of bacteria. Simpler techniques worked more effectively. *The Lancet* amplified these comments in an editorial, taking the view that cleaning up hospitals would clean up wounds, and that therefore Lister was seriously misleading surgeons.

> Mr Savory alleges that the Listerian plan of dressing does not afford the protection it pretends to afford, that it conceals the wound from proper inspection, that it postpones and prolongs repair, and is moreover irritating both locally and constitutionally. But the graver evil may attend its adoption. 'It is preferable to a pestilential atmosphere'; and if operations were compulsory in such an atmosphere, probably Lister's mode of dressing might be found to be as safe as any other. *But the surgeon's duty, under ordinary circumstances, is not to find what are the most dangerous conditions under which he dare operate; it is rather to*

> *discover the causes of this pestilence and banish them as far as possible from his field of action.*[93]

Savory's and Lister's statistics featured large in two meetings of the South London District of the BMA in December 1879, expressly held to debate the value of the antiseptic method. Both *The Lancet* and the *BMJ* carried extensive coverage of the meetings. Lister gave an extended presentation in which he compared his results with Savory's. Savory, he pointed out, had inherited the antiseptic practice of Callender, so that he used carbolic washes and lint even though he did not use the carbolic spray. Lister admitted that, on the face of it, the Bartholomew statistics were impressive, and his own mortalities were in fact slightly greater. In a further analysis of his results Lister showed how his figures were not comparable.[94]

At the second meeting the critics of Lister gave their opinions. These surgeons, unlike Lister, were prepared to implicate a range of factors in the cause of disease and argued that directing attention to hospital fevers would make for healthy wounds. Progress on this front, they claimed, had already produced impressive results. Jonathan Hutchinson, from St Bartholomew's, made this point, for, he noted, 'during the development of Listerism, other and very important hospital reforms were in progress. Gradually every hospital was provided with an isolation ward, and cases of erysipelas and gangrene were promptly removed from proximity with the healthy'.[95] Sir James Paget took a similar view:

> In the last twenty years, we have had the complete sanitation, so far as the sanitary art has yet extended, of all our hospitals in which our patients are contained. Then we have had amongst us the whole system of skilled nursing . . . A patient ought to be cured with as little risk to life as possible.[96]

That using the Listerian method involved some risk was accepted by some of Lister's supporters at this meeting and they owned that the full antiseptic apparatus was not always desirable. As Mr Morant Baker put it,

> was it necessary to use that mode of treatment that has been called 'Listerism'? or that which Mr Hutchinson calls

> the 'spray and gauze' system? He would answer no . . . there were many cases in which the system in fullest sense was unnecessary, and it had evils of its own, more particularly in the direction of carbolic acid poisoning, of infiltration in the wound tightly confined under antiseptic dressings, and of concealed recurrent haemorrhage.[97]

Enter the micrococci

In 1879 what was eventually to become a serious issue for the Listerians made its appearance. In that month the medical press carried a report of a paper delivered to the Pathological Society by Watson Cheyne. Cheyne discussed German claims to have found small spherical organisms, micrococci, in antiseptic dressings.[98] Cheyne's response was not encouraging to those inclined to accept such conclusions as significant. On the basis of his own investigations, Cheyne said, such micrococci were harmless. He added that it also seemed 'quite certain that if there are noxious forms of micrococci, they are rare'. The evidence was that in 'unhealthy wounds' and in 'erysipelas', (rod-shaped) bacteria were to blame. The micrococci found in septic wounds and acute abscesses, he explained, were secondary colonizers of unhealthy tissues and were 'not essential to the inflammatory process'. He added 'when the antiseptic treatment is thorough organisms are either completely absent or, where . . . present they belong to the class of [harmless] micrococci'.[99] Lister, who was at the meeting, added various comments endorsing Cheyne's opinions.

Unlike Pasteur's views, which seem to have been supported predominantly by the relatively small group of Listerians, German work was taken up across the medical spectrum. A germ theory of infection, as opposed to the germ theory of putrefaction, found a more receptive audience.[100] One of the most significant features of the German work was the model employed for understanding disease. Whereas Lister's model was the decomposition of organic fluids in glassware, the German model was the transmission of disease from living animal to living animal.[101] The Listerians themselves were very alert to this work; it was after all increasingly being perceived as the most up-to-date scientific contribution to medicine. Since the Listerians presented themselves as being in the vanguard of scientific medicine, they either had to challenge German work or take it on board; it could not be ignored. At first they challenged the work on micrococci, adopted the account of the causes of specific fevers and retained their own theory of wound sepsis. Later they subordinated this latter theory to a general theory of infection.

In 1880 Cheyne produced a translation of Robert Koch's *Etiology of Traumatic Infective Disease*, which had appeared in German in 1878. Koch's work was performed entirely on animals and was intended to elucidate the nature of the great fevers, such as epidemic septicaemia and erysipelas, which were associated with local sepsis. In brief Koch's conclusions were that, in animals, diseases analogous to human ones could be produced; these were specific, parasitic, transmissible by inoculation and were always associated with micro-organisms, frequently micrococci. Abscess formation was also caused by micrococci and specific bacteria were responsible for specific clinical and pathological configurations. Koch's work made no use of the putrefactive model, although he used 'putrid products' initially to inject the experimental animals. He pointed to parasitic *invasion* of the tissues of perfectly healthy animals as the cause of the symptoms.[102] Cheyne's translation was without commentary on the significance of this material.

In England, Lawson Tait, although not an ardent advocate of German views, had long criticised Lister's putrefactive model. In February 1880 *The Lancet* carried a report of a meeting which was

> occupied by the reading and discussion of a paper contributed by Mr Lawson Tait, in which he aimed at proving that in his own practice the adoption of antiseptic precautions had not apparently influenced the results obtained in ovariotomy. For whilst admitting the truth of the germ theory of putrefaction, he maintained that the practice of antiseptic precautions delayed the healing of wounds, and was accompanied by more constitutional disturbance than careful methods followed without the details of Listerism.[103]

Tait, one of Lister's most persistent critics, always maintained that whatever the process was which occurred when wounds became septic, it was in no way similar to the putrefactive changes seen in dead material, or to the fermentation observed in Pasteur's or Lister's flasks. He admitted to a germ theory of these processes, but denied it had any relevance to the explanation of sepsis in the living body.

March 1880 saw an anonymous review of the *Chirurgie Antiseptique* of Lucas-Championnière in the *Medical Times.* The reviewer was a champion of the antiseptic method and, given his detailed understanding of Lister's position, was probably Watson Cheyne. Noteworthy was his chastising of Championnière for extending Lister's theory of pus formation and suggesting that, by some direct means, germs could stimulate pus production. He noted that Championnière

> falls into more than one error . . . he assigns to . . . organisms a *double action* – 'they not only provoke the formation of pus, but they also cause that pus to putrefy'. Such an assertion in a work which professes to be a *résumé* of Mr Lister's views is scarcely pardonable, and if Dr Championnière will refer to Mr Lister's writings he will find it stated that it is by causing putrefaction of the discharges in the first instance that these organisms induce suppuration. *Mr Lister nowhere states that they can cause suppuration without a preceding putrefaction.*[104]

This seems an absolutely correct representation of Lister's views if putrefaction is understood to include non-odiferous fermentation. It was a view also held by Cheyne at this time (see below).

By the early 1880s the Listerians had failed to convince the surgical community of the superiority of their methods; what then occurred was an interesting *volte face.* Having for over ten years deemed other surgical results inferior, Listerians began to acknowledge that other techniques were as successful as their own. In doing this, however, they began to claim this was so because, unknowingly, all other practices were based on Listerian truths. At the Cambridge meeting of the BMA in August 1880, a Kilmarnock surgeon, John McVail, presented a series of excellent statistics. His patients' wounds had been treated with lint spread with lard or with 'blood dressing'. Lister was reported as replying

> There was . . . great truth in a remark . . . that every good surgeon was, whether consciously or unconsciously, an

> antiseptic surgeon. In this respect, the improvements of surgery had been improvements in antiseptics. Scrupulous cleanliness, frequent changes of water-dressings or poultices, as distinguished from leaving water-dressings on for a long time together, were antiseptic means – that was to say, means tending to guard against the evil effects of septicaemia. Drainage, so as to prevent accumulations in the wound, dependent openings, the open treatment of wounds, all operated as antiseptic agencies. Free ventilation, so as to ensure as pure air as possible, was also an antiseptic measure. Even judicious selection of cases for operation might be said to be antiseptic.[105]

To Lister's speech the surgical elder statesman Erichsen

> confessed he was somewhat staggered when he heard that under the word antiseptic were to be now included every possible hygienic and other precautions taken in the hospital, even to the exclusion of unfit cases for operation. Used in that sense, the word simply lost all significance.[106]

Lister then described experiments which he had performed on ox blood in which the power of fresh (that is, living) serum to resist putrefaction had been revealed to him. On the basis of these experiments Lister claimed that McVail's dressing 'was a kind of antiseptic dressing'.[107] Lister then acknowledged again that there might be organisms which did not produce odour yet which did produce septic 'mischief'. The following, he argued, was the corollary:

> That if they were still to use the words septicity and antiseptics, they must enlarge the scope of these words, and that the word septic change was not necessarily one which produced a putrefactive stink; and so antiseptic treatment must include all treatment tending to guard against all these organisms, whether or not they tended to produce a putrefactive odour.[108]

In August 1880 Lister delivered an address, 'On the relation of micro-organisms to disease'. This paper is an important publication in the history of Listerism. In it Lister took cognizance of Koch's work. But in doing so Lister was by no means taking the same isolated position as he had when he championed Pasteur's theory of putrefaction fifteen years earlier. German germ theory had been well reported and was looked upon favourably by the medical establishment. Lister represented himself as having anticipated Koch, not as being his champion. Lister reported that Koch's work (then recently translated by Cheyne and about to be published) had shown that, in addition to the morbid effects of the absorption of putrid matter (a chemically toxic process), there could also exist in animals septicaemia, spreading gangrene and erysipelas characterised respectively by the presence of large numbers of rod-shaped bacilli, and two sorts of micrococci in the blood. The diseases were transmissible experimentally and were analogous to anthrax. This observation was conjoined with a recognition of the uniqueness of Koch's method, 'the animal body . . . was converted by Koch into a pure cultivating apparatus'.[109] Lister also reported that the bacterium of fowl cholera grew in broth without producing putrefaction, yet caused the disease when injected. He observed,

> The growth of the organism occasions no putrefaction in the liquid; so that this is a good example of a bacterium which is most destructive as a disease, but which is at the same time entirely destitute of septic property, in the primitive sense of that term as equivalent to putrefactive.[110]

It is important to note what was being done here. Koch's work was being added on to the putrefactive model, the latter was not being dropped. There was a distinction, which Cheyne was shortly to make more explicit, between a (German) germ theory of infection and a (Listerian–Pasteurian) germ theory of putrefaction. The cause of wound sepsis for Lister was putrefaction (whether or not odiferous), and the systemic symptoms of septicaemia and pyaemia were still decreed to be caused, in most cases, by the absorption of toxic chemicals. However, in addition to this cause Lister acknowledged that, in animals at least, micrococci and bacilli injected locally entered the body and could be transmitted experimentally, setting up a fever in a second animal. By inference there was a similar human condition: 'thus it has been shown by Koch that septicaemia may exist as a deadly blood disease, caused by the development of micro-organisms, equally distinct from pyaemia and from the chemically toxic effects of septic products'.[111] Lister can be read here as endorsing (in some instances) a specific aetiology model of the epidemic diseases of hospitals, a model which he had earlier rejected in favour of an environmental theory.

By 1881 Lister had retreated from the diffuse airborne origins of sepsis to the view that it originated in concentrated accumulations of organisms on, for instance, hands and surgical instruments. Experiments demonstrated, he said, that 'putrefaction . . . is due rather to septic matter in a concentrated form than to the diffused condition in which it exists either in water or in air'. This conclusion, which his own experiments had once repudiated, now suggested the question, 'Is the spray really necessary?'[112] The answer was shortly to be no, and the spray was abandoned. In this paper, which he delivered to the International Medical Congress where the most distinguished medical audience ever gathered was in attendance, Lister also described a series of experiments on a live donkey. These were designed to examine the microscopic changes in a clot surrounding putrefying material introduced into a vein of the animal. Lister reported that he had long held the view that an undisturbed blood clot had 'a special power of preventing the development of septic bacteria'. This, he recounted, he had once 'ascribed to the white corpuscles'.[113] However, his current experiments had shown him that when putrid matter was introduced into the living animal it was surrounded by a clot 'teeming with cells of new formation'. Microscopy showed that what these cells constituted 'was in fact neither more or less than pus'. Lister reported that this validated experiments which he had made in 1864 and which

> proved in the clearest manner that a blood clot . . . under septic influence, [is] liable to a genuine suppuration . . . which is no mere . . . accumulation of white cells . . . but consists of a growth of living corpuscles multiplying by endogenous cell development.

His present experiments, Lister claimed, also showed that the new cells originated from a 'proliferation of elements of the tissues of the wall of the vein' in which the clot was formed. This was a version of his long-standing view that pus was the product of local cell proliferation stimulated by putrefactive products. It was a nutritive-proliferative model of pus formation, similar to the one used by Simon describing the origin of pus in granulations. Lister was claiming originality on the grounds that he had discovered the process occurring *in a clot.* Although he recognised that some workers had suggested that pus was formed by white cell migration he observed that, even if pus was formed from such white cells, they were not 'mere emigrated white corpuscles' but 'they had sprung from them as a new and altered progeny'.[114] This work represents a change in tone. For years having pointed out the ever-present menace of putrefactive organisms Lister was increasingly stressing 'the *power* of an undisturbed healthy coagulum in the vicinity of living tissues to resist the development of putrefactive bacteria'.[115] This was not a new concept; from early on Lister had regarded the resisting power of healthy tissue as one of his principles. It is important to iterate, however, that what healthy tissues could resist were *putrefactive* bacteria. This 'power' of resistance Lister now found in the 'multitude of new living elements' and was proven by the fact that in the pus he had found 'only a single bacterium'.[116] It was, of course the power of tissue to recover and heal when left relatively untouched, or simply cleansed, that his opponents insisted made minimal surgical interference desirable. Indeed, what followed could have been taken by his opponents as an admission by Lister that this was the best course to follow. Lister noted, 'Our principle' explains the possibility of first intention healing under 'the apparently clean water dressing'. A little further on this principle had become 'our new principle' and it explained 'the *rationale* of the rules of the older surgery in aiming at union by the first intention'. Lister, however, was not about to subordinate the antiseptic 'principle' to the 'principle' that the healthy coagula could resist germs; he added, 'it would . . . be a grievous thing if our desire for simplicity should induce us in any degree to relax our efforts to carry out the strict antiseptic principle, the strenuous endeavour so to deal with wounds as to prevent from first to last the development in them of pathogenic organisms'.[117]

Traditional simplicity versus Listerian complexity was the theme of a *The Lancet* editorial summing up and commenting on the surgical section of the Congress. It noted, 'in the main the old classical principles were reasserted'. All the surgeons present agreed that first intention healing should be the goal after surgical incisions. However, in complex wounds, while 'some surgeons' urged that the same techniques should be adopted as in simple ones, another school 'concentrates their attention – in some cases their sole attention – upon the prevention of access of "germs"'. *The Lancet* added,

> the divergence in practice has recently become greater, for while the one school of surgeons look upon primary union [first intention healing] of a wound as the surest safeguard against septic mischief, the other school confident in its own power of preventing septic mischief, will forego the primary union of a wound in attaining this end.

Statistically, *The Lancet* said, there was nothing to separate the two schools. It pointed out, however, that Lister's so-called followers had in fact adopted many of the techniques of the other school. Thus Esmarch, the author of 'brilliant statistics . . . dresses his cases far more after the fashion of Mr Gamgee than that of Mr Lister'. It concluded,

> The danger has been that the 'system' should blind some of its followers to the fact that Nature works along certain lines or according to certain principles, all of which must be understood by the successful surgeon; and surely when primary union of a wound is dispensed with in order that the 'system' may be carried out, this danger has become real indeed![118]

In a footnote to his 1881 paper to the Medical Congress, Lister had recorded, 'The term "pathogenic bacteria" has been introduced by the German pathologists to signify bacteria which give rise to disease in the animal body by developing within it'.[119] It would be a mistake, however, to conclude from this that Lister had now embraced totally a theory which posited all pathological action as owing to germs 'developing within' the body. He absorbed and employed German work piecemeal, specifically rejecting aspects of it. Thus in 1881 Lister praised Koch's 'beautiful results' but expressed a 'note of warning' against exaggerating the relations between micro-organisms and disease. We know, he said, that 'Acute inflammation is certainly very often caused by the products of decomposition', but it was 'exaggerated' to suggest 'that all inflammation is caused by micro-organisms, and that suppuration, whether acute or chronic, is always due to similar agencies'.[120] Equally important was the inflammation caused by the nervous system. In this address Lister discussed the work of Alexander Ogston of Aberdeen who had raised the increasingly pressing question of whether micrococci had some role in pus formation. Ogston had claimed that acute abscesses were 'loaded with micrococci' and that chronic abscesses were free of them. Lister, however, argued that the cocci were not the cause of suppuration. He claimed that the inflammation that preceded suppuration was often accidentally caused, for example by a 'chill', and 'We can hardly suppose that the accident of exposure to cold could lead directly to the development of micrococci'.[121] Similarly antiseptic management of acute abscesses gave the same results as in chronic cases. Hence, Lister said, he took the part of Mr Cheyne who had stated that 'micrococci are . . . a mere accident of these acute abscesses'. The bacteria merely found the pus 'a congenial soil'.[122]

In 1882 Watson Cheyne's massive *Antiseptic Surgery* appeared. It represents the high-water mark of early Listerism. Cheyne offered a definition of antiseptic surgery as first described by Lister.

> The causes of fermentation are . . . solid particles . . . It is thus evident that in order to prevent putrefaction it is only necessary to prevent the access of these particles . . . It is on this principle that the *Aseptic Surgery*, as introduced by Mr. Lister, is based.[123]

Cheyne defended his use of the term aseptic, claiming that he was using it 'to indicate this [Listerian] form of antiseptic surgery, because . . . there are many different forms of treatment which come under the term "antiseptic"'. Lister's alone was founded on a 'true principle'.[124] In conformity with Lister's (and all other surgeons') views, Cheyne noted that, after operations, pus produced by inflammation was undesirable. When present, however, it did not necessarily indicate the action of septic organisms. For instance, discussing wound drainage he observed that, if the discharges do not exit freely, 'they give rise to tension, and tension gives rise to inflammation, and the latter, if allowed to go on long enough, to suppuration'.[125] On the issue of the micrococci Cheyne's position appeared rather more equivocal than previously. In acute abscesses, Cheyne agreed with Ogston, micrococci were 'always present'. But, he added, 'if the abscesses be not opened for some time, these organisms will be found to have died'.[126] Cheyne proposed to leave the question of the cause of abscesses unresolved, although his presentation of the evidence would probably have suggested to the reader that he did not consider that micrococci were implicated. Cheyne admitted to being puzzled by the discovery of micrococci in wounds treated aseptically. He concluded that wound discharges containing very dilute carbolic formed a 'particularly favourable medium' for micrococci, which then 'become more able to live in fluids containing a larger proportion of carbolic acid, and . . . eventually reach the wound'.[127] The dangerous rod-shaped bacteria which produced putrefaction, however, could not tolerate carbolic. What Cheyne was arguing here needs emphasising, in view of the way in which the theories and practices of modern surgery are read into early Listerian texts. At this time, Listerian antiseptic or indeed aseptic surgery, as it was now being styled, was, because it was still based on the germ theory of putrefaction, consistent both with *the growth of micrococci in wounds and pus production.* Interestingly, although Lister was becoming more cautious at this time about affirming the pathogenic power of atmospheric dust, Cheyne still seemed to have held it to be very important.[128]

Using his orthodox Listerian definition of the causes of wound sepsis Cheyne then embraced as effective a whole range of previously disparaged surgical practices. He noted that antiseptic surgery was 'no longer surgery which only *excludes* the causes of putrefaction'. It was possible to take 'a much wider view of the meaning of the term "Antiseptic Surgery"'. It included '*all those methods of wound treatment in which, wittingly or otherwise, the growth and fermentative action of the lower forms of organisms (bacteria) are more or less impeded*'.[129] Cheyne then demonstrated that nearly all current surgical techniques produced this result: free drainage, irrigation, open treatment, perfect rest. Thus Cheyne, like Lister, admitted to the success of other techniques but, in doing so, claimed them to be based on Listerian truths. Cheyne reviewed these techniques and explained in a number of ways the success of methods once vilified. By some techniques he was puzzled: 'The favourable results of constant irrigation in preventing septic diseases are very remarkable'.[130] Cheyne then pronounced what was once anathema to be the epitome of modern surgery, 'the open method is an advanced method of antiseptic treatment'. Using this technique, he explained, 'the discharges dry up, and become more concentrated, and thus become unfit soil for the growth of bacteria'.[131] In addition the free admission of oxygen retarded putrefaction. The success of Gamgee's rest and approximation treatment was explained by the fact that 'the *living tissues, when in a healthy state,* have the power of preventing the development of organisms in their immediate vicinity'.[132]

Cheyne explained in detail the practice of Listerian surgery. Surgical incisions were stitched and, Cheyne noted, 'if the wound remains aseptic, union by first intention may be expected'.[133] Carbolic was used to cleanse both instruments and the wound. The oiled silk protective coated with copal varnish and the carbolic-impregnated dressings were still the cornerstone of management. Discharge was acknowledged to be an important problem and drains were mandatory. In compound fractures, surgical incisions for fracture realignment and in most joint operations healing by organisation in a clot was the rule.

Cheyne's *Antiseptic Surgery* also situated Lister's work with respect to the theory of infective disease. They were presented as parallel intellectual developments. He noted,

> antiseptic surgery is simply a struggle with the causes of putrefaction. I have not mentioned the germ theory of infective disease at all. *That has no essential bearing on the principles of antiseptic surgery.* All that is required of antiseptic surgery is to prevent the occurrence of all kinds of fermentation. The germ theory of infective disease is, I say, an independent view, and not part of those principles at all. It is from mixing up of these two theories that the confusion, and much of the difficulty, in accepting the principles of antiseptic surgery, have arisen.

The germ theory of infective disease explained the specific fevers. It did not encompass wound decomposition. In saying this Cheyne ridiculed the opinion of an unspecified surgeon (without doubt Lawson Tait) who had claimed that it was ludicrous to argue from putrefaction 'in a dead infusion of beef' to living tissues because, this surgeon said, 'there is not the slightest particle of evidence that they [germs] do produce any change whatever upon *living* tissues'. Cheyne then explained that this benighted surgeon had also argued that there was even less evidence that 'blood poisonings, even when they are of an undoubtedly local origin, have the slightest analogy to those [changes] seen in a putrefying dead infusion.' This, said Cheyne, 'simply shows that the author is confusing together the two germ theories – that of putrefaction with that of infective disease'.[134]

Interestingly (and infuriatingly), Lister and, to a lesser extent, Cheyne published little over the next six years, a period in which the germ theory of putrefaction was slowly subordinated to the germ theory of infection. By the middle of the decade, however, it is clear the issue of the micrococci had to be dealt with if Lister was still to be father to *the* germ theory. In September and early October 1884 Cheyne published an account of his own and other recent work on micrococci. Cheyne reassessed the question of the significance of micrococci found in aseptic wounds and his own earlier view that such organisms were harmless. He reported Ogston's opinion that all micrococci were the same and all produced suppuration.[135] On the basis of his own work Cheyne concluded that not all micrococci were dangerous and that harmless forms did not become pathogenic when growing in a wound.[136] Cheyne then addressed the issue of whether micrococci were the sole cause of suppuration and Ogston's denial of the existence of 'what Sir Joseph Lister has termed antiseptic suppuration'. He conceded that in some cases micrococci were the 'primary cause' of suppuration but 'in most instances' their action was 'preceded by inflammation'. Micrococci, however, were generally necessary for the inflammation to proceed to suppuration. It was not, he concluded, always the same species of micrococcus that was associated with suppuration. Cheyne denied, however, that all suppuration was caused by micrococci. Chemicals and tension could set it up, he noted: 'I see a necessity in admitting the existence of "antiseptic suppuration"'. It was 'difficult to decide', however, whether tension alone was sufficient or whether micrococci were exploiting this situation.[137]

Shortly after this Lister published an 'Address on corrosive sublimate as a surgical dressing'. This difficult paper seems open to a variety of readings but it indicates that Lister was now also abandoning a germ theory of putrefaction as the sole explanation for wound sepsis. Lister declared that in rare cases pus production was directly stimulated by micrococci or 'some unusual organism'. He explained that he had recently observed 'several instances of deviation from the typical course' of wound healing. After a mastectomy in which the wound had failed to heal, pus had appeared after two days and not the usual four of the 'pre-antiseptic days'.[138] Although Lister still deemed 'genuine putrefaction' as the regular source of problem in wounds, in these abnormal instances the pus was 'undoubtedly of septic character'.[139] It was, he said, septic 'in the sense in which we now use the term septic, that is to say dependent upon the development of micro-organisms, although no smell was perceptible'.[140]

Some sense of the state of surgical theory and practice at this time can be found in the Bradshaw Lecture, 'Antiseptics in surgery', given in 1885 by John Wood. In his review of wound healing Wood stressed hygiene, the patient's constitution, drainage and the use of local applications 'calculated to prevent suppuration and putrefaction, and promote quick healing'. Wood did not utterly disapprove of the spray but digressed on the 'drawbacks' of the 'Listerian combination', notably carbolic poisoning and irritation of the skin.[141] The tone of the address was to give Lister limited credit for introducing an effective chemical antiseptic into the great array of resources that had to be mobilised in order to heal wounds by first intention. Commenting on Wood's lecture, the *Medical Times* concluded, 'Indeed, Mr. Wood might shortly have described successful antiseptic surgery as careful co-optation of the parts, free drainage, and absolute cleanliness'.[142]

How far chemical antisepsis was perceived in some quarters as a limited part of surgical cleanliness can be judged from a review of a book on obstetrics, which appeared in the *BMJ* in 1888. Significant is the assumption that a clean environment was a precondition of healthy healing whether in a wound or in the post-partum uterus. The author noted,

> it is necessary to bear in mind that cleanliness is after all the most powerful antiseptic we can employ – cleanliness, that is, of atmosphere, of persons, and of instruments. With it chemical antiseptics, the use of which is not unattended with danger, may be safely dispensed with; without it all such agents are useless, or nearly so.[143]

The next significant Listerian publication was Watson Cheyne's *Suppuration and Septic Diseases* of 1888. In this work Cheyne began the final abandonment of the germ theory of putrefaction or at least its total subordination to a germ theory of infection, which was now agreed to apply to wounds. The balance had shifted in favour of the micrococci as the most significant cause of wound sepsis. To have resisted this view any longer would have placed the views of the Listerian party outside the growing consensus on the role of bacteria in disease. Cheyne argued that putrefactive bacteria, if they gained access to wounds, did sovery quickly, producing the smell of decay. They produced chemicals in decomposing tissue (putrescine and cadaverine) which could debilitate the patient, set up local inflammation and enable the pyogenic cocci to gain access. It was pyogenic cocci, however, which were implicated in pus production. He explained how they often entered wounds without any prior putrefaction.[144] Lister's 'great principle', that putrefaction was the cause of all wound mischief, had finally been abandoned. Pyogenic cocci, once harmless invaders, were now the most serious culprits in the production of sepsis. Ogston's claim that cocci were the cause of abscesses was acknowledged to be a 'great landmark'.[145] Pyogenic cocci, Cheyne noted, were usually present on the surgeon's hands and instruments. Airborne contamination, for twenty years the prime fear of Listerians, was a 'rare occurrence'. Pyogenic organisms, Cheyne explained, 'spread in by growing in the discharge which is lying between the dressings and the skin'.[146] Thus if a dressing was left for several days pyogenic organisms ultimately reached the wound. Dressings left on for long periods, soaked in wound discharges and carbolic were a feature of early Listerian practice, indeed a feature to which Lister drew attention. The notion that pus was hyperplastic tissue response to putrefaction was now also deserted. Pus formation only occurred when pyogenic organisms invaded the body.[147] Pus comprised micrococci and repelling leucocytes which 'oppose the spread of the organisms'.[148] The effects of mechanical and chemical irritation on the tissues (formerly 'antiseptic suppuration') were to produce 'what the one set of observers calls pus, [and] the other set. . . fibrinous exudation'. Thus the pus which, admittedly, occurred in Lister's wounds and was said by him and Cheyne to be caused by chemical means and tension, was redefined, since now pyogenic cocci alone were acknowledged as the cause of suppuration. The former 'antiseptic pus' was not pus at all. To admit that it was would have been to admit that the Listerian wounds of those days were infected. Cheyne explained that strictly 'true creamy pus' only appeared when micro-organisms were present. The 'pus' formed by carbolic was not pus; he observed, 'I suspect that the antiseptic can only increase the amount of exudation and the number of leucocytes, and thus cause at most a semi-purulent discharge'.[149] These arguments, it should be noted, could have been equally well applied to 'laudable pus'. This substance which, from current (largely Listerian) perspectives, appears to condemn all past surgeons who praised its presence could be reconstructed differently. Laudable pus which, after all, in Paget's and Simon's accounts was not the product of inflammation, could be reconstructed as 'fibrinous exudation'. Its actual status is not the issue here. The point is that the adoption of Listerian perspective has informed all accounts of alternative practices. Laudable pus was real pus but Lister's pus was not.

Cheyne now repudiated various practices which were once central to Listerian antiseptic surgery and which had been used as evidence of its efficacy. He questioned the value of employing antiseptics in wounds 'which have become septic'. The harm they did to the granulation tissue was greater than any benefit they might convey:

> where strong irritating antiseptics are employed, unless they are able to kill all the micro-organisms present in the wound, and thus render it aseptic, the result of their injection might be . . . that they will injure the granulation wall and thus produce a weak spot in which the pyogenic cocci present in the wound can develop.[150]

In his preface to the book Cheyne included a brief history of Listerian antisepsis. Although not inaccurate in detail it suggested that the new object of surgical opprobrium, pus, was from the beginning the focus of Lister's attention. It also implied that the suppurative consequence of putrefaction was more important than putrefaction itself. Yet for Lister suppuration was a nutritive *response.*

> Sir Joseph Lister's earliest views may be summed up as follows: – It is the putrefaction of the discharges of the wound that leads directly or indirectly to suppuration and septic diseases.

Lister's putrefactive germ theory was then described and, Cheyne continued, Lister then 'found that the application of . . . strong carbolic acid . . . was in some cases followed by suppuration'. Lister thus 'came to the conclusion' that the antiseptic irritation caused the suppuration. In other cases, he noted, Lister held that suppuration followed the 'tension' of pent-up discharges. All this seems an accurate representation. Cheyne then added,

> Cases however occurred from time to time in which wounds suppurated without any reason for supposing that either tension or irritation of the antiseptic were at work . . . it *thus became evident* that in some cases, at any rate, the organisms which caused suppuration were not necessarily the same as those which caused putrefaction.[151]

The phrase 'it thus became evident' is noteworthy, for it implies that without reference to any other views, without any interpretive work and on the basis of appearances alone, Lister realised that suppuration was not related to putrefaction and was produced by different organisms. That is, he anticipated German infective theory which Cheyne then described at length. This, as we have seen, was not so. Confronted by odourless suppuration (which Lister only very rarely discussed) Lister subordinated it to his pathological principles. It was produced by non-odiferous fermentation in wound products by highly plastic organisms. These fermentative products stimulated inflammation and its consequent tissue hyperplasia, which was suppuration. Only in the early 1880s, in the light of German work, did Lister declare that suppuration could be produced by species-specific micrococci independent of putrefaction. In 1884 he was still reporting cases of sepsis without putrefaction as extremely unusual.[152]

This account of antiseptic surgery, suggesting that Lister had anticipated German views, was continued by Lister himself in, of all places, Berlin in 1890. Here Lister described the work of Metchnikoff who had suggested that pus was composed, primarily, of migrating white cells acting as defensive phagocytes ingesting invading bacteria. Lister recounted his donkey experiments which he had reported to the London Congress in 1881. He explained how he had introduced putrid matter into a donkey's vein and found, after a few days, it was surrounded by a multitude of cells. He added, 'I supposed that these cells must have been in some way or other the antibacteric agents but how, I could not imagine. The phagocyte theory clears up the mystery.'[153] Lister presented his work as a necessary anticipation of Metchnikoff's: identical in essence but lacking the detail provided by the phagocyte work. But in 1881 Lister had invoked his experiments to show how healthy tissues *could not be invaded* by putrefactive bacteria, not what the tissue response was to invasion by infective organisms. Lister had no such concept. The work employed the nutritive model of suppuration and was used to show that pus was composed of immature cells produced by rapid local tissue proliferation. Indeed he was at pains to point out how his work refuted a simple theory of white cell migration.

In 1891, in 'On the principles of antiseptic surgery', published in a German journal, Lister recalled another aspect of the history. He claimed that soon after commencing carbolic treatment his wards were not only rid of unpleasant, odiferous, putrefying wounds but also of odourless hospital diseases. This, he said, 'naturally suggested' the idea that 'erysipelas and odourless forms of suppuration' were caused by microbes, 'each disorder, having, probably its own specific organism'.[154] This again is a reading of the infective theory of disease back in the 1870s. In fact, in the early days Lister had suggested that the hospital fevers were caused by 'putrid exhalations' and later he argued that they originated in fermentations caused, not by specific organisms, but by highly plastic, locally-produced microbes. Odourless suppurations, we know, were also held to be caused by chemical and mechanical stimulation and nervous irritation. The phrase 'naturally suggested' like Cheyne's 'it became evident' implies no significant human mediation was necessary in converting the germ theory of putrefaction to the germ theory of infection. Nature spoke unequivocally. The written evidence, however, is that only on reception of Koch's work did Lister acknowledge species-specific, non-putrefactive disease.

By the end of the century modern germ theory could be presented as an unfolding of Listerian ideas. Surgical practice fitted into the same mould. In 1903 Cheyne was noting how 'aseptic method' was a 'natural development of Listerism'.[155] It is important to stress that we are not suggesting there was any attempt at deliberate deception on the part of the Listerians here. The discovery of current scientific theories in earlier versions at the expense of their local contextual meanings is a feature of all scientific endeavour. It is a way of presenting science as a continuous, cumulative development. Lister and Cheyne 'naturally' saw the past like that. It was only an extension of what had been happening for thirty-odd years. Lister represented each bit of theory change as a more precise articulation of what he knew all along.

By the 1890s Lister's name had become firmly linked by the medical community at large to asepsis and infective germ theory. The germ theory of putrefaction had fallen into desuetude. To our knowledge Lister never used the term again. A book reviewer in the *BMJ* of 1891 chided an author as follows:

> In the glossary we read "sepsis the condition of putrefaction". This is not the case; septic infection may take place without putrefaction, and *mere* putrefactive change does not cause septicaemia.[156]

Listerian antiseptic surgery, if not Lister's own practice, was changing too. The spray had been dropped. Dry aseptic gauze, in some cases impregnated with an antiseptic, was increasingly used as the only dressing. The protective slowly declined in use. Godlee recorded this, noting (perhaps inadvertently) that this decline was a consequence of the abandonment of other Listerian practices:

> improved dressings and improved technique, especially the more sparing use of antiseptic materials at operations and consequent diminution of discharge, have, however, rendered a protective less necessary than formerly. It has thus almost passed out of use, and its meaning has been forgotten, but the term survives and is applied, now to one material now to another, according to the whim of the pharmaceutical chemist.[157]

As far as modes of healing were concerned, first intention became the general goal. Apposition of the skin was seen as the surest safeguard against sepsis.[158] But in very severe fractures, or when the 'surfaces of the wound cannot be brought together', healing by blood clot was permitted.[159] The use of drains diminished, being cited as a source of infection.[160]

It was, however, the Listerians' account of the past which was taken as an accurate record. By the early twentieth century Lister could even be credited with being the author of the reform of hospital architecture. As one author put it,

> If you visit a large hospital to-day, the influence of Lord Lister's antiseptic and aseptic principles is very marked . . . Enter the new aseptic operating theatres, for instance, of St Thomas's Hospital, and what do you find? The walls are of white marmorite, a substance that is beautifully clear and hard, the invention of a clever Belgian; white enamel looks down at you from the ceiling; mosaic meets your eye on the floor. The tiers of seats at the back are of solid white marble, so that no dust shall collect in any hollow, crack or crevice. The sinks and taps are specially adapted for their purpose of harbouring no dust or microbes, and the whole room is a paradise of cleanliness.[161]

The reasons why the Listerians had triumphed cannot be dealt with here. They are linked to much wider issues, especially the Listerians' espousal of a variety of causes: laboratory science, university and hospital-based medical education, animal experimentation, Darwinian evolution, cerebral localisation: that whole network of related ideologies that comprise late Victorian naturalism. Lister and most of his supporters were, through and through, the champions of these causes. As medicine moved in the direction defined as desirable by the Listerians, in part because of their wider reforming activities, recent rapid change could be identified as being based on their labours. The 'revolution' in surgery was presented as their achievement and attributed to their employment of basic science. Given the heroic style of Victorian thought, and of Victorian science in particular, it is not surprising that Lister was endowed by his followers with the attributes of hero and revolutionary. Indeed he cast himself in that mould. German germ theory and asepsis, the theoretical and practical pillars of modern surgery, were adopted by the Listerians whose own theories and practices might have led to a quite different sort of surgery; equally successful perhaps, but different. The practices and goals of aseptic surgery – simplicity of dressing and first intention healing – had their origins as much or more in the natural school as they did in Lister's work.[162] German germ theory was quite unlike the germ theory of putrefaction which Lister employed for twenty-five years. Yet both theory and practice were then, as now, regularly traced to early Listerian formulations.

In a paper in *The Lancet* of 12 September 1891 Lawson Tait spotted this curious lineage and he tersely referred to the use of antiseptics as a 'strange phrase of surgical eccentricity'.[163] Shortly afterwards he gave an interesting historical summary:

> The old word 'phlogiston,' and the theories attached to it [were] . . . an elaborate system of quackery. Yet the terms employed in connexion with it, such as 'antiphlogistic,' survived as everyday terms in the legitimate practice of medicine and surgery so late as my own pupillage, and this survival depended entirely upon the fact that they had absolutely changed their meanings and conveyed no sense of the purport which they had in their early invention. So it is now with the word 'antiseptics,' and [surgeons now use] . . . that word as applied to practice and theory alike in a way which is perfectly different from the method of its use twenty and fifteen years ago . . . Lister's antiseptic doctrines and practice were based upon a conception altogether false . . . A belief that the phenomena which were induced by the admission of germs to a dead infusion of hay or of beef were paralleled by the pathological processes of inflammation, and that the aim and object of the treatment of our surgical operations and surgical wounds were to be the chemical destruction or mechanical exclusion of germs . . . The Listerism of twenty and fifteen and twelve and ten years ago is dead. Each wave of altering principle and different detail killed the wave in front of it . . . To the young school of graduates and dentists who use the word 'antiseptics' in a sense altogether new and outside the discussion of which I am speaking, my words may seem strange and startling, but they are strange only because the line of practice which I advocated at the time is now being universally adopted . . . For my own part, to hear the men who wildly proclaimed the necessity of performing surgical operations under a cloud or a stream of potent chemical germicides, declaring now that the essence of their doctrine and their practice was, not the destruction of germs, nor their exclusion, but simple scrupulous cleanliness, is, to say the least of it, startling.[164]

Epilogue

The representatory tradition begun by Lister and Cheyne was continued by the biographers and has been accepted ever since. The germ theory of putrefaction has been elided into the modern pathology of inflammation. Putrefaction has become suppuration, healing in a clot has become first intention healing. In particular the term 'infection' has usefully served to conflate early Listerism and modern theory. In fact the earlier biographers were much more accurate in their accounts than later ones. The most substantial and still highly readable account of Lister is the biography by his nephew, Rickman Godlee, published in 1917. Godlee addressed Lister's early work on inflammation, which he represented as follows:

> That putrefaction or decomposition – which for him were then synonymous terms – caused suppuration and wound infection; and that wound infection did not occur without suppuration.[165]

Once again suppuration is identified as the danger. In addition, the introduction of the term 'infection' here invites a modern gloss. Lister, however, rarely used the term in the early days.

Although brief the most accurate account of Lister's pathological views is that in Watson Cheyne's biography:

> As a matter of fact, Lister overrated his first success because at that time he looked on the presence or absence of *putrefaction* as the criterion of failure or success – and most of the cases were free from putrefaction. It was not till later that he adopted *suppuration* as a truer criterion.[166]

How much later, however, Cheyne does not say, for suppuration was explained away in Lister's wounds until the 1880s. Besides, both Cheyne and Godlee emphasised the point that Lister's achievement was his recognition that the source of surgical mischief was 'germs'. The nature of these germs, however, was not explained. Once again the reader, without further guidance, would simply identify them with modern concepts. But Lister's germs of 1867 were quite different from the germs of today. His support of the germ theory of putrefaction was relatively unusual. His support of Koch was, possibly, less ardent than that of some of his contemporaries. By the time of Hector Cameron's biography of 1949 the story had become further collapsed: 'Infection and suppuration of wounds, [Lister] . . . became convinced, must be due to the entry into the wound of hosts of minute, living, airborne organisms, comparable to yeast'.[167] More recent accounts have continued to employ what now may be fairly called Listerian historiographical assumptions. Cartwright's careful and informative sketch of 1968 came close to seeing the vast differences between 1867 and 1900, but still presented the change as a simple and necessary development.[168] Fox makes a great deal of the difference between asepsis and Listerian antisepsis but has no account of the historical process by which the one was considered to be the father of the other. Granshaw's account is a detailed historical picture of the various views on antisepsis that surgeons adopted, but the degree of transformation that went on in Listerian theory is missing.[169]

In conclusion, therefore, we have argued that a history of the theories and practices employed by the Listerians can be written as a history of meaning change. Using this approach it is possible to see how Lister's supporters and biographers have been able to describe his surgery of 1867 as 'revolutionary'. For if the ideas of the 1890s are read into Listerian ideas of the 1860s his work does look fundamentally different from that of his contemporaries. Undeniably there was a major transformation, a revolution even, in surgery between the late 1860s and the 1890s, but it is possible to see it, not as deriving from a single sudden innovation engineered by a small group (the Listerians) but as the accumulation of many small deviations from intellectual and practical routine among the surgical community *as a whole*. This analysis of the 'Listerian revolution' endorses Barnes's interpretation of Kuhn.[170] In adopting this view we bring ourselves in line with other recent historical work which sees a 'revolution' in science not as an innate, necessary or essential event but as a term which is deployed, as one historian has noted, 'by interested parties, historical actors or historians, seeking to explain the process [of change]'. Listerism perfectly illustrates this historian's view that a case for 'revolution can almost always be made out by selectively stressing certain aspects of change at the expense of others'.[171]

Acknowledgements

We are grateful to Christopher Hamlin, Michael Worboys and John Pickstone for comments on an earlier draft of this paper.

Notes and references

1. Nicholas J. Fox, 'Scientific theory choice and social structure: the case of Joseph Lister's antisepsis, humoral theory and asepsis', *History of Science*, vol. 26 (1988), pp. 367–97; Lindsay Granshaw, '"Upon this principle I have based a practice": the development and reception of antisepsis in Britain, 1867–1890', in John Pickstone (ed.), *Medical Innovations in Historical Perspective* (Macmillan, London, 1992).

2. For the most part this paper will dwell on the works of Lister and Cheyne. However, many other surgeons identified themselves with Lister's views in the period under discussion. For convenience we will use the term Listerians.

3. Richard B. Fisher, *Joseph Lister* (MacDonald & Jane's, London, 1977), pp. 131–2.

4. Fielding H. Garrison, *An Introduction to the History of Medicine*, 4th edn (W. B. Saunders Co., Philadelphia, 1929), p. 589.

5. Rickman John Godlee, *Lord Lister* (Macmillan, London, 1917), p. 137, our emphasis.

6. But see Granshaw, 'Development and reception' and David Hamilton, 'The nineteenth-century surgical revolution: antisepsis or better nutrition?', *Bulletin of the History of Medicine*, vol. 56 (1982), pp. 30–40.

7. J. Paget, 'Wounds', in T. Holmes (ed.), *A System of Surgery*, 4 vols (John W. Parker, London, 1860–4), vol. 1, p. 583.

8. Ibid., p. 584.

9. Ibid., p. 598.

10. Ibid., p. 586.

11. Ibid., p. 588.

12. Ibid., p. 594.

13. The term primary union was sometimes used synonymously with first intention healing. This creates problems since Lister also used primary union to describe all non-granulating healing. The context of the debates, however, always makes clear which meaning was applied and will be pointed out in what follows.

14. On the taxonomy of pus see Holmes Coote, 'Abscess', in Holmes, *System*, p. 143.

15. John Simon, 'Inflammation', in Holmes, *System*, p. 90.

16. Ibid., p. 30.

17. Nutrition was the fundamental classifying category in mid- and late nineteenth-century pathology. Tissue changes evidenced too much of it, too little, morbid forms, etc. See T. Henry Green, *An Introduction to Pathology and Morbid Anatomy* (London, 1871). On the history of inflammation as a necessary healing process which could get

out of hand, see L. J. Rather, *Addison and the White Corpuscles* (Wellcome Institute of the History of Medicine, London, 1972).

18. Margaret Pelling, *Cholera, Fever and English Medicine 1825–1865* (Oxford University Press, Oxford, 1978); John M. Eyler, *Victorian Social Medicine: the Ideas and Methods of William Farr* (Johns Hopkins University Press, Baltimore, 1979); Christopher Hamlin, 'Providence and putrefaction: Victorian sanitarians and the natural theology of health and disease', *Victorian Studies*, vol. 28 (1985), pp. 382–411; *What Becomes of Pollution: Adversary Science and the Controversy on the Self-Purification of Rivers in Britain, 1850–1900* (Garland, New York, 1987); *A Science of Impurity: Water Analysis in Nineteenth Century Britain* (Adam Hilger, Bristol, 1990); cf. John Crellin, 'The dawn of the germ theory: particles, infection and biology' in F. N. L. Poynter (ed.), *Medicine and Science in the 1860s* (Wellcome Institute of the History of Medicine, London, 1958), pp. 57–76. Despite the anachronism this is an extremely useful paper.

19. William Savory, 'Some statistics of pyaemia', *St Bartholomew's Hospital Reports*, vol. 3 (1867), pp. 17–85: 73.

20. *British Medical Journal*, vol. ii (1864), p. 195.

21. Robert Liston on hospital gangrene, in *Elements of Surgery*, 2nd edn (Longman, London, 1840), p. 235.

22. *British Medical Journal*, vol. ii (1864), p. 195.

23. Spencer Wells, 'Some causes of excessive mortality after surgical operations', *British Medical Journal*, vol. ii (1864), pp. 384–8: 385.

24. See Hamlin, *Pollution*, pp. 93–107.

25. James Watson, 'Carbolic acid', *Edinburgh Medical Journal*, vol. 9 (1864), pp. 625–7.

26. Joseph Lister, *The Collected Papers of Joseph, Baron Lister*, 2 vols (Clarendon Press, Oxford, 1909), vol. 2, p. 270.

27. Ibid., p. 272. Lister was distinguishing the reparative and pathological aspects of inflammation by invoking different mechanisms. See Rather, *Addison*.

28. Ibid., vol. 2, p. 2.

29. Ibid., p. 1.

30. Ibid., p. 2.

31. Ibid.

32. Lister's pronouncements on the ability of germs to invade living tissue offers space for multiple interpretations. When discussing wounds, in most contexts he insisted on the power of living tissue to resist germs. This later became a 'principle' (see below). He never made clear, however, whether the 'putrid exhalations' which could cause, say, erysipelas were living agents which entered the body or were chemical products.

33. Lister, *Works*, vol. 2, pp. 2–3.

34. Ibid., p. 75.

35. Ibid., p. 5.

36. Ibid., pp. 34, 32.

37. Ibid., p. 37.

38. On the inadequacy of this as a description see Hamlin, *Pollution*.

39. Lister, *Works*, vol. 2, p. 37, emphasis in original.

40. Ibid., p. 2.

41. Ibid., p. 39. This is an extremely good example of the difficulties of interpreting contemporary views of suppuration. Lister seems to have been appealing to some general surgical criterion by which suppuration was used as an indication of something amiss.

42. Ibid., pp. 40–1.

43. Ibid., p. 45. See note 32 above.

44. Ibid., pp. 47, 50.

45. Ibid., pp. 54, 57.

46. Just before this time, Lister seems to have regarded granulation as identical to the process of organisation occurring under a scab, for he described how in one case the dressing fell off, 'disclosing a small superficial granulating sore, without the slightest suppuration, just as in ordinary healing by scabbing', *Works*, vol. 2, p. 7.

47. The details of the dressings used by Lister were changed considerably by him over the years but the central assumption remained: a massive germicidal layer must be placed between the wound and the air and the wound must also be protected from the germicidal layer.

48. Lister, *Works*, vol. 2, p. 74.

49. Ibid., p. 82. Lister here denominated his technique as producing 'primary union', that is union without granulation.

50. Ibid., p. 148.

51. Ibid., pp. 142, 143, 146.

52. *British Medical Journal*, vol. ii (1874), p. 383.

53. Isabelle M. Z. Elliott and J. R. Elliott, *A Short History of Surgical Dressings* (The Pharmaceutical Press, London, 1964) makes this quite clear if the book is read without privileging Lister. See also Granshaw, 'Development and reception'.

54. 'Carbolic acid in the London hospitals', *Medical Times and Gazette*, vol. ii (1867), pp. 575–6: 576. See also *The Lancet*, vol. ii (1867), pp. 277, 299, 575, 787; *British Medical Journal*, vol. ii (1867), pp. 472, 556. For a good review of responses see Granshaw, 'Development and reception'.

55. *The Lancet*, vol. ii (1867), p. 502.

56. *Medical Times and Gazette*, vol. ii (1868), p. 465.

57. *British Medical Journal*, vol. ii (1869), pp. 152–3, our emphasis.

58. Lister, *Works*, vol. 2, pp. 479, 482. It is significant that Lister uses the phrase 'living organisms *developed* from germs'. At this time he had a view of micro-organisms as very plastic and tentatively proposed that septic organisms were the buds of yeasts. *Works*, vol. 1, pp. 275–307, 309–34. The word 'germ' carried a connotation of its original meaning as germinal or original. The 1869 paper may well have been a response to John Hughes Bennett, *On the Atmospheric Germ Theory and Origin of Infusoria* (Adam & Charles Black, Edinburgh, 1868). Bennett, professor at Edinburgh, proposed that the 'germs [which] were the cause of putrefaction', were 'imaginary', p. 24.

59. Lister, *Works*, vol. 2, p. 147.

60. Ibid., p. 149.

61. Ibid., pp. 148–9.

62. Ibid., pp. 123–4, 135–6. The similarity of this to Edwin Chadwick's reduction of disease to a single determining cause and a denial of the significance of multiple accessory causes (diet, ventilation, cleanliness, etc.) is striking.

63. Holmes Coote, 'On the treatment of wounds', *St Bartholomew's Hospital Reports*, vol. 6 (1870), pp. 113–17: 113–14.

64. Lister, *Works*, vol. 2, pp. 166–7.

65. Ibid., pp. 172–98, 175–7, 183.

66. *Edinburgh Medical Journal*, vol. 15 (1870), p. 177.

67. Edward Lund, *Antisepticity in Surgery*, (J. E. Cornish, Manchester, 1872), p. 8.

68. *British Medical Journal*, vol. ii (1873), p. 146.

69. *The Lancet*, vol. ii (1873), p. 184, our emphasis.

70. Ibid., p. 432.

71. Ibid., p. 470.

72. Lister, *Works*, vol. 1, p. 277.

73. Ibid., pp. 309–10.

74. Ibid., p. 306.

75. Ibid., p. 333.

76. Ibid., p. 304.

77. Ibid., p. 277.

78. *The Lancet*, vol. ii (1875), p. 743.

79. *Medical Times and Gazette*, vol. ii (1875), p. 575.

80. Lister, *Works*, vol. 2, p. 254.

81. Ibid., p. 219.

82. Ibid., p. 265, our emphasis. See also note 27.

83. T. Longmore, *Amputation; an Historical Sketch* (Bell & Bain, Glasgow, 1876), p. 24.

84. *The Lancet*, vol. ii (1875), p. 597.

85. Sampson Gamgee, 'Wound treatment', *The Lancet*, vol. ii (1878), p. 869.

86. Sampson Gamgee, 'Absorbent and medicated surgical dressings', *Lancet*, vol. ii (1880), pp. 127–8.

87. William Roberts, 'The doctrine of contagium vivum', *Medical Times and Gazette*, vol. ii (1877), p. 142, emphasis in original.

88. Ibid.

89. Ibid. The hospital fevers, Roberts noted, although they appeared to be similar to the specific infections, were in fact quite different. They were produced when putrefactive organisms modified by local conditions became parasitic on living tissues. He observed,

> To me it appears that, under a certain concurrence of conditions in and about the wound, a modification takes place in the vital endowments of the septic organism, whereby it acquires a parasitic habit, which enables it to breed in tissues of degraded vitality, or even in the healthy tissues, and in this way to produce the infective endemic pyaemia which we sometimes witness in the wards of our large hospitals.

This was a view not so different from that elaborated by Lister a few years earlier.

90. Lister, *Works*, vol. 1, pp. 335–8.

91. Lister, *Works*, vol. 2, pp. 443, 446, 447.

92. William Savory, 'Prevention of blood poisoning in the practice of surgery', *British Medical Journal*, vol. ii (1879), pp. 211–12.

93. *The Lancet*, vol. ii (1879), p. 246, our emphasis.

94. *British Medical Journal*, vol. ii (1879), pp. 906, 1000; *The Lancet*, vol. ii (1879), pp. 850, 902.

95. *British Medical Journal*, vol. ii (1879), pp. 1001–2.

96. Ibid., p.1002.

97. Ibid., p. 1004.

98. W. Watson Cheyne, 'On the relations of organisms to antiseptic dressings', *Transactions of the Pathological Society*, vol. 30 (1879), pp. 557–82. On the history of micrococci in this period see the valuable paper by Leonard G. Wilson, 'The early recognition of streptococci as causes of disease', *Medical History*, vol. 31 (1987), pp. 403–14. Our perspective on Cheyne's perceptions is quite different from Wilson's.

99. *The Lancet*, vol. i (1879), p. 703.

100. For a measure of the warm reception of German work see 'Report . . . by the Pathological Society . . . [on] pyaemia septicaemia and purulent infection', *Transactions of the Pathological Society*, vol. 30 (1879), pp. 1–188.

101. On the increasing use of this model see W. F. Bynum, '"C'est un malade": animal models and concepts of human disease', *Journal of the History of Medicine*, vol. 45 (1990), pp. 397–413.

102. Robert Koch, *Investigations into the Etiology of Traumatic Infective Diseases*, translated by W. Watson Cheyne (The New Sydenham Society, London, 1880), pp. 64–5.

103. *The Lancet*, vol. i (1880), p. 250.

104. *Medical Times and Gazette*, vol. i (1880), p. 355, our emphasis.

105. *British Medical Journal*, vol. ii (1880), p. 340.

106. Ibid., p. 342.

107. Ibid., p. 341.

108. Ibid.

109. Lister, *Works*, vol. 1, pp. 388–9. On the problem of interpreting Lister's views on the possibility of 'germs' invading the body see note 31.

110. Ibid., p. 391.

111. Ibid., p. 389.

112. Ibid., vol. 2, p. 279.

113. Ibid., p. 280. We are not aware of where, if at all, in print Lister had earlier ascribed the antibacterial power of the blood to white corpuscles. Curiously, however, if he did ever hold that view he was retreating from it in spite of the fact that Cohnheim's work on white corpuscle migration was gaining approval. Lister, as far as we know, did not refer to Cohnheim's work until some years later. On the white cell theory see Rather, *Addison*.

114. In a footnote Lister also claimed that, in 1864, he was the first

to recognise that new cell formation in coagula was a healthy restorative process and that in certain circumstances, as, for instance, when adjacent to putrefying matter, this process simply became pus formation.

> The development of cells of new formation in organising coagula within the living body, first ascertained, so far as I am aware, by myself in 1864, has been the subject of various observations of late years, especially by German pathologists, as, for example, Tillmanns. That this cell development may, under some circumstances, go on to genuine suppuration is a fact I believe not hitherto published by any pathologist, though the truth of the occasional conversion of coagula into pus has always seemed to me sufficiently apparent from the naked-eye appearances of suppurative phlebitis and the beautiful experiments of Cruveilhier. (Ibid., p. 285).

This is an interesting recollection in the light of his earlier claim that he had not had time to investigate organisation in coagula (see note 82) and that in the early 1860s he seems to have regarded granulation and organisation as the same (see note 46).

115. Ibid., pp. 282–5, our emphasis.

116. Ibid., pp. 284–5.

117. Ibid., pp. 288–9.

118. *The Lancet*, vol. ii (1881), pp. 424–5. Primary union here means first intention healing.

119. Lister, *Works*, vol. 2, p. 289.

120. Ibid., vol. 1, pp. 399–400.

121. Ibid., p. 407.

122. Ibid., pp. 408–9. Wilson, 'Early recognition', calls this paper an 'embarrassing lapse on the part of the great man', and notes 'He cited no experiments' (p. 410). But he could have done so; Cheyne's experimental work was held to refute German views.

123. W. Watson Cheyne, *Antiseptic Surgery* (Smith, Elder & Co., London, 1882), p. 51, emphasis in original.

124. Ibid.

125. Ibid., p. 76.

126. Ibid., pp. 256, 258.

127. Ibid., p. 263.

128. Ibid., p. 266.

129. Ibid., emphasis in original.

130. Ibid., p. 274.

131. Ibid., p. 276.

132. Ibid., p. 282, emphasis in original.

133. Ibid., p. 85.

134. Ibid., pp. 287–8, our emphasis except *principles.*

135. W. Watson Cheyne, 'Report on micrococci in relation to wounds, abscesses and septic processes', *British Medical Journal*, vol. ii (1884), pp. 553–6.

136. Ibid., pp. 599–604.

137. Ibid., pp. 644–8.
138. Lister, *Works*, vol. 2, p. 293.
139. Ibid., pp. 293, 300.
140. Ibid., p. 293.
141. John Wood, 'Antiseptics in surgery', *British Medical Journal*, vol. ii (1885), pp. 1095–7, 1147–9.
142. *Medical Times and Gazette*, vol. ii (1885), pp. 845–6.
143. *British Medical Journal*, vol. ii (1888), p. 195.
144. W. Cheyne, *Suppuration and Septic Diseases* (Young J. Pentland, Edinburgh, 1889), pp. 56, 82. By this time not to have accepted the by-now extensive German work on the micrococci would have left the Listerians very isolated; see Wilson, 'Early recognition'.
145. Cheyne, *Suppuration*, p. ix.
146. Ibid., p. 91.
147. Ibid., p. 14.
148. Ibid., p. 22.
149. Ibid., pp. 27–9.
150. Ibid., p. 54.
151. Ibid., pp. vi–viii, our emphasis.
152. See note 138 above.
153. Lister, *Works*, vol. 2, p. 334.
154. Ibid., p. 341. This paper was first published in *Virchow – Festschrift*, Bd. iii (1891).
155. W. W. Cheyne, 'Aseptic and antiseptic surgery', *The Lancet*, vol. i (1903), p. 347. Cheyne was actually being mildly critical of what he saw as an expensive, elaborate, surgery which dispensed with antiseptics.
156. *British Medical Journal*, vol. i (1891), p. 970.
157. Godlee, *Lister*, pp. 217–18.
158. C. B. Lockwood, *Aseptic Surgery in Theory and Practice* (Harrison & Sons, London, 1904), p. 33.
159. William Johnson Walsham, *Surgery: Its Theory and Practice*, 6th edn (J. & A. Churchill, London, 1897), pp. 95, 172–3.
160. Lockwood, *Aseptic Surgery*, p. 36.
161. F. M. Holmes, *Surgeons and their Wonderful Discoveries* (London, S. W. Partridge & Co. [1902?]), p. 50.
162. Fox, 'Scientific theory', spots this but the historical process is not identified. Granshaw, 'Development and reception', does so too but the significance of Lister's changing theory is missing.
163. Lawson Tait, 'Details necessary in the performance of abdominal section', *The Lancet*, vol. ii (1891), p. 597.
164. Ibid., p. 896.
165. Godlee, *Lister*, p. 163. Godlee's biography is revealing. It is a celebration of the triumphal entry of basic science into medicine. Although it was published during the war Godlee was still prepared to hint at the superiority of German university education (p. 331). Godlee perceived and prized exactly what the Listerian triumph entailed.
166. W. Watson Cheyne, *Lord Lister and his Achievement* (Longmans, London, 1925), p. 19.
167. Hector Charles Cameron, *Joseph Lister: the Friend of Man*

(Heinemann, London, 1949), p. 60.

168. F. F. Cartwright, 'Antiseptic surgery', in Poynter, *Medicine and Science*, pp. 77–104.

169. Fox, 'Scientific theory'; Granshaw, 'Development and reception'.

170. For the model of revolution and change employed here see Barry Barnes, *T. S. Kuhn and Social Science* (New York, Columbia University Press, 1982), pp. 83–90.

171. John A. Schuster, 'The scientific revolution', in R. C. Olby, G. N. Cantor, J. R. R. Christie and M. J. S. Hodge (eds), *Companion to the History of Modern Science* (Routledge, London, 1990), pp. 217–42: 222–3.

7

From conservative to radical surgery in late nineteenth-century America

Gert H. Brieger

At the semi-centennial celebration of the American Medical Association in 1897 Dr William W. Keen, one of the country's leading surgeons, summarised the state of his field and neatly framed the subject of this paper:

> Two dramatically opposing tendencies are prominent in modern surgery; radical interference with disease so that there is now scarcely an organ or portion of the body not within our reach; yet on the other hand, a remarkably conservative tendency in cultivating remedial rather than radical surgery.[1]

For Keen's contemporaries his distinction between conservative and radical may have been clear enough. Yet in the last decades of the nineteenth century radical could also mean conservative in the sense of complete or finally curative: conservative of life. Although in this quotation Keen seems to have opposed radical to conservative, or even operative to non-operative, he was well aware that the operative approach was often the more conservative choice if using the tools of the new surgery of his day. In what follows I will show the historical connections of the conservative and the radical approaches to surgical therapies in nineteenth-century America. I shall argue that by the late nineteenth century, because of scientific developments in surgery, the tradition of maximum conservation of the integrity of the body was seen as compatible with the notion of the complete cure of disease and malformation. Thus both conservative surgery and the radical treatment of hernia, thyroid tumours, cancer of the breast and prostatic hypertrophy became common approaches in the new scientific surgery of the early twentieth century. Furthermore, this new surgery, I shall suggest, moved away from the drama and theatricality of the operation itself to the drama of the results.

In the following pages I shall relate some of the developments in surgical practice to surgical thought in the six or seven decades following the advent of anaesthesia. Surgical thinking is far more difficult to describe than are the more readily visible and manifest surgical practices. To find a means of assessing surgical thought we must resort to the modes of medical and surgical discourse common at the time. It will be important therefore to develop definitions of the words or the notions that were then in use. I will confine myself to only three terms; all, as I hope to show, are important to each other and crucial to our understanding of the role of surgery in the medical practices of the late nineteenth and early twentieth centuries. I use the term 'medical' here and throughout the following discussion to signify medicine, the medical profession, and medical practices as a whole. I generally do not use medical to signify non-surgical or non-operative modes of therapy. So when I speak of the medical profession, I mean to include all varieties of doctors, surgical as well as non-surgical.

The three specific terms I shall discuss in some detail are conservative, radical and heroic, each connected to a whole set of notions. I will trace their interconnections, and end by attempting to bring them together in the work and the thought of one of the most influential of American surgical teachers, William Stewart Halsted.

Conservative surgery

Turning first to the idea of conservation and conservative as they were applied to medical practices in the last century, we will see that it was the surgeons who were credited with the introduction of this mode of medical thought. Conservative, in the *Oxford English Dictionary* definition, means characterised by a tendency to preserve or keep intact or unchanged. It was mainly in this preservative sense that the notion of conservative surgery was used in the middle of the nineteenth century. Specifically the term was first applied to resection of parts of bones, leaving sufficient periosteum behind for healing to take place.

Resection rather than amputation was the hallmark of conservative surgery. This preservative approach to sepsis and injury of bones, common occurrences in the experience of physicians in the middle of the nineteenth century, would later come to have an even more profound effect upon both surgical technique and surgical thinking. Despite what the term indicates, the appearance of a conservative point of view had a dramatic consequence for widening the basis of surgery as therapy. Amputation was no longer inevitable in injury or sepsis. No longer was the image of the surgeon to be tied to either heroic feats or to a cut and slash daring with which it had so often been associated.

The classic visual representation of conservative surgery is the 1875 painting by Thomas Eakins of Samuel D. Gross, with bloody scalpel in hand, removing a piece of bone from the femur of his patient, in full view of his class of students. I have discussed this representation extensively elsewhere but a few points bear repetition.[2] The conservative surgery of the bones of the arm or leg, although created prior to anaesthesia, was vastly assisted by it. As Theodor Billroth aptly noted about resection of a piece of bone, 'the operation is a very violent one, and the chiselling, sawing, and hammering about the bony case appear horrible to a looker on, especially as the operation may require a great deal of time. An amputation is a trifle in comparison with it.'[3]

Samuel D. Gross gave credit for the concept of conservative surgery to Dr Philip Syng Physik, an early nineteenth-century Philadelphia surgeon.[4] Be that as it may, as early as 1837, nearly a decade prior to the introduction of ether in Boston, Dr Robley Dunglison was writing about a new approach to surgery. Dunglison, of whom Gross said he was the most intelligent of his medical community, taught at the universities of Virginia and Maryland and for over three decades at the Jefferson Medical College in Philadelphia along with Gross.[5]

In 1837 Dunglison published a well-received guide for medical students of the day. In it he described new and improved surgical instruments that allowed operations unknown in the eighteenth century to be performed, now with some hope of success. The surgeon, for instance, no longer had to stand idly by while patients afflicted with aneurysms of major arteries inevitably died. Today we are so accustomed to see surgery as based on science, that we forget a similar view existed virtually throughout the nineteenth century. Dunglison, 150 years ago, held that much of the progress of surgery was owing to the 'discoveries of modern science'.[6] It was by no means only in the operative part of surgery of the time that surgical advance occurred. 'The skilful and benevolent surgeon', Dunglison explained to prospective medical students, 'has more gratification in saving a limb which has been doomed to the knife, than in his most brilliant operations.'[7]

By the middle of the nineteenth century more thoughtful surgeons were becoming concerned by the way in which some physicians and medical students were exploiting the potential drama of major surgical intervention rather than practising careful conservation. Henry J. Bigelow, a leading Boston surgeon and teacher, pointed out that 'Animal sense is always fascinated by the presence of animal suffering'. The surgeon, Bigelow warned, was all too prone to encourage an undue appreciation of surgery, an attitude too readily accepted by the public.[8]

Similarly, John Watson, one of the surgeons to the New York Hospital, in a lecture to the clinical students there in 1846, voiced a growing sentiment among surgeons who were the teachers and the authors of surgical books and papers. They often cautioned their students about the morbid appetite for surgical operations. 'Surgery', Watson ended his lecture, 'is a good thing, a useful, an excellent thing in its way; but too much of it is a great evil. And the sooner you find this out for yourselves, the better for your patients.'[9] The true reputation of a surgeon, Stephen Smith (another New York surgical teacher) wrote a decade and a half later, was now based not on the number of limbs amputated, but on the number saved from amputation.[10] The goal of this conservative surgery was to prevent deformity and to save arms and legs. Samuel Gross drew the specific parallel between prevention and conservation:

> the discovery has been made that the true function of medicine is to prevent rather than to cure disease. Surgery, during the last thirty years, has achieved some of its proudest triumphs in preventing pain, and in saving limb and life.[11]

One of the earliest references I have found to notions with the specific name 'conservative surgery' appeared in an editorial of the *New York Medical Gazette* in 1853. Here the unnamed writer claimed that it was the duty of the surgeon to cure, not merely to cut. The conditions which prompted this three-and-a-half-page closely printed editorial were graphically described.

> No department of our profession attracts so much eclat from the populace, nor awakens the ambition of the medical tyro to such an extent, as do the *operations of surgery*. By the former they are looked upon as evidences of bravery, daring, and skill, just in proportion to their desperate character, and without the least reference to their necessity or propriety, or even to their fatal results. The more bloody, and even the more uniformly fatal, the higher is the huzza of the ignorant and vulgar multitude for the surgeon, so called, who figures in these "deeds of blood". Hence, students and junior practitioners will often run miles to witness a capital operation, and ransack neighborhoods and cities to find patients whose surgical diseases will furnish them opportunities to *cut*, or to witness *cutting*, performed by others. And they too become partakers in the popular idolatry of the *mere operators*, whose frenzy for the use of scalpel and saw, mallet and chisel, and even the red hot iron, upon the living bodies of their victims, becomes a passion, which too often degrades surgery into human butchery. And the ambition to learn surgery upon the living body, instead of the dead subject, and thus share the ephemeral reputation of being called surgeons, too often seduces students from the diligent cultivation of the *science* of surgery, which includes the whole of medicine among its principles, into the degrading pursuit of the mere *art*, which requires little study, and promises distinction among the ignorant multitude, though at the expense of self-respect and all professional character worthy of possession.[12]

This call for principles of surgery that could constitute its science was more frequently heard in the following decade, a period of bloody wars in the Crimea and between the northern and southern states in America. By 1861 Stephen Smith could claim that conservative surgery was the 'problem of our time', by which he meant that all surgeons should practise it whenever possible.[13] Smith's Bellevue Hospital colleague Austin Flint wrote most extensively about conservative medicine as a whole in the next few years. To surgeons Flint gave the credit for popularising the need for a conservative medicine.

'The conservative surgeon', Flint wrote in 1862, 'aims to preserve the integrity of the body . . . He weighs carefully the dangers of operations so as not to incur too much risk of shortening life by resorting to the scalpel.'[14] Flint clearly related the conservative practices of the careful surgeon to those of his colleagues who treated by means of medications only. These too must not be prescribed in a merely routine way with an unsparing hand. Not only might a limb be preserved, but life itself might be spared.

Radical surgery

The second term that requires brief definition is 'radical'. Derived from the Latin word for root, radical is often contrasted to conservative. I will attempt to show that there was an evolution from a conservative to a radical surgery. Here I simply mean radical as complete, in the attempt to cure the patient of disease. The idea was to get at the root of the problem, thereby achieving a radical or a permanent cure. I do not mean radical in the way it was sometimes used around 1890 to signify merely an eagerness to operate, while 'conservative' in that context was associated with a hesitancy to do surgery.

In the last decade of the nineteenth century the surgical literature is filled with discussions of the merits and techniques of the radical approach. After Reginald Fitz published his classic paper on appendicitis in 1886, this disorder became the typical example of the radical form of surgery.[15] Operation was to occur early, and the inflamed appendix was to be totally excised. But the radical approach was also used in the treatment of thyroid tumours, prostatic and uterine diseases, cancer of the breast and in the repair of inguinal hernias. We are referring then to a surgical philosophy that can only be understood in the context of the developments in cellular pathology and in bacteriology, both of which have been admirably discussed by Peter English.[16] Radical surgery also developed in the context of an ever-increasing specialisation, even among surgeons. Orville Horowitz of Philadelphia, for instance, in a review of 150 cases of radical operations for prostatic hypertrophy in 1904, noted that 'It must not be forgotten that, in the present day, surgery is divided into many special branches; hence the general surgeon does not have an opportunity to see and operate on many prostatic cases.'[17]

Conservatism in an age of radical surgery was a paradox not lost on the surgical writers around the turn of the century. The most common way to reconcile these seemingly different surgical philosophies was to distinguish clearly between rashness and boldness. Careful diagnosis and a full understanding of the underlying disease processes, together with the aid of the new laboratory methods, were the prerequisites for the judicious use of the knife. Many surgeons claimed that it was compatible with conservative surgery to destroy certain parts of the body in order to save others. According to this view, the judicious use of surgery in the treatment of disease was the hallmark of progressive medicine and surgery. Both conservative as well as radical surgery were thus viewed as progressive in the best sense of that term.

The notion of a radical conservatism was clarified by Maurice Richardson, an eminent Boston surgeon and Harvard teacher. Writing in the *Journal of the Wisconsin State Medical Society* in 1900, Richardson asked what the word conservatism meant when applied to acute abdominal episodes such as inflammation of the gall-bladder or the appendix. For some, he admitted, the conservative was synonymous with medical treatment or palliation. 'But', Richardson continued,

> the word may be used in quite a different way to express a line of surgical treatment called radical; when by operation under the most favorable circumstances the patient is subjected to a slight risk that he may avoid the possibilities of much greater dangers in the future. Such a line of treatment is true conservatism, – a conservation of life at the least possible risk.[18]

In discussing the proper approach to the patient with an acutely inflamed appendix, a disorder he agreed was now in 1900 being seen commonly, he stressed that the first symptoms may be caused by perforation. So the appendix should be removed at the earliest opportunity. 'I am fully convinced, therefore', Richardson claimed, 'in the treatment of acute appendicitis the only place for radicalism is in the very beginning.'[19]

Heroic surgery

The theme of the hero and of heroic deeds is most often associated with Greek mythology, with literature, and military history. Storytellers from Homer to the space age have used dangerous and bold adventures, in war or in peace, as the stuff of heroic epics. During the American presidential debates of 1988 candidates were asked about their heroes. In 1840, Thomas Carlyle published his *On Heroes, Hero-worship, and the Heroic in History*. Carlyle began by claiming that for him history was the story of the world's great men. These were the leaders of other men and of thought. It was an infinitely profitable thing, Carlyle maintained, to spend time in their company.[20]

One of the most sustained and subtle accounts of the origins of heroes in western thought is Joseph Campbell's *The Hero with a Thousand Faces*. In tracing the mythological beginnings of the hero and concluding with a brief note on the hero today, Campbell points out that the symbols and the facts of modern science and technology have replaced the timeless web of our earlier symbols. He claims that there is no hiding place for the gods 'from the searching telescope and microscope', but also that the society that once supported such gods is no more.[21] But in the realm of modern medicine, until quite recently, those who were perceived to be testing themselves most severely, those who ventured the greatest risks and garnered the highest rewards, were often those who practised by the hand, the surgeons.

The American historian Dixon Wecter, nearly half a century ago in his book *The Hero in America*, pointed out that hero-worship answered an urgent need.[22] The fan and the autograph hunter, he claimed, were native to America, and homage to heroes, whether they explored outer or inner space or won athletic contests, became a vital part of American politics and patriotism. Throughout our history we have had our political heroes – Washington, Jackson, Kennedy – our physical heroes, and our entertainer heroes. We have also had our medical heroes. Witness the publicity about such developments as a vaccine for polio or an artificial heart. Although Carlyle believed that the history of the world was the story of its great men and women, a century and a half later we no longer write the history of medicine and surgery from such a perspective.

What is, however, very much a part of the history of surgery is how surgeons viewed themselves and how they were seen by others. For many, surgeons and non-surgeons, there were and still are heroic aspects to the craft. Surgeons performed great and noble deeds that required bravery, boldness, nobility, fortitude and strength, all attributes of the hero as well. In 1850 the Boston surgeon Henry J. Bigelow was quite specific in describing the surgeon as hero. He wrote,

> The surgeon, with the public, is associated with surgical operations; and his notoriety is in measure with the belief which the world may entertain of the number or magnitude of the operations he may perform. Singular as it may seem, a surgical operation, even in the medical world, is apt to be looked upon with an undue appreciation; and even eminent physicians concede an unquestioned position to a skilful operating surgeon. So true is this, that for acquiring the notoriety which is a nucleus for surgical practice, a surgeon had better sometimes be known as the hero of extraordinary operations which have proved unsuccessful, even fatal, than as a follower of the usual routine of ordinary treatment.[23]

Bigelow warned his medical students that as a result of this view there was an arbitrary importance attached to surgical operations that was unwarranted, but unfortunately all too frequently fostered by surgeons themselves.

In his early and most explicit formulations about conservative medicine, Austin Flint in 1862 echoed the sentiments of Bigelow:

> During the last quarter of a century a change has taken place in medical sentiment as regards surgical operations. New and grand achievements in surgery seemed formerly to be the leading objects of personal ambition. To borrow a fashionable expression, they were decidedly the rage. Boldness in the use of the knife was the trait in the character of the surgeon which was most highly admired. The history of surgery during the first third of the present century is characterized by the introduction and frequent performance of numerous formidable operations. It was customary to speak of them as brilliant, and the daring surgeon enjoyed somewhat of the *éclat* which belongs to

> the hero of the battlefield. This analogy was implied when one of the greatest of our American surgeons wishing to distinguish his most brilliant exploit styled it his Waterloo operation. The change that has taken place is marked. We hear now comparatively little of terrible operations and of that sort of heroism which is associated with bloody deeds. What would once have been considered as a degree of courage to be admired is now stigmatized as rashness. It is an equivocal compliment to say of a practitioner that he is a bold surgeon.[24]

A similar change, Flint asserted, was occurring in medical practice. Heroic practice, he pointed out, was formerly a common expression that denoted the use of powerful remedies pushed to an enormous extent. Now, he claimed, diseases were being managed with little or no medication. This was the revival of the trust in nature's powers to heal. Conservatism was becoming the leading principle of medicine as well as of surgery. Heroic, depletive therapy was being moderated, as Flint noted, by a change in American medical practice that was well underway by the second quarter of the last century.

We do not have to search long to find that surgeons today still use the vocabulary once associated with a heroic image of their predecessors. To cite but one example from a recent issue of the *Journal of the American Medical Association*, Dr Bobby Alford commented on a 1906 landmark article by George Crile. Crile described his method of excision of cancers in the region of the neck, a procedure that for decades has been known as a radical neck dissection. The aim is to dissect carefully the lymphatic drainage from the face, tongue or mouth. Crile, in his description of 132 such operations, referred to them as block dissections. Only in the discussion was the notion of a radical or a less radical operation raised. Certainly by 1906 radical surgery was already being widely discussed, though the term may not yet have found truly common usage. At any rate, in 1987, Dr Alford's comment following the reprint of Dr Crile's landmark article carried the title, 'The heritage of the radical neck dissection'. In his discussion of it, Alford spoke of Crile in heroic terms. He called him imaginative and bold, and said that Crile's work revealed courage, determination, and conviction. I am not questioning Alford's conclusion that 'legions of patients throughout this century have benefited from his [Crile's] ingenuity and astuteness'.[25] I am commenting on one aspect of our medical discourse that still retains the language of the bold, conquering hero. As Dixon Wecter has described it in his chapter on how we choose our heroes, 'bravery, honesty, strength of character are the stuff for hero-worship'.[26]

William S. Halsted

Returning to one of the original meanings of conservative as tending to preserve or to conserve, it will be apparent that the technique and the philosophy of William S. Halsted is a key to our understanding of the developments in American surgery in the early decades of the twentieth century. What makes Halsted so central to this story of the transition from conservative to radical surgery is that he, as much as any surgeon of those years, typified both approaches, and was at the same time one of the most influential teachers of surgery of the period. Halsted was the epitome of the conservator in surgery. He followed the principles of careful and gentle handling of all tissues, meticulous control of bleeding, use of the finest possible sutures and the approximation of tissues with the slightest possible tension. All these distinguished Halsted's teaching and his methods in the laboratory and in the operating room.[27] Halsted's close friend, the French surgeon René Leriche, concisely summarised Halsted's place as a founder of an entire school of surgery, 'which may be described as the surgery of safety; of a technique which sacrificed everything to the immediate and future success of the operation and the welfare of the patient'.[28] Halsted's school was destined to endure because, as his Baltimore protégé J. M. T. Finney pointed out, the work was built on the solid foundation of understanding the relationship of anatomy and physiology.[29]

Here is not the place for an extended discussion of the genesis of Halsted's conservative or preservative approach to his surgical work. Some have speculated that his severe cocaine addiction prior to coming to Baltimore, and perhaps his lifelong dependence on morphine, so affected his personality and his approach to life that his surgical style was influenced. It is an intriguing hypothesis. What is important to note, though, is that Halsted viewed the careful control of bleeding as central to conservative surgery which he regarded as having been made possible by anaesthesia. He related the general reaction against bleeding as a therapeutic measure to a former reckless waste of blood during operations. Technical advances, such as the leg bandage introduced by Esmarch that allowed surgeons to operate on an artificially bloodless limb, came into use in the 1870s, a time when resort to the lancet for the treatment of fevers and other ailments was already much decreased. The preserving of the patient's blood was thus a key aspect of conservative surgery, one especially important in the decades before the ready availability of human blood for transfusion and replace- ment of blood lost from injury or operation.

As the Halsted school of meticulous surgery grew and flourished, so too did the new approach to diseases of the breast, the thyroid, the uterus, the prostate gland and to the treatment of hernia. Halsted and his students and co-workers at the Johns Hopkins Hospital introduced the radical approach to the surgery of all these organs as well as to the technique of hernia repair. The Baltimoreans were not necessarily the first nor the only surgeons writing about radical cures, radical extirpations, or radical approaches in the years around 1900. Halsted himself is closely associated with the radical surgery for cancer of the breast, with that for thyroid nodules and with an improved method for hernia repair. His student Hugh Young developed the new approach through the perineum for surgery of the prostate, and the members of Howard Kelly's department of gynaecology advocated a radical approach to the diseases of the uterus.

It was in Halsted's operating rooms that rubber gloves were used to guard against infection. The exact priority rights for the introduction of rubber gloves need not detain us here. One of the first surgeons to make routine use of them was Halsted's young associate, Joseph C. Bloodgood. Many years later Bloodgood recalled that

> Gloves in Halsted's operating room were in constant use by two members of the operative group and occasionally used by Halsted himself in operating upon joints, yet it was seven years (1896) before it became the practice of everyone who cleaned up for the operation to wear these gloves as a routine.
>
> The moment this routine use of gloves was adopted the suppuration of closed wounds, for example in inguinal

hernia, fell from more than 9 percent to less than 0.5 percent.[30]

Halsted, in a letter to Henry Pritchett in late 1910, summarised clearly the events of the previous twenty years:

> Consider the every-day, urgent problems which have been confronting the surgeon – problems involving the life of the patient – and which each actively engaged surgeon has in great part had to solve or try to solve for himself. The recognition and treatment of appendicitis, of affections of the bile passages, of the pancreas, of the kidneys. The devising of the various forms of intestinal suture, the cure of hernia, of cancer, of exophthalmic goitre. The treatment of the enlarged prostate gland, recognition and treatment of diverticula of the bladder and oesophagus, of ulcer and cancer of the stomach. The management of hemorrhage, the surgery of the arteries and veins, and in general the entire surgery of the abdominal, thoracic and cranial cavities, I might almost say of the whole body. Twenty years ago we did not know how to close an abdominal wound, nor how to make one. And as to technique, surgeons throughout the world operated, little more than ten years ago, not only without gloves or other protection, but in their every day clothes, covered usually by a rubber apron taken from a hook and used day after day and week after week without sterilization.[31]

Halsted was too reticent a man to point out to Pritchett that much of the capsule history of recent surgery he provided had taken place in his own surgical service owing to the work he and his young disciples were then carrying on. Of interest here is that Halsted, who could easily serve as the epitome of the early radical surgeons, in the closing passages of this remarkable letter that spelled out his surgical philosophy very fully, said, 'I trust that it may ultimately be said of the surgeon that he looks to the physician for encouragement in operating, to himself for restraint; that his aim is the study of disease to the end that he may cure without the knife.'[32]

Such were the tenets of the so-called new medicine of the early twentieth century. In Boston Reginald Fitz questioned some of the surgical tendencies from a medical point of view.

He was especially keen to point out that doctors needed to pay far more attention to their patients' subsequent history and not merely to the immediate success of an operation. Surgical wisdom, Fitz believed, was as evident in restraint from operating as in successful operations.[33] In any case, surgeons in the years around 1900 were insisting on clean operations and healing without suppuration. They expected good results from their handiwork. This change in the emotional climate surrounding operations – both for the surgeon and for the patient – was the new characteristic of surgery. No longer was the drama of the operation nor the technical skill or the virtuosity of the surgeon on centre stage. The theatricality of surgery was changing. Even the place of surgery was less often referred to as the theatre. The more prosaic term operating room was finding increased usage, as the focus shifted increasingly from the operation itself to the results that were achieved.

This focus upon the relief of pain or on the ultimate cure of disease rather than upon the drama of the surgical procedure was one of the distinguishing elements of the so-called new surgery of the early twentieth century. The old surgery had been based upon an anatomical approach to pathology. With the advent of cellular pathology and then the developments in microbiology, the new surgery came to be based mainly on physiology. From a twentieth-century perspective it now seems that in the older surgery it was art that predominated and, in the new, science. As surgery emerged from empiricism to a practice based upon both observation *and* scientific experiment, the evolution of a conservative surgery into a radical one does not seem in the least contradictory. Such a transition was, in the context of the developments in the sciences of medicine, a very natural one.

Notes and references

1. W. W. Keen, 'Address in surgery', *Journal of the American Medical Association*, vol. 28 (1897), pp. 1102–10: 1109.

2. G. H. Brieger, 'A portrait of surgery, surgery in America, 1875–1889', *Surgical Clinics of North America*, vol. 67 (1987), pp. 1181–216.

3. T. Billroth, *Lectures on Surgical Pathology and Therapeutics*, translated from 8th edn, 2 vols (New Sydenham Society, London, 1878), vol. 2, p. 210.

4. S. D. Gross, 'A century of American medicine 1776–1876: Part II Surgery', *American Journal of the Medical Sciences*, vol. 142 (1876), pp. 431–84; p. 484.

5. S. D. Gross, *Autobiography*, 2 vols (George Barrie, Philadelphia, 1887), vol. 2, p. 329.

6. R. Dunglison, *The Medical Student* (Carey, Lea, & Blanchard, Philadelphia, 1837), pp. 166–9.

7. Ibid., p. 167.

8. H. J. Bigelow, *Introductory Lecture* (B. B. Mussey, Boston, 1850), p. 21.

9. J. Watson, 'A lecture on practical education in medicine', *New York Journal of Medicine*, vol. 8 (1846), pp. 7–23: 23.

10. S. Smith, 'Conservative surgery', *American Medical Times*, vol. 3 (1861), pp. 295–6.

11. S. D. Gross, *The Glory and the Hardships of the Medical Life* (P. Madeira, Philadelphia, 1875), p. 29.

12. 'Conservatism in surgery', *New York Medical Gazette*, vol. 4 (1853), pp. 462–5: 462.

13. Smith, 'Conservative surgery', p. 295.

14. A. Flint, 'Conservative medicine', *American Medical Monthly*, vol. 18 (1862), pp. 1–24; p. 1 reprinted in part in G. Brieger, *Medical America in the Nineteenth Century* (Johns Hopkins University Press, Baltimore, 1972), pp. 134–42.

15. R. H. Fitz, 'Perforating inflammation of the vermiform appendix; with special reference to its early diagnosis and treatment', *Transactions of the Association of American Physicians*, vol. 1 (1886), pp. 107–36. See also C. McBurney, 'Experience with early operative interference in cases of disease of the vermiform appendix', *New York Medical Journal*, vol. 50 (1889), pp. 676–84. An extensive historical review is by D. Smith, 'A historical overview of the recognition of appendicitis', *New York State Journal of Medicine*, vol. 86 (1986), Part I, pp. 571–83; Part II, pp. 639–47.

16. P. English, *Shock, Physiological Surgery, and George Washington Crile* (Greenwood Press, Westport, Conn., 1980), esp. ch. 2.

17. O. Horowitz, 'The best method of operating to effect a radical cure of senile hypertrophy of the prostate gland: based on the study of 150 radical operations', *New York Medical Journal*, vol. 80 (1904), pp. 246–9; 292–6; 341–4.

18. M. H. Richardson, 'Conservatism in surgery', *Transactions of the State Medical Society of Wisconsin*, vol. 34 (1900), pp. 328–51: 330.

19. Ibid., p. 345.

20. T. Carlyle, *On Heroes, Hero-Worship, and the Heroic in History* (Chapman & Hall, London, 1840).

21. J. Campbell, *The Hero with a Thousand Faces*, 2nd edn (Princeton University Press, Princeton, 1968, paperback reprint, 1972), p. 387.

22. D. Wecter, *The Hero in America* (Charles Scribner's Sons, New York, 1941).

23. H. J. Bigelow, *Introductory Lecture*, p. 20.

24. A. Flint, 'Conservative medicine', in Brieger, *Medical America*, p. 135.

25. G. Crile, 'Excision of cancer of the head and neck', *Journal of the American Medical Association*, vol. 258 (1987), pp. 3286–93; B. R. Alford, 'The heritage of the radical neck dissection', ibid., pp. 3294–5.

26. Wecter, *The Hero in America*, p. 486.

27. G. W. Heuer, *Dr. Halsted, Bulletin of the Johns Hopkins Hospital*, vol. 90, no. 2, supplement (1952).

28. Quoted in R. Matas, 'In memoriam – William Stewart Halsted', *Bulletin of the Johns Hopkins Hospital*, vol. 36 (1925), pp. 2–27: 10.

29. J. M. T. Finney, 'A personal appreciation of Dr. Halsted,' *Bulletin of the Johns Hopkins Hospital*, vol. 36 (1925), pp. 28–33.

30. J. C. Bloodgood, 'Halsted thirty-six years ago', *American Journal of Surgery*, vol. 14 (1931), pp. 89–148: 93.

31. W. S. Halsted to H. S. Pritchett, 8 November 1910, General File No. 80, Carnegie Foundation Archives.

32. Ibid.

33. R. Fitz, 'The border land of medicine and surgery', *Boston Medical and Surgical Journal*, vol. 156 (1907), pp. 655–62.

8

Knowledge of bodies or bodies of knowledge? Surgeons, anatomists and rectal surgery, 1830–1985

Lindsay Granshaw

Introduction

In nineteenth-century medicine, specialists grouped themselves around a number of structures and functions of the body. This paper focuses on those surgeons who came to regard their understanding of the rectum as an area of special expertise and a means to status and prosperity.[1] Their interpretations of rectal anatomy played a vital part in the way they marked themselves out as specialists. According to them, their knowledge meant that rectal surgery was safe in their hands, not in those of general surgeons or general practitioners.[2]

Far from increased study of the rectum leading to agreed 'facts' and 'truths', those writing specialist surgical texts and those writing anatomical texts, whether for fellow anatomists or for medical students, produced different accounts, largely ignoring the others' point of view. The different groups sought to address different questions and constructed their knowledge for different uses. They saw little reason to pay attention to each other. Thus there was no single medical notion of rectal anatomy. The specialists refined and developed their area, generating a body of knowledge which was orientated towards therapeutic intervention rather than academic or pedagogical ends. Although in the medical schools, and perhaps in the profession more generally, it was claimed that the anatomy taught in the dissecting room underlay the surgeon's work, in practice what was learned in medical school bore little relation either to the clinical anatomy of general surgeons or yet again to the distinctive accounts of the specialists.

Specialisation

From the first, specialists sought to mark themselves out as having special – and different – knowledge. Specialisation in medicine was very much a nineteenth- and twentieth-century development, largely resisted by the medical profession as a whole. Those in positions of power, wealth and prestige tried to remain there and ensure that their friends and relations followed in their footsteps. Those who were lower down sought to challenge them, and specialisation was one of their weapons. Specialisation had, of course, long existed and frequently served as a route to prosperity for those on the medical and social periphery. However, in the nineteenth century specialisation gained an institutional foothold that it had lacked before.[3]

There had been travelling 'quacks' who, for example, specialised in the treatment of fistula, but they were not known for passing their information on.[4] There had been tracts devoted to rectal problems before the nineteenth century, but none of their authors would have claimed to be a rectal specialist. Percivall Pott had written a book on fistula in 1765 but he also wrote on other maladies.[5] Thomas Copeland wrote an important work on diseases of the rectum and anus which was first published in 1810 and reissued twice in the next eight years. During the same period, however, he also wrote on diseases of the hip joint, wrist, knees and spine.[6] William White, a practitioner in Bath in the early years of the nineteenth century, seems to have been one of the first identifiable (orthodox) specialists on digestive and rectal ailments, publishing on that subject alone. His work, *Observations on the Contracted Intestinum Rectum*, was first published in 1812 and subsequently revised and reissued three times between 1815 and 1822 as *Observations on Strictures*.[7] Such publications served to advertise specialists' expertise both to patients and other practitioners who might refer cases to them. Publishing in an orthodox manner also helped to dispel the image of secrecy which associated specialisation with quackery.

The institutional basis of rectal specialisation in Britain came to be the Fistula Infirmary, later St Mark's Hospital, founded in London in 1835 by Frederick Salmon. Salmon originated from Bath, but then walked the wards in London, at St Bartholomew's Hospital. He failed to gain a position there due to the nepotism of the surgeon whom he hoped to replace.

When a position at the Aldersgate Street Dispensary evaporated over a dispute with the governors, Salmon did what a number of medical entrepreneurs were now doing: he established his own institution. The model on which these (to the established profession) upstart and medically irrelevant institutions were based was a dispensary for eye and ear diseases, established in 1804. Moorfields' Eye Hospital, as it later became, spawned replicas in major towns and cities around the country, and eventually played a part in establishing the speciality of ophthalmology.

Before he established his hospital, Frederick Salmon had published two books on rectal disease. His work on stricture (dedicated to William White) went through four editions between 1828 and 1833. He also published a book on prolapse in 1831, as well as some lectures on rectal disease.[8] In his works, Salmon cited cases which reflected his apparent ability to attract patients: businessmen, merchants and lawyers, from Britain and overseas, seemingly consulted him. Some patients, he reported, had done the rounds of various hospitals and surgeons, to no avail until they came to him. Salmon did not publish again after he founded his hospital; he no longer needed such advertisement. Neither did he see his specialised hospital as a vehicle for disseminating published material or building a speciality for other surgeons. Frederick Salmon's publications, like the foundation of his hospital, were a means by which he established himself on the path to prosperity.[9] In justifying his specialisation he argued that his particular area was not adequately studied by the rest of the profession and merited greater concentration. Like other specialists, he defined new problems, proposed new solutions and at all times emphasised that danger would ensue to patient and practitioner if specialist help was not enlisted. From the prosperity that accompanied specialisation, and the demand for specialist hospital admission, it is clear that patients responded to these claims.

Salmon published at a time when Parisian clinical ideas were being promulgated by those who portrayed themselves as in the vanguard of medicine. The rejection of written authority, the correlation of post-mortems with symptoms recorded before death, and the study of pathological specimens were characteristic of the Paris clinics and Salmon promoted such ideas in his writings. He emphasised that surgeons were too apt to rely on the authority of others instead of judging from their own observations. He claimed to have undertaken a number of post-mortems and collected pathological specimens (although when later embroiled in a controversy his specimens went unaccountably missing). Salmon saw it as appropriate to begin his books with an anatomical description. In natural theological terms, Salmon expressed great admiration for the rectum: 'the entire arrangement of the part, as respects its form, muscular structure, and general anatomy, evinces a design far beyond the intervention of human ingenuity'.[10] Despite his claims to be describing rectal anatomy on the basis of his own investigations and despite his emphasis on avoiding authority, Salmon's description was, in fact, borrowed from older texts. Galen had described the muscles surrounding the rectum from dissections of Barbary apes, and his detailed account remained the chief authority throughout the Middle Ages. Vesalius' written description was based on Galen, although he included a drawing from his own dissections. In the seventeenth century, Riolan in his description multiplied the muscles, labelling the levators. The work of these and other authors formed the basis of Salmon's view. Although in much simpler form, his description cannot be seen as significantly divergent from anatomical texts of his time.[11]

Salmon was successfully establishing himself as a leading rectal authority, through his practice and publications, when his position was suddenly threatened by a Dublin surgeon, James O'Beirne. The latter challenged views which Salmon and others held on the mechanism of defaecation.[12] More importantly for Salmon, O'Beirne also implicitly criticised a major element of Salmon's work. The most common rectal affliction which Salmon identified was 'stricture'; strictures were to be found at a defined point in the rectum, and were held to result from neglect of proper attention to the necessary balances of the body. As did other surgeons, Salmon treated strictures mechanically with dilators of various sizes. On the basis of his anatomical account, O'Beirne attacked this approach and declared that Salmon and others were, in fact, stretching part of the normal rectum. The controversy was acrimonious and the outcome interesting. While anatomical texts regarded O'Beirne's descriptions as a contribution to their field, Salmon's view on stricture predominated among surgeons.[13] They were not ready to abandon the management of what they identified as a major ailment. It was only when the specialists themselves had identified numerous other rectal problems that stricture began to disappear as a category of rectal complaint.

By the middle of the nineteenth century there was a growing band of rectal specialists. One of the significant features of their speciality – like that of others – was the extent to which they used the knife. Surgery offered the best chance of cure, they emphasised, but only when undertaken by a specialist. A major area of their work was the treatment of rectal fistula, in which the contents of the bowel made a track to the skin. The successful treatment of fistula was increasingly stressed by specialists as the dividing line between themselves and non-specialists. The specialists claimed that only *their* skills were sufficiently highly developed for fistula to be cured operatively without causing incontinence.

Laying open a fistula with a knife in fact had been standard practice for centuries, although creams and pessaries had been used as well. James Syme, writing in 1838, thought that such laying open was very straightforward, and was surprised that not all surgeons had yet adopted that practice. He also wondered why the 'slight incision' required was performed in hospital theatres 'with all the pomp and circumstance of a great operation'.[14] Syme may have been keen to see this as a simple surgical operation, but Salmon, the rectal specialist, took such intervention much further. He performed not a slight incision but cut the length of the fistulous track. As one commentator put it, this 'necessarily involves an extent of incision at least three times that usually employed'.[15] Salmon also added a T-shaped cut beyond the external opening of the fistula to prevent premature healing of the outer part of the wound before the track had healed. Another St Mark's rectal specialist, William Allingham, later noted that if this was carried to excess, incontinence could result, but that 'there can be no hesitation in saying that Mr Salmon cured many cases by this means where other surgeons had failed'.[16]

The treatment of haemorrhoids was also claimed as their field by potential rectal specialists, and here again Salmon emphasised greater surgical intervention than did his contemporaries. Prominent surgeons such as James Syme, Benjamin Brodie and Astley Cooper recommended ligation of piles rather than excision. Cooper had earlier lost patients after haemorrhoidal excision. Salmon, however, recommended ligation followed by quite extensive excision – described as a 'deep gash' by a medical writer at the time.[17] In the treatment of fissure, too, Salmon made 'very free and deep incisions'.[18] Once again, the rectal specialist could be relied upon to offer more extensive surgical intervention than his generalist counterparts, claiming that not only did rectal problems require such treatment, but also that he was particularly skilled in carrying them out.

St Mark's surgeons

Salmon's hospital flourished, as also did his private practice. Only when he was nearing retirement at the end of the 1850s did he appoint other surgeons (who might otherwise have been competitors) to the staff of St Mark's. The four whom he appointed were not, as he had been, outsiders. They were already on the road to successful practices. They either used the hospital as a stepping-stone to other, higher-status institutions or remained at St Mark's and made their fortunes in the speciality. This came to be the pattern in the upper reaches of surgery. Whereas the early and mid-nineteenth century specialists tended to be regarded as somewhat peripheral, and to be discouraged, from about the 1860s onwards it became appropriate for those aspiring to the top of the profession to spend some time at specialist hospitals on the way up, to be seen to acquire specialist skills, even if they often later emphasised that they were general surgeons. Although most sought a teaching hospital position, or held multiple positions, some remained at the specialist hospitals. It was the latter who defined and promoted the area in which they worked as a speciality, publishing on the subject and describing new diseases, treatments and instruments.[19]

Of Salmon's immediate successors, William Allingham stood out. He was the first St Mark's surgeon to publish a book on rectal disease while holding an appointment at the hospital. First published in 1871, with six subsequent editions between 1873 and 1901, the last three co-authored with his son, Herbert, *The Diagnosis and Treatment of Diseases of the Rectum* proved very influential.[20] Allingham emphasised the need for thorough grounding in his subject: 'Thoroughly well informed as the majority of general practitioners are on most professional subjects, rectal disease is one on which much uncertainty prevails'.[21] He added that 'It is not uncommon for me to hear gentlemen who come to St Mark's Hospital to see the practice say they know next to nothing about diseases of the rectum'.[22]

This he observed was most unsatisfactory, particularly as many rectal maladies in their early stages were curable by simple means, often without recourse to operation. Allingham emphasised his unique position: he had had for years 'unusual opportunities for observing diseases of the rectum'. He would not have 'usefully occupied' his position if he failed to publish his experience 'for the benefit of my professional brethren'.[23] Unlike Salmon, Allingham did not publish introductory anatomical and physiological descriptions for his readers. It was his special skills in treatment that he emphasised: he claimed that he had more to say than other writers on rectal disease such as the general surgeons and anatomists, Syme, Curling and Quain. Allingham explained that he had decided against using illustrations in his book: he argued that if a reader was very familiar with this part of the body then perhaps sense might be made of the illustration, but otherwise not. It was a telling point. Although ostensibly intended to inform general practitioners, he was implying that they could not have sufficient knowledge of the rectum to be given specific advice on diagnosis and treatment. The only course of action he left open to them, therefore, was to refer patients to a specialist like himself.

Allingham also stressed that he intended to avoid 'the domain of theory' so that he could disseminate a clear and applicable knowledge 'of a very prevalent class of disease'.[24] He emphasised physical examination and diagnosis, stressing that 'great information' could be gained from examination with 'the instructed and practised finger'.[25] Naturally, the specialist would be best placed to make correct diagnoses. Allingham placed more emphasis on physical diagnosis than on the use of instruments to elucidate rectal problems. Each chapter in his book was a description of a different disease, with a detailed account of treatments, followed by examples of his cases that he considered particularly successful or instructive. In the 1888 edition of his book Allingham emphasised that 'the essentially practical character' of the book was maintained, with 'anatomical and pathological questions only being considered when important in diagnosis or treatment'.[26] It was implied that treatment required more than textbook anatomical knowledge; a specialist, it was assumed, knew from experience the conformation of the part.

The expansion of the field in the later nineteenth century was reflected in differences between Salmon's and Allingham's books. For example, specialists were multiplying the number of rectal diseases and diagnosing patients as suffering from them in changing proportions. Of those who had come to Salmon's hospital in 1835–6, 26 per cent were diagnosed as suffering from stricture, 20 per cent from piles and 18 per cent from fistula.[27] Salmon used thirteen types of disease to classify his patients. By the 1860s, Allingham classified twenty-two types of affliction among patients at St Mark's, with fistula accounting for 30 per cent of patients, piles 24 per cent and stricture only 4.5 per cent.[28]

In the treatment of fistula, rectal surgeons agreed among themselves that fistulous tracks needed to be laid open along their whole length. When operating for this condition in the early 1870s William Allingham did not administer a general anaesthetic (like Salmon he found that the patient bled more under anaesthetic), although he might spray the anal region with ether so that the operation 'otherwise exquisitely painful' might be almost painless.[29] Perhaps not surprisingly he reported that he was frequently asked by sufferers if a fistula could be cured without 'the use of the knife', since they had seen advertisements by individuals 'who pretended to cure fistula and other diseases of the rectum without cutting or laying up'.[30] To him, however, rectal diseases were among 'the most satisfactory in the whole range of surgery' since they were particularly amenable to cutting operations.[31] Allingham described those who claimed to cure fistula without surgery as 'advertising quacks'. He had found the poor less likely to be swayed by such quacks, as (he claimed) they had too little time to waste on them; they wanted cures, and were readier to submit themselves to a knife at an early stage. It was not only so-called quacks who were apparently at fault. Allingham also accused general surgeons in their private practice as well as at hospitals such as St Thomas's and St Bartholomew's, of dealing unsuccessfully with fistula. Allingham urged speedy surgery, warning that cases treated conservatively would be unsuccessful and thence bring discredit and disgrace to the practitioner.[32] On the other hand, Allingham, like other rectal specialists, also warned that surgery for fistula carried with it dangers both to the operator and to the patient. He included cautionary tales of surgeons who had taken their division of the rectal muscles too far up the bowel, resulting in that ultimate disgrace of the surgeon, an incontinent patient. It was absolutely crucial, the specialists argued, for one of their number to undertake such work, not a general surgeon or general practitioner. Underpinning the specialists' case was their claim to unique experience, and their clinical knowledge of the rectum.

By the turn of the century there were a number of rectal specialists, in particular in Britain, France and America. St Mark's had been joined by a rival in the 1880s, the Gordon Hospital, which flourished until it was linked to the Westminster Hospital on the establishment of the National Health Service. At both hospitals textbooks were produced which continued to be directed at GPs and specialists. The number of journal articles the specialists were producing increased markedly: they were now more obviously addressing their own field rather than informing general practitioners of their skills. With the development of antiseptic and then aseptic methods, opening the abdomen was becoming 'the new frontier' for many of these surgeons. Despite their forays into these new areas, most cases treated by the rectal specialists continued to be problems such as haemorrhoids and fistula.[33]

Rectal anatomy

In developing their speciality, rectal surgeons emphasised that they possessed more useful knowledge of the rectum than their generalist counterparts, including knowledge of the conformation and functioning of the rectum. Differences can be seen not only in treatment, but also in perceptions of the body, between the specialists and those working in other areas. Much of the specialist surgeons' interest focused on continence, which featured hardly at all in anatomy texts. The promise of the preservation of continence was a potent weapon in the specialists' armoury. If they alone could cure diseases *and* keep a patient continent, then their place ahead of general surgeons, general practitioners and irregulars was assured. It was widely agreed in the second half of the nineteenth century that the sphincter muscles were responsible for continence. Rectal specialists showed a keen interest in the relationship of the internal and external sphincters to each other, although they did not agree among themselves. There was consensus that the sphincters lay one above the other: from the anus, the surgeon first encountered the external sphincter, then the internal sphincter. They also agreed, in an oft-repeated phrase, that surgical division should not be taken 'too high up'. Every experienced specialist surgeon knew what that meant, and if a surgeon did not know, he should pass his endangered patient on. The differences among themselves centred on whether it was the internal or the external sphincter which was important for continence, and therefore to what extent either muscle was being divided in a surgical operation.

The specialists showed no sign of finding anatomical texts useful in resolving their differences. The anatomists were interested in the pelvic region as a whole (not just the last part of the rectum) and the embryological and evolutionary relations of the muscles, particularly the levators, which it was agreed lay above the sphincters.[34] In the context of this interest, Meyer in 1861 used the term 'pelvic diaphragm' to include the levators and their surrounding area, a notion the surgeons did not pick up.[35] Nineteenth-century anatomists increasingly used animal anatomy to elucidate human anatomy. Such an emphasis on comparative anatomy brought its own controversies, but they were controversies in which again the clinicians had little interest. Thus Straus-Durckheim in 1845 argued that the levator ani in man corresponded to two tail muscles in carnivores.[36] It was a view which gained a strong foothold among anatomists.[37] Anatomists also discussed what parallels could be drawn between humans and animals, and what could be learned from embryological development.

The emphasis in anatomy texts for medical students were somewhat different, but still did not look at the body in the same way as the surgical specialists. Henry Gray had first published his *Anatomy, Descriptive and Surgical* in 1858, and this became the standard British textbook on anatomy for over a century, used particularly by first-year medical students. A Fellow of the Royal Society, as well as surgeon at St James's Infirmary, Gray followed his detailed anatomical descriptions with a section on 'surgical anatomy'. In neither section relating to the rectum was the subject of continence addressed, although the sphincters and levators were described. In Gray's view, the lowest portion of the rectum, terminating at the anus, was 'invested by the Internal sphincter, supported by the Levatores ani muscles, and surrounded at its termination by the External sphincter'.[38] In his surgical section Gray reported that the internal sphincter was divided in the operation for fistula and in some cases of fissure, the object being 'to keep the parts at rest and in contact during the healing process'.[39] Neither his treatment nor his explanation tallied with those of the rectal specialists. In most instances they warned against dividing the internal sphincter, since this was seen as the higher muscle, and the higher the division the more danger it carried, and the reason they gave for laying open fistulae was to clean out the track. Gray did not mention risk of incontinence or how to avoid it, and neither was there any account of how continence was achieved. Subsequent editions did not elaborate further.[40]

Even the perspective of Gray's diagrams of the rectal region was at right angles to those of the rectal specialists. For example, in the 1901 edition of *Gray's Anatomy*, of the six drawings of muscles in the rectal region, five were horizontal cross-sections, showing a slice through the body as if looking from above or below. (The remaining diagram was a sagittal section, as if slicing through the body sideways.) The muscles were shown in the diagram as a sling or sack across the pelvis, and their topographical relations to the pelvic bones were portrayed. None of the drawings labelled separately the two sphincters which were usually identified by the surgeons as so important. They were simply named together as 'sphincter ani'.[41]

While Gray's illustrations were *horizontal* cross-sections of the pelvis as a whole, to illustrate how the muscles related to the pelvic bones, the rectal surgeons illustrated their texts with *vertical* cross-sections of the rectum alone, as if looking from the front of the subject. The vertical cross-section allowed the surgeons to show how far up they could safely operate, and what landmarks there were in the rectum indicating the point above which no surgery should go if continence was to be maintained. As might be expected, the muscles the rectal specialists marked were those which they identified as important for continence. Thus, the internal and external sphincters were marked individually.

It might be assumed that an anatomical account explicitly directed at intending surgeons rather than first year medical students would be similar to those of the rectal specialists. However, this was not the case in, for example, Treves's *Surgical Applied Anatomy*. In Treves's account, the anatomy of the rectum was not related in a detailed way to surgical practice. Frederick Treves, a distinguished general surgeon at the London Hospital, first published his book in 1883. It proved very

Figure 8.1 The perineum, as pictured in *Gray's Anatomy* (1901) showing a horizontal cross-section.[42]

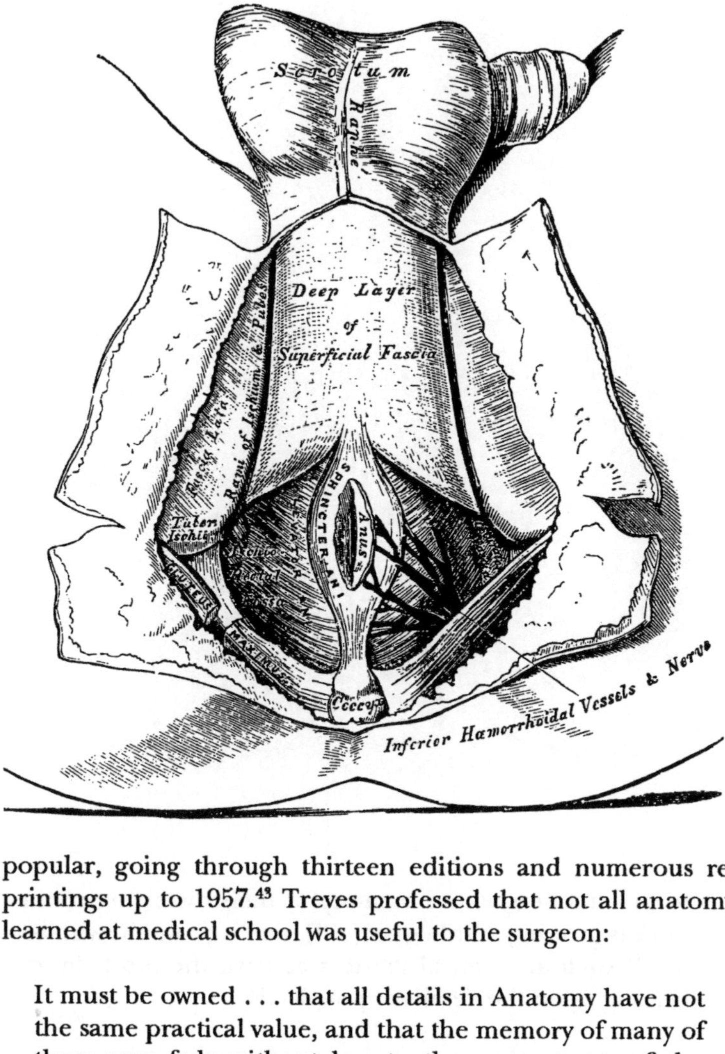

popular, going through thirteen editions and numerous reprintings up to 1957.[43] Treves professed that not all anatomy learned at medical school was useful to the surgeon:

> It must be owned . . . that all details in Anatomy have not the same practical value, and that the memory of many of them may fade without loss to the competency of the practitioner in medicine or surgery.[44]

He intended his work to be used by students preparing for their final examination in surgery, but also expressed the hope that it would be of use

Figure 8.2 'Diagrammatic representation of the lower part of the rectum and its immediate surroundings', showing a vertical cross-section, according to Goodsall and Miles (1900).[45]

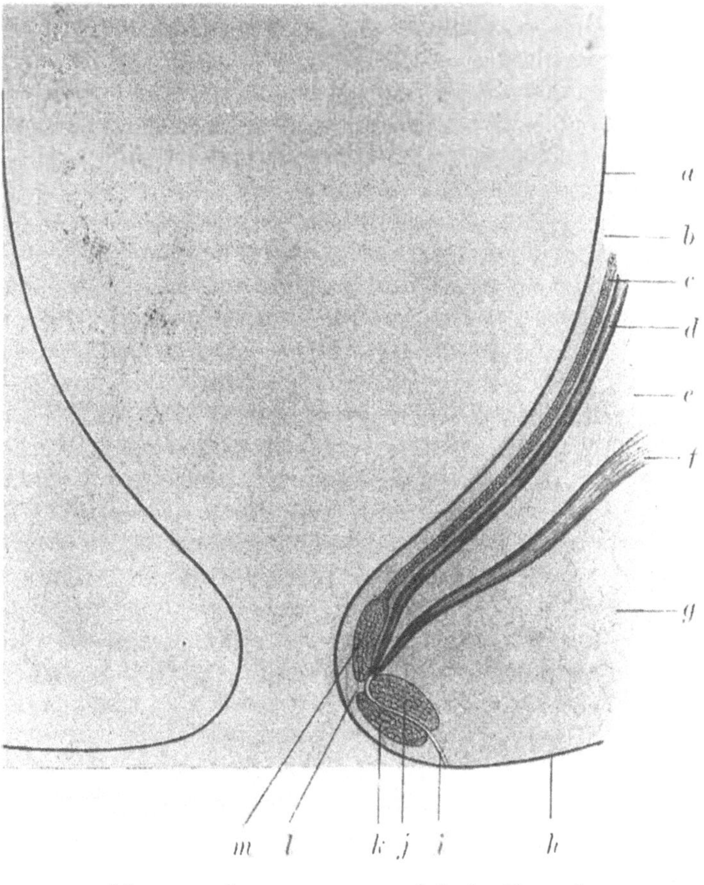

> to practitioners whose memory of their dissecting room work is growing a little gray [*sic*!], and who would wish to recall such anatomical matters as have the most direct bearing upon the details of practice.[46]

In the 1883 version, Treves gave an extended account of the perineum, and afflictions that might befall it. He explained that what some termed Hilton's white line marked the interval between the internal and external sphincters. It was an important point if it was assumed that the external but not the internal sphincter could be severed without affecting continence.

However, he did not spell this out as his reasoning, and although he mentioned a few rectal operations, he gave no details of how these might relate to the anatomy that he had described, despite doing so with urological procedures.[47] When discussing examination of the rectum, he suggested that the entire hand, if small, could be introduced into it, a claim rebutted by rectal specialists such as the Allinghams, who explained that this jeopardised continence. Neither did they like the idea of violently dilating the anus to deal with fissure.[48] Treves included two diagrams of this area: one a horizontal cross-section, the other a vertical view, but the aim here seemed chiefly to show the urinary organs. Although Treves's 1888 edition mentioned fistula, explaining that it usually occurred within an inch of the anus (a point expanded upon slightly in the 1892 edition), he still gave no account of a mechanism of continence.[49] By 1901 Treves declared that nearly all fistulae were within half an inch rather than an inch of the anus, gave a little more information on the structure of the rectum, and mentioned one operation for cancer, but otherwise did not elaborate on rectal diseases and their treatment in relation to anatomy.[50]

Although texts on anatomy, whether surgical in orientation or otherwise, indicated little interest generally in the rectal region, the work of Peter Thompson, later Professor of Anatomy at Birmingham, was subsequently seen by rectal surgeons as a significant intervention. As senior demonstrator of anatomy at Owens' College, Manchester, he published *The Myology of the Pelvic Floor* in 1899. Thompson's diagrams were almost all along the classical anatomy textbook lines, horizontal cross-sections. His aim was to illuminate by comparative anatomy the study of the muscles of what, following the latest anatomy texts, he called the pelvic floor, the muscle sling which ran from the pelvic bones. He argued that these muscles had received too little attention from the anatomist although the gynaecologist and obstetrician (no mention of rectal surgeons) regarded them as supremely important. Johnson Symington had, in 1889, described as the 'anal canal' the third part of the rectum, that is, below the pelvic floor and running to the anus, and Thompson accepted this new description.[51] Thompson was interested in the actions of the pelvic floor as a diaphragm, thus not only in the conformation of this region but also its function. He wrote that muscles formed a sling around the lower part of the rectum acting as a levator of the pelvic floor. By its action the rectum could be raised, and also it exerted 'an important sphincter action on the bowel, and assists the anal sphincters in guarding the rectal opening'.[52] This sling was highly developed in anthropoids, while this was not the case in other animals. He pointed to similar conclusions among other anatomists. Looking at the pelvic muscles, he suggested that the ischio-anal muscle was not a tail muscle but rather probably derived during embryological development from the primitive sphincter cloacae, although he accepted that two others, the ilio-coccygeus and pubo-coccygeus, were tail muscles. Although Thompson had emphasised the role of the pelvic sling, and in particular the levator muscles, in bowel function, his work was no guide to which muscles could safely be severed in surgery. The surgeons' sights remained different: their focus remained on the sphincters and their division. There was little interest in the levators and the pelvic floor.

The difference can be seen in an almost contemporary rectal surgery textbook by Goodsall and Miles. David Goodsall, a surgeon at St Mark's, and Ernest Miles, from the Gordon Hospital, published their book, *Diseases of the Anus and Rectum*, in two parts, in 1900 and 1905.[53] They began with a forty-page account of the anatomy of the 'peri-rectal' region. They stated that as a preliminary to the study of the diseases of the rectum and anus,

> it is essential that we should possess an accurate knowledge of the anatomy of the perineum, first, because diseased conditions can only be accurately determined by comparison with the normal; and, secondly, because intimacy with the relative position and importance of the several structures met with in the region enables us to carry out operative procedures with such precision as will ensure that our interference is extensive enough for the complete cure of the disease, and just so limited that no more damage than is absolutely necessary for the purpose is inflicted upon the structure concerned.[54]

Each part of their anatomical account concluded with a paragraph on the 'surgical importance' of the preceding information. Goodsall and Miles agreed that the levator ani muscles were important in controlling defaecation, arguing that operations should avoid damaging these muscles 'lest the power of expulsion be impaired'.[55] After describing the internal sphincter, they noted in the section on 'surgical importance' that 'Partial injury to this muscle causes great impairment of the power of control; while complete division, even on one side, frequently leads to permanent rectal incontinence'.[56] The external sphincter, embracing the terminal portion of the rectum, was responsible for the voluntary closure of the anal orifice. However, complete division of the external sphincter did not permanently diminish its power of control, 'unless the main trunk of its nerve is divided'; this ran very deeply, along the levator ani, and was likely to be out of harm's way.[57] For them therefore, though the pelvic floor might be important for defaecation, it was the sphincters which must be highlighted for surgeons because they could inflict damage on these which would cause incontinence. They considered that it was the higher (internal) sphincter which was the most important muscle here.

Goodsall and Miles used diagrams from anatomical texts including that of Quain. But differences in interpretation can be found between these diagrams, their own diagrams later in the book, and the text itself, both in the section on anatomy and in their descriptions of different diseases. This can be seen, for example, in their use, or lack of it, of the term 'anal canal'. An illustration used by Goodsall and Miles from Quain labelled the anal canal. They themselves explained that the section which was embraced by the levators and the internal and external sphincters made the rectum into a narrow canal, therefore termed the anal canal.[58] Despite this reference to a feature which anatomical texts identified, they did not use the concept at all in their own diagrams or in their descriptions of individual diseases and treatments. Although apparently acknowledging the 'invention' of the anal canal, in practice Goodsall and Miles did not find it a useful concept and it was ignored. The authors used the simple diagrams that they had drawn themselves to explain to fellow specialists the safe extent of division of the muscles. Unlike previous descriptions, they showed the internal sphincter lying *above* the levator ani, the sling-like muscle or muscles. They depicted the levator ani as joining a longitudinal muscle which ran down between what were described as the superficial and the deep portions of the external sphincter.[59]

The rectal specialists to a great extent based their claims to expertise on their practical skills and the clinical knowledge these incorporated. Thus one surgeon working at St Mark's in the first third of the twentieth century, J. P. Lockhart-Mummery, emphasised that, in his *Diseases of the Rectum and Anus* (1914), he was providing a 'practical guide' to the treatment of diseases of the rectum and anus.[60] St Mark's offered 'unrivalled opportunities' for studying such diseases. He declared that

> It is much regretted that while numbers of doctors from America, the Colonies, and abroad generally attend the practice of this hospital, the number of English doctors who avail themselves of the clinical material to be found there is deplorably small.[61]

He estimated that nearly half of the population suffered from rectal ailments at some period of their lives, and that 'Surgery of the rectum has now become quite as much a speciality as gynaecology, ophthalmology, or laryngology.' However, although there were specialists attached to teaching hospitals, no general hospital had yet appointed a proctologist or provided special teaching in rectal surgery. Lockhart-Mummery was as much a medical entrepreneur as Salmon, and a great proselytiser for rectal surgery: he was one of the prime movers in the establishment of a specialist society which was quickly absorbed as a subsection of the Royal Society of Medicine. It is of value, therefore, to see what this fierce advocate of rectal surgery regarded as appropriate in his textbook. Lockhart-Mummery had no section at all on anatomy: the only chapters in addition to those on specific diseases were on examination and diagnosis, antiseptic technique and diet, and anaesthesia. Neither did he, in general, introduce anatomical sections into his descriptions of treatment. He did not find it useful to include illustrations from anatomical texts, and in fact was not consistent in the way that he portrayed the body in his own simple diagrams used to illustrate treatment. For example, at the top of one page he had a diagram which showed the levator joining the external sphincter, while a second diagram lower down the page showed the levator joined to the internal sphincter. The operative consequences for a non-specialist who did not know his way around the region from experience in the oper- ating theatre with the specialists could have been considered drastic.[62]

Lockhart-Mummery brought out an updated version of his book as *Diseases of the Rectum and Colon* in 1923. He now began with a chapter on the anatomy of the rectum and colon, followed by one on large bowel physiology. In discussing the rectum, he noted that the point at which the colon joined the rectum was 'arbitrary' and that some anatomists made the rectum 'very much longer' than the one that he was describing. However, he argued that there were good reasons for adopting his description. At the place that he indicated, the moveable colon became fixed and was thus a clinically recognisable point. Like Goodsall and Miles earlier, he mentioned the term 'anal canal', being happy to ascribe it to the lower section of the rectum, yet like them he did not use the term elsewhere in his book. In direct contrast to Goodsall and Miles, however, Lockhart-Mummery was dogmatic that it was the external sphincter 'upon which complete continence . . . alone depends'.[63] The internal sphincter, he declared, was not capable of fulfilling the same function, 'and is comparatively unimportant'.[64] Thus, although the rectal specialists were agreed that the sphincters were important for continence, and that surgical division of the muscles should not go too high up, there was no consensus among them on their relative arrangement and exactly how continence was achieved.

The Milligan and Morgan resolution

In the 1930s, two St Mark's surgeons, E. T. Campbell Milligan and Clifford Naunton-Morgan, addressed the subject of disputed muscle arrangements, seeking to put treatments on what they saw as a sound anatomical basis. These surgeons now found Peter Thompson's account, published a generation earlier, useful in their endeavour.[65] To anatomists, they were simply introducing to the surgical community what was already known. A later anatomist wrote that the value of the Milligan and Morgan paper on the 'Surgical anatomy of the anal canal' lay 'in the way it brought [Thompson's] work to the attention of the surgeon'.[66] He cast strong doubt on the surgeons' originality, suggesting that 'the lineage of several passages and illustrations is clear'.[67] To surgeons, on the other hand, Milligan and Morgan had contributed a classic paper, still referred to, original in its content, changing and clarifying practice. William Gabriel, from St Mark's, noted that 'There is no doubt that [this] work on the anal musculature has had profound influence towards improving the general standard of rectal surgery'.[68] The specialists were indebted to his colleagues' 'enthusiasm for anatomical exactness'.[69] As another rectal surgeon put it in 1984, 'The first serious study of the anatomy of the anal musculature from the surgical point of view was made by Milligan and Morgan.'[70]

Milligan and Morgan undertook some anatomical dissections of their own, but used Thompson as their starting point. At several points, however, they modified his account to make it more useful to surgery; these modifications were ignored or rejected by the anatomists. They also made observations on patients under anaesthesia, arguing that the muscles appeared differently in conscious, anaesthetised and dead subjects, and that, therefore, conclusions drawn by anatomists from cadavers were not necessarily useful to surgeons working on anaesthetised patients.[71] Milligan and Morgan explicitly addressed the relative arrangement of the internal and external sphincters. By this time surgical drawings were gradually changing to show the internal sphincter reaching to a lower level and the external running alongside it to a certain degree. Milligan and Morgan argued that the two muscles were, in fact, largely parallel, and were internal and external to the anal canal rather than superior and inferior to the anus itself. Thus between 1830 and 1930 these muscles had been rotated 90 degrees in relation to each other. The new account was generally accepted by their colleagues, at least at this time. If the sphincters were largely parallel, divisions in the lower reaches of the anal canal involved dividing *both* sphincters. This fitted the point that rectal specialists had always made: surgical division should not be taken 'too high up'. However, surgeons no longer had to choose whether they thought that it was the internal or the external sphincter which would be severed at this higher level and was therefore the one that must be responsible for continence. (Although placing the sphincters in this new arrangement, Milligan and Morgan did continue to show the external sphincter curving beneath the internal at its lowest level.)

However, Milligan and Morgan now shifted surgical emphasis away from the relative importance of the internal and external sphincters and looked again at the levator ani. They argued that one part of the levator ani, in conjunction with part of the internal sphincter, formed a ring which could be distinctly felt at operation. It was this 'ano-rectal ring' which was crucial in maintaining continence. If the surgeon kept his finger on that ring and did not sever it, the patient would not be rendered incontinent. They now accepted the existence of the anal canal, but not the conformation described by anatomists. The latter placed its upper limit at the valves of Morgagni, which was in keeping with its apparent embryological development. Milligan and Morgan placed its upper end higher, at their newly described 'ano-rectal ring'.

By this time many of the rectal specialists, for example Miles and Lockhart-Mummery, had made their reputations and fortunes through cancer operations. The work by Milligan and Morgan in contrast applied to less heroic procedures for piles and fistula. It brought them their own kind of recognition. Thus an Australian surgeon visiting St Mark's in the 1930s remembered as a high point not Lockhart-Mummery's work but Milligan's operation for haemorrhoids:

Figure 8.3 Milligan and Morgan on ano-rectal musculature.[72]

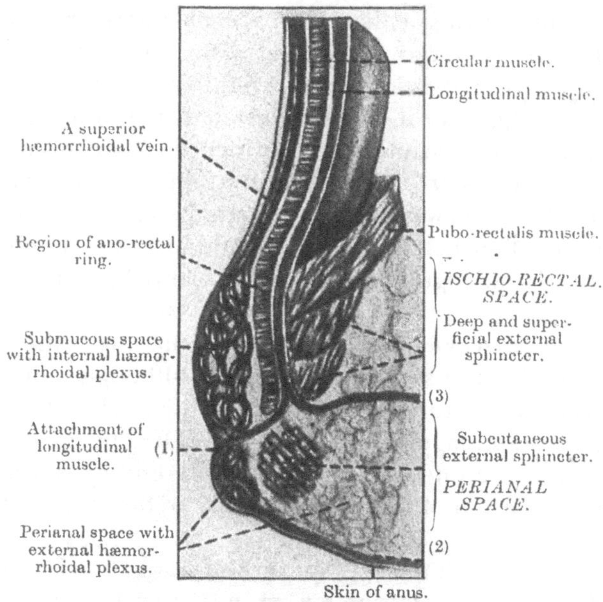

> Up till the time I saw Milligan perform this operation I always considered haemorrhoidectomy a mess, a nasty little operation done at the end of the list, which you preferred to do quickly and hoped no one was watching.[73]

When he saw Milligan performing the operation, 'with every anatomical structure clearly demonstrated', it became 'a surgical art form'.[74] As Gabriel put it in 1945:

> In the operative treatment of internal haemorrhoids only one method will be described, namely ligature and excision by the technique described by Milligan and co-workers in 1937. This method is correct anatomically and is a great advance on what was usually known as Salmon's operation.[75]

Those at St Mark's competed with each other to see who could make the end result look most pleasing, and the following couplet was devised: 'If it looks like a clover the trouble is over, if it looks like a dahlia, it is surely a failure.'[76]

However enthusiastic the surgeons, the anatomists rejected certain aspects of Milligan's and Morgan's work. They disagreed that the external sphincter curved below the internal and they also continued to argue that the anal canal was shorter than the one that the surgeons described.[77] The surgeons responded that they regarded it as better to end the anal canal at the ano-rectal ring, since it could be distinctly felt while operating and was crucial in maintaining continence. There was no value to the surgeons in using the anatomists' embryological criterion. Function was more important than form, a difference in interpretation between surgeons and anatomists which was publicly acknowledged by surgeons. As Gabriel put it,

> the anal canal extends from the ano-rectal ring to the anal margin; this is a surgical description, although morphologically the rectum extends down to the level of the anal valves of Morgagni or, as some consider, to the lower border of the internal sphincter, representing as it does the termination of the circular muscle of the rectum.[78]

The way in which the application and adaptation by Milligan and Morgan of Thompson's work was used can be seen in

Gabriel's own texts. The first edition of his *Diseases of the Rectum* in 1932 had no section on anatomy and its first chapter was on 'rectal diagnosis'. He added a section on 'surgical anatomy' to the second edition of his book, published in 1938, but incorporated only a little of his two colleagues' work. The third edition, published in 1945, took this much further, taking far more from Milligan and Morgan as well as three drawings from Thompson. Also in this edition Gabriel mentioned the 'pelvic diaphragm' which he now regarded as of 'practical importance', marking as it did for surgeons the point at which the anal canal began and the rectum ended, significant because 'the anal canal differs markedly from the rectum both in its function and in its intimate relationship with the anal sphincters.'[79] Thus, in the aftermath of the Milligan and Morgan resolution of some of the anatomical problems which had concerned rectal surgeons, the anatomists' notion of the pelvic floor as a diaphragm, with the horizontal cross-sectional perspective this implied, was beginning to be seen as useful by those surgeons.

Convergence?

In the post-war period, there was something of a closer relationship between anatomists and surgeons, perhaps mediated by physiologists. By the 1960s there was an increasing number of joint publications between clinicians, anatomists and physiologists. Some surgeons in the 1950s had attempted to synthesise their colleagues' work with that of the anatomists, following on from Milligan and Morgan. However, considerable differences in emphasis can be seen. For example anatomists at the time were dissecting and classifying the pelvic muscles in increasing detail. One of their number, Wendell-Smith, later criticised the extent of this enterprise: 'This type of analysis was carried to the lengths of absurdity by Uhlenhuth (1953) who described six components, and twenty-three different elements, in a single pubococcygeus muscle'.[80] Another commentator, trying to simplify Uhlenhuth's material for surgical use, declared that he had used some of his illustrations but 'for practical considerations [presented] a somewhat simpler if not strictly academic arrangement of this anatomy'.[81] The notion that the anatomist's work was simply 'academic', with all the negative connotations that this implied, was rejected by

Wendell-Smith even though he had been critical of the detail into which Uhlenhuth had gone.[82] He certainly did not have a high opinion of surgeons' contributions to his field: 'misinterpretations continue, largely because the investigators are inadequate anatomists'.[83] Thus in 1958 when one leading surgeon (a future President of the Royal College of Surgeons) drew on contemporary anatomical work to address in briefer form the subject of muscle layering, his account of 'Modern concepts of the anatomy of the ano-rectal region' was judged by Wendell-Smith to have produced a 'topological impossibility'.[84] Despite new interest by the surgeons in the work of the anatomists, the latter at least did not necessarily judge the two fields to have converged in any meaningful way.

The vexed question of whether the external sphincter, though accepted as mainly in parallel with the internal, finally curved beneath it, was resolved after controversy among the surgeons rather than because of disagreement expressed by anatomists. Adapting the Milligan and Morgan description, surgeons eventually agreed that the crucial point was the difference in the appearance of the sphincters in conscious, anaesthetised and dead subjects. For example, when a patient was under anaesthetic, the external sphincter relaxed and it was the internal sphincter which appeared below it. In conscious subjects new electromyographical tests were invoked as the arbiter to demonstrate that the muscles were in fact parallel. This fitted the anatomists' conclusions from dissections on the dead, conclusions which had formerly not been regarded by the surgeons as relevant to their treatment of the living.

Electromyography was becoming a tool which was shared by anatomists, clinicians, physiologists and neurologists. In 1953, for example, Floyd and Walls (later Professor of Anatomy at University College, London) had used electromyographic techniques to demonstrate that the external sphincter was continually active rather than inactive at rest, a point of relevance to others working in related fields.[85] From St Mark's, clinicians Parks, Porter and Melzak contributed in 1962 to work now seen as relevant both to the clinic and physiologists on the reflex in normal and spinal man.[86] From the 1960s numerous other papers, usually co-authored across fields, published the results of using such techniques.

Bernard Wood, Professor of Anatomy at the Middlesex Hospital, saw other changes, too, which led to a convergence between anatomy and surgery. He perceived changes in his own field which made anatomists' knowledge more applicable within surgery. *Gray's Anatomy* had been overtaken in the 1960s by Last's and Grant's textbooks, and their emphases were on function rather than form. They influenced those who used their texts, but also reflected a more general shift in their field. Against this background, anatomists had begun to review their conception of ano-rectal muscles. The idea of muscles as pulleys not as static forms was more amenable to surgical adoption, Wood suggested.[87]

A major reason for increased interest by surgeons from the 1960s in normal anatomy and physiology was their definition of a new set of diseases, 'pelvic floor disorders'. Pelvic floor disorders were defined in such a way that they demanded a multidisciplinary approach. Instead of concentrating on the muscles of the anal canal, surgeons were now looking to the 'pelvic floor', the sling of muscles between the pelvic bones, through which the anal canal passed at the ano-rectal ring and which was now seen as crucial to continence, taking this privilege away from the sphincters alone. Electromyography had been used to study normal function, and from that disordered function. Electromyographical tests now become part of what was required in diagnosis, although solutions might still be surgical in a more traditional sense.

Among the afflictions now gaining attention, rectal prolapse, which had long been described and treatments proffered, was newly explained. Incontinence too was newly focused upon, no longer simply as something surgeons might produce by their actions, but rather as one in a range of pelvic floor disorders. In 1959, for example, Gabriel had introduced a new chapter in his text on anal incontinence, listing what he claimed was a fairly exhaustive catalogue of causes, such as post-operative problems or physical trauma.[88] By the 1980s it was routine to include anal incontinence as a chapter in colo-rectal textbooks, but now the list of causes had extended significantly.[89] To one writer in 1985, the newly defined condition was estimated to afflict one person in a thousand.

> Since incontinence is felt to be shameful, patients are reluctant to discuss it with their intimate relatives and their medical advisers. There are therefore difficulties in appraising its true nature and the extent of the problem.

> This is further compounded by an apparent lack of professional interest.[90]

Gabriel's emphasis had been on physical trauma or operative damage resulting in the severance of muscles, but those working on the pelvic floor in the 1970s and 1980s were more interested in nerve damage. Thus, in 1984 Snooks, Setchell, Swash and Henry (a surgical researcher, an obstetrician, a neurologist and a colo-rectal surgeon) examined faecal and urinary incontinence after childbirth, concluding that it resulted from damage to the innervation of the pelvic floor muscles.[91] Not only was their focus nerve damage, they were also highlighting a problem which had not previously been considered to exist, at least not in textbooks on rectal surgery, and that was incontinence after childbirth.

The anatomists had long taken a horizontal or almost three-dimensional approach to their study. Surgeons now began to do the same. Although their drawings continued to emphasise the muscles of the anal canal, they now began to talk of the 'pelvic floor', the mechanisms by which it operated and how it could be corrected when disordered. Anatomists and physiologists might continue to complain of lack of scientific rigour among the clinicians, but they needed to collaborate with them if they were to make tests on live patients on exposed muscles during surgery.

The first British book to bring together articles from surgeons, anatomists and physiologists on colo-proctology was published in 1985. It was co-edited by Michael Henry and Michael Swash, a colo-rectal surgeon and a neurologist. Interestingly in the foreword John Goligher, prominent surgeon and author of the main contemporary textbook on colo-rectal surgery, envisaged a problem over language and mutual understanding in the title of the new book, *Coloproctology and the Pelvic Floor*: 'For many readers the question that will immediately arise on first contemplating this book is exactly what is meant by the term "pelvic floor"'.[92] Clearly there was as yet no common surgical agreement that this was a useful anatomical expression (even though adopted by anatomists a century earlier) or of what it might mean in clinical terms. Goligher noted that uncertainty also remained on the precise mechanisms of anal continence, defaecation and colonic propulsion.[93]

In the new textbook the anatomist Bernard Wood argued

that his anatomy colleagues had previously lacked interest in the general area: 'the anal canal, the pelvic floor, and, to a lesser extent, the rectum are structures which have been sadly neglected by non-clinical anatomists'.[94] He thought that there were several reasons for this. 'The region is inaccessible, difficult to fix and bony reference points are few.'[95] What might be seen as the 'normal' relationships between its components were maintained by muscle tone so that post-mortem appearances did not necessarily reflect *in vivo* relationships. There were also morphological differences between the neonate and the adult. Given the anatomists' greater interest in the relationship of anatomy to embryological development, contrasted with the surgeons' concern that their knowledge of (largely) adult anatomy assisted their operative skills, this difference was significant. Wood also pointed to the continued differences over the anal canal: 'it is clear from the literature that there are two anal canals; a longer (approximately 4–4.5 cm) "surgical" or "clinical" one, and a shorter (approximately 2 cm) "anatomical" or "embryological" one'.[96] He urged convergence over this, questioning the embryological truth of the anatomists' description. He also suggested that the surgical 'long' anal canal, terminating at the ano-rectal ring, was in fact a 'useful physiological concept, even though its proximal limit is not marked by any apparent epithelial or developmental boundary'.[97] Wood noted that there were yet more definitions of the anal canal but that 'mercifully they have attracted few adherents'.[98] Despite Wood's attempts to reconcile anatomists and surgeons over this and other matters, or at least to explain one to the other, and despite the attempt by Henry and Swash to integrate the anatomical, physiological and surgical contributions from their colleagues, the differences between the various groups remained apparent between the various chapters. Later chapters on particular diseases and treatments, for example, did not necessarily apply information from earlier chapters on anatomy and physiology.

Conclusion

Anatomists and clinicians both form part of the medical profession, yet, as the case of rectal surgery and anatomy illustrates, their approaches, and their theoretical and practical concerns have been and in many ways still are quite different. They seem, almost literally, on different planes, sometimes without a common language. Bodies of knowledge did not equate with knowledge of bodies. At times there was convergence, when ideas were borrowed from the other side. Usually these were ideas long accepted in the other camp, yet ignored by the other group at the time. The ideas were then adapted so that they were more useful to the second group but in ways which were then unacceptable to their originators. The different institutional and social settings of the authors of anatomical and specialist surgical texts play a large part in explaining such divisions. They were addressing different audiences and different questions and on both sides – where they showed any interest in the other – there was a feeling that the others had got it wrong.

Acknowledgement

Figures 8.1, 8.2 and 8.3 are reproduced by courtesy of Wellcome Institute Library, London.

Notes and references

1. This paper, first given to a symposium at the Wellcome Institute, grew out of a study of specialised hospitals and the history of colo-rectal surgery. Lindsay Granshaw, *St Mark's Hospital, London: a Social History of a Specialist Hospital* (King's Fund Historical Series, London, 1985).

2. I am grateful to Bernard Wood, Professor of Anatomy at the Middlesex Hospital, for pointing out the different ways in which anatomists and surgeons had viewed the rectal region, and why that might be so, when I sought elucidation from him about the changing views of rectal surgeons in the early part of the twentieth century.

3. See Lindsay Granshaw, '"Fame and fortune by means of bricks and mortar": the medical profession and specialist hospitals in Britain, 1800–1948', in Lindsay Granshaw and Roy Porter (eds), *The Hospital in History* (Routledge, London, 1989), pp. 199–220.

4. See for example Martin van Butchell, in Granshaw, *St Mark's Hospital*, pp. 3, 5.

5. Percivall Pott, *Remarks on the Disease, Commonly Called a Fistula in Ano* (Hawes, Clarke & Collins, London, 1765).

6. Thomas Copeland, *Observations on some of the Principal Diseases of the Rectum and Anus* (J. Callow, London, 1810; 2nd edn, 1815; 3rd edn, 1818).

7. William White, *Observations on the Contracted Intestinum Rectum and the Mode of Treatment* (Wood and Cunningham, Bath, 1812); William White, *Observations on Strictures* (H. Gye, Bath; 2nd edn, 1815; 3rd edn, 1820; 4th edn, 1822).

8. Frederick Salmon, *A Practical Essay on Stricture of the Rectum* (James Bullock, London, 1828a; 2nd edn, 1828b; 3rd edn, 1829; 4th edn, Whittaker, Treacher & Arnot, 1833); Frederick Salmon, *Practical Observations on Prolapsus of the Rectum* (Whittaker, Treacher & Arnot, London, 1831).

9. For Salmon's views on the medical establishment, and his feeling that the Royal College of Surgeons and leaders within the profession were selfishly looking after themselves without regard to the middle ranks of the profession among whom he then perceived himself to be, see his *Oration of the Necessity for an Entire Change in the Constitution and Government of the Royal College of Surgeons, Delivered before the Medical Society of London, March 8 1833* (Whittaker, Treacher & Arnot, London, 1833).

10. Salmon, *Stricture* (1828a), p. 8.

11. For a history of the development of views on pelvic and rectal anatomy, see C. P. Wendell-Smith, 'Studies on the morphology of the pelvic floor', PhD thesis, University of London. I am grateful to Professor Wood for giving me a copy of the historical section of this thesis.

12. Salmon, *Stricture* (1833), pp. 6–8; James O'Beirne, *New Views of the Process of Defaecation and their Application to the Pathology and Treatment of the Diseases of the Stomach, Bowels, and other Organs* (Hodges & Smith, Dublin, 1833); 'Review of O'Beirne, 12. *Process of Defaecation*', *London Medical and Surgical Journal*, n.s. vol. 3 (1833), pp. 253–6, 284–7; 'Mr Salmon on the functions of the rectum', *London Medical and Surgical Journal*, n.s. vol. 3 (1833), p. 376; 'Mr Salmon's reply to Dr O'Beirne', *London Medical and Surgical Journal*, n.s. vol. 5 (1834), pp. 110–13.

13. *Gray's Anatomy* (1980).

14. James Syme, *On Diseases of the Rectum* (Adam & Charles Black, Edinburgh, 1838), pp. 1–2.

15. 'The London practice of medicine and surgery', *Medical Times and Gazette*, n.s. vol. 14 (1857), p. 261. After the introduction of general anaesthesia into surgery, Salmon, if implored, would use it in private work, but never in hospital practice, claiming that the patient bled more when anaesthetised.

16. William Allingham, *The Diagnosis and Treatment of Diseases of the Rectum*, 7th edn (Baillière, Tindall & Cox, London, 1901), p. 51.

17. 'St Mark's and other hospitals', *Medical Times and Gazette*, n.s. vol. 14 (1857), p. 386.

18. 'London practice of medicine', p. 261.

19. Granshaw, 'Fame and fortune'.

20. William Allingham, *Fistula, Haemorrhoids, Painful Ulcer, Stricture, Prolapsus, and other Diseases of the Rectum. Their Diagnosis and Treatment* (J. & A. Churchill, London, 1871; 2nd edn, 1873; 3rd edn, 1879; 4th edn, 1882); *The Diagnosis and Treatment of Diseases of the Rectum*, 5th edn edited and revised by Herbert Allingham (J. & A. Churchill, London, 1888; 6th edn, 1896; 7th edn, 1901).

21. Allingham, *Diseases of the Rectum* (1871), p. v.
22. Ibid.
23. Ibid., p. vi.
24. Ibid., p. vii.
25. Allingham, *Diseases of the Rectum* (1871), p. 5.
26. Allingham, *Diseases of the Rectum* (1888), p. v.
27. *List of Subscribers* (1837), p. 11.
28. Allingham, *Diseases of the Rectum* (1871), p. 3. Non-specialists, in fact, professed themselves astonished that fistula seemed so prevalent in the Allinghams' experience. The Allinghams later withdrew this table from their book, indicating that there was a difference between hospital (i.e. poor) and private patients; there were several diseases, such as piles, 'to which hospital patients pay little or no attention, but which in well-to-do people are a source of great trouble' (Allingham, *Diseases of the Rectum* (1901), p. 3). Fistula, therefore, disproportionately brought the poor to hospital.
29. Allingham, *Diseases of the Rectum* (1873), p. 11.
30. Ibid., p. 17.
31. Ibid., p. v.
32. Ibid., pp. 41 and 42.
33. Granshaw, *St Mark's Hospital*, pp. 138–9. Methods abounded among specialists and non-specialists alike for treating piles – including clamp and cautery, crushing and removal of the whole 'pile-bearing' area. The Allinghams and their colleagues at St Mark's rebutted most of these practices as ineffective, dangerous, or likely to produce stricture or incontinence.
34. Thus in 1843 Jean Cruveilhier, professor of pathological anatomy in Paris, had discussed fusion of the fibres of the levator ani with the longitudinal muscle coat of the rectum and referred to the levator ani muscle as a constrictor of the rectum like the external sphincter. J. Cruveilhier, *Traité d'anatomie descriptive* (Labé, Paris, 1843), quoted in Wendell-Smith, 'Pelvic floor', p. 25.
35. G. H. Meyer, *Lehrbuch der Anatomie des Menschen* (Leipzig, 1861), quoted in Wendell-Smith, 'Pelvic floor', p. 30.
36. H. Straus-Durckheim, *Anatomie descriptive et comparative du chat* (Paris, 1845) quoted in Wendell-Smith, 'Pelvic floor', pp. 30–1.
37. This was challenged by R. H. Paramore, 'The Hunterian lectures on the evolution of the pelvic floor in non-mammalian vertebrates and pronograde mammals', *Lancet*, vol. i (1910), pp. 1393–9, 1459–67, who thought that these muscles had more to do with the closure of the pelvic outlet than with tail movements. Paramore's own background was in surgery, hence perhaps his relation of this controversy back to human function.
38. Henry Gray, *Anatomy: Descriptive and Surgical* (John W. Parker & Son, London, 1858), p. 612.
39. Ibid., p. 710.
40. For example *Gray's Anatomy*, 5th edn (1869), pp. 623, 731; *Gray's Anatomy*, 9th edn (1880), pp. 645, 766; *Gray's Anatomy*, 14th edn (1897), pp. 987, 1139.
41. Ibid., pp. 368–75.

42. *Gray's Anatomy* (1901), p. 370.
43. Frederick Treves, *Surgical Applied Anatomy* (Cassell & Co., London, 1883). Subsequent editions were published in 1888, 1892, 1901, 1907, 1911, 1918, 1926, 1934, 1939, 1947, 1952 and 1957.
44. Ibid., p. viii.
45. D. H. Goodsall and Ernest Miles, *Diseases of the Anus and Rectum* (Longmans, Green & Co., London, pt 1 1900), p. 61.
46. Treves, *Surgical Anatomy*, p. ix.
47. Ibid., p. 377.
48. Ibid., pp. 374, 412; Allingham, *Diseases of the Rectum* (1901), pp. 13–14.
49. Treves, *Surgical Anatomy*, 2nd edn (1888), p. 379; Treves, *Surgical Anatomy*, 3rd edn (1892), p. 386.
50. Treves, *Surgical Anatomy*, 4th edn (1901), pp. 384, 414–18.
51. J. Symington, 'The rectum and anus', *Journal of Anatomy and Physiology*, vol. 23 (1889), pp. 106–15.
52. Thompson, *Myology*, p. 87.
53. D. H. Goodsall and Ernest Miles, *Diseases of the Anus and Rectum* (Longmans, Green & Co., London, pt 1 1900, pt 2 1905).
54. Goodsall and Miles, *Diseases of the Anus and Rectum* (1900), p. 1.
55. Ibid., p. 14.
56. Ibid., p. 22.
57. Ibid., pp. 5–7.
58. Ibid., pp. 19–20.
59. Ibid.
60. P. Lockhart-Mummery, *Diseases of the Rectum and Anus: A Practical Handbook* (Baillière, Tindall & Cox, London, 1914), p. v.
61. Ibid.
62. Ibid., p. 185.
63. P. Lockhart-Mummery, *Diseases of the Rectum and Colon, and their Surgical Treatment* (Baillière, Tindall & Cox, London, 1923), p. 4.
64. Ibid.
65. E. T. C. Milligan and C. Naunton-Morgan, 'Surgical anatomy of the anal canal, with special reference to ano-rectal fistulae', *Lancet*, vol. ii (1934), pp. 1150–6, 1213–17.
66. Wendell-Smith, 'Pelvic floor', p. 36.
67. Ibid.
68. William B. Gabriel, *The Principles and Practice of Rectal Surgery*, 3rd edn (H. K. Lewis & Co., London, 1945), p. v.
69. Ibid., p. 8.
70. John Goligher, *Surgery of the Anus, Rectum and Colon*, 5th edn (Baillière Tindall, London, 1984), p. 9.
71. Milligan and Morgan, 'Surgical anatomy of the anal canal'.
72. E. T. C. Milligan, 'The surgical anatomy and disorders of the perianal space', *Proceedings of the Royal Society of Medicine*, vol. 36 (1943), p. 365.
73. W. W. Davey, 'E. T. C. Milligan, 1886–1972: a great Australian', paper presented to the Royal Australian College of Surgeons, 1983.
74. Ibid.
75. Gabriel, *Rectal Surgery* (1945), pp. 84–5.

76. Davey, 'A great Australian'.

77. See for example Wendell-Smith, 'Pelvic floor'.

78. Gabriel, *Rectal Surgery* (1945), p. 2.

79. Ibid.

80. Wendell-Smith, 'Pelvic floor', p. 37, on E. Uhlenhuth, *Problems in the Anatomy of the Pelvis* (J. B. Lippincott, Philadelphia, 1953).

81. R. V. Gorsch, *Proctologic Anatomy*, 2nd edn (Williams & Wilkins, Baltimore, 1955) as quoted in Wendell-Smith, 'Pelvic floor', p. 40.

82. Wendell-Smith, 'Pelvic floor', p. 40.

83. Ibid., p. 45.

84. Ibid., p. 40, on A. Parks, 'Modern concepts on the anatomy of the ano-rectal region', *Postgraduate Medical Journal*, vol. 34 (1958), pp. 360–6.

85. W. F. Floyd and E. W. Walls, 'Electromyography of the sphincter ani externus in man', *Journal of Physiology*, vol. 122 (1953), pp. 599–609, as quoted in Wendell-Smith, 'Pelvic floor', p. 41.

86. A. G. Parks, N. H. Porter and J. Melzak, 'Experimental study of the reflex mechanism controlling the muscles of the pelvic floor', *Diseases of the Colon and Rectum*, vol. 5 (1962), pp. 407–14.

87. In earlier draft but not final version of B. A. Wood, 'Anatomy of the anal sphincters and pelvic floor', for M. M. Henry and M. Swash (eds), *Coloproctology and the Pelvic Floor* (Butterworths, London, 1985).

88. Gabriel, *Diseases of the Rectum* (1959), pp. 133–59.

89. See, for example, John Goligher, *Surgery of the Anus.*

90. D. A. Mandelstam, 'Faecal incontinence, social and economic factors', in Henry and Swash, *Coloproctology*, p. 217.

91. S. J. Snooks, M. E. Setchell, M. Swash and M. M. Henry, 'Injury to innervation of pelvic floor musculature in childbirth', *Lancet*, vol. ii (1984), pp. 546–50.

92. John Goligher, 'Foreword', in Henry and Swash, *Coloproctology*, p. v.

93. Ibid.

94. B. A. Wood, 'Anatomy of the anal sphincters and pelvic floor', in Henry and Swash, *Coloproctology*, p. 3.

95. Ibid.

96. Ibid., p. 9.

97. Ibid., p. 10.

98. Ibid. The nature of the anal canal itself, even when its upper level was agreed upon, remained an area of contention, according to Wood. Its epithelial lining changed part way along. A number of expressions had been used over the years to describe where this occurred: the pecten, Hilton's white line, the ano-rectal, anocutaneous or mucocutaneous or dentate line. In their works, some surgeons suggested procedures at, say, the dentate line. But according to Wood and others this 'line' was far from clear. The transition from skin continuous with that outside the anus to epithelium of a different nature did not take place at the same level at all points around the circumference of the canal wall. Thus there were different epithelial relationships on longitudinal sections produced by anatomists. Nevertheless surgeons used the line as a marker because the anal valves at this level were usually visible in a patient about to be operated upon.

9

Experiment and experience in anaesthesia: Alfred Goodman Levy and chloroform death, 1910–1960

Christopher Lawrence

Science and the clinic

Chloroform is rarely used as an anaesthetic these days, but from late in 1847, when James Young Simpson introduced the agent, until the 1950s it was widely employed. From its early use to its abandonment chloroform anaesthesia was known to be associated with fatalities. An excellent account of the history of theories of chloroform death has been given by Duncum, who terminates her study with a synopsis of the work of Alfred Goodman Levy who, she notes, in 1911, 'showed ventricular fibrillation to be the cause of death in lightly chloroformed subjects'.[1] Similar observations can be found in many of the other better histories of anaesthesia. Levy's experiments are often designated as 'classic' and the impression can be easily formed that, as Sykes put it, they 'explained the mystery of chloroform death' and 'sealed the fate of chloroform as an anaesthetic'.[2] Bryn Thomas, although describing Levy's work as 'the final blow' to chloroform, added 'anaesthetists were slow to recognise that this was so'.[3] This paper addresses the question of why, when Levy had apparently demonstrated a lethal relationship between chloroform and the heart in 1911, did British anaesthetists still continue to employ the drug (it was less popular in North America for a variety of reasons). In brief, I argue that Levy's so-called classic experiments were rarely seen as such by practising anaesthetists, who found them simplistic and inconsistent with their clinical work. Levy's experiments were not originally acclaimed by the anaesthetic community, but by laboratory scientists and clinicians concerned to promote the basic sciences in medicine. In particular experimental pharmacologists and members of a group designated 'new cardiologists' were quick to indicate their favourable perceptions of Levy's work. Levy's experiments only attained their undisputed 'classic' status when chloroform was displaced by other drugs and practising anaesthetists no longer displayed an interest in its clinical effects. By the late 1940s the high status which the experiments had long been accorded in basic science texts was no longer contested by an anaesthetic community unfamiliar with, or uninterested in, the drug.

The anaesthetists I am discussing, it should be noted, were not hostile to, or suspicious of, the new basic sciences as some clinicians of an earlier generation had been.[4] But they did not, in general, endorse straightforward extrapolation from the results of a few experiments on cats or dogs to what they saw as complicated clinical situations, where experience was deemed to have an important evaluative role. Basic scientists, however, found experiments and clinical situations analogous, and adopted an approach that might be termed reductionist. From their perspective, experiments were unproblematic demonstrations in the laboratory of the pathophysiological basis of clinical phenomena. Clinicians were more synthetic in their approach, stressing that apparently similar clinical events might have different explanations and that imponderable factors might have a part to play. Sometimes they adopted an overtly teleological view of symptoms. From their perspective, experiments illuminated only aspects of a clinical problem.

Early work on chloroform death

The first reported chloroform fatality occurred in January 1848 and others soon followed. Controversy over the cause of death ensued. A significant text in the debates was John Snow's *On Chloroform* of 1858, for it continued to be cited as authoritative in the twentieth century and was used by Levy to endorse his arguments. Snow invoked clinical experience and animal experiments to sustain his conclusions. Snow described two forms of chloroform death. The first, he said, occurred only in experimental animals. It was gradual and characterised by increasingly deep narcosis terminating in respiratory failure while the heart continued to beat. In the clinical situation, he observed, such deaths were not seen, since removal of the vapour when the signs of narcosis appeared ensured recovery. This effect, slow chloroform narcosis, was recognised by all clinicians and is not the primary focus here. It was the second form of chloroform death on which controversy centred. Clinically, Snow noted, suddenness of the fatality was the hallmark of this form of death. Snow, along with most other observers, acknowledged that this phenomenon could occur very early in chloroform administration, indeed at its inception. In such situations, Snow concluded, death was caused by the direct action on the heart muscle of a sudden overdose of chloroform leading to 'cardiac syncope, or arrest of the action of the heart'.[5]

In spite of its recognised dangers chloroform continued to be used. It had numerous advantages over ether and other agents, most notably ease of administration and rapidity of action. Over the next fifty years various British medical bodies set up committees to examine and pronounce on the mechanism of chloroform death. There was much disagreement although, in England at least, many anaesthetists endorsed Snow's view; abrupt death under chloroform was owing to the sudden direct action of a large dose of the agent on the heart muscle. There was, however, also support for the view that death was caused by chloroform acting indirectly, stimulating the vagus or cardioinhibitory nerves, slowing and then stopping the heart. Some advocates of this view held that an injection of atropine, to produce blocking of the vagus nerves, should be given routinely before administering chloroform.[6]

This view was rejected by J. A. MacWilliam, Professor of the Institute of Medicine at Aberdeen. In 1890 on the basis of experiments, chiefly on cats, MacWilliam reported that chloroform caused a 'more or less sudden enfeeblement and dilation of [the heart]' and that 'Section of both vagi does not obviate the weakening and dilating influence of chloroform upon the heart'.[7] During the 1890s chloroform was the object of a great deal of investigative activity. In part this was in response to the Hyderabad Commission, which concluded that all forms of chloroform death were owing to respiratory depression and that the drug was without significant cardiac action. Details of this episode are unimportant here since the conclusions were never widely accepted in England. Significant, however, is the work that the Commission stimulated.[8]

In the last decade of the nineteenth century various physiologists including Walter Gaskell, Leonard Hill and Charles

Sherrington presented evidence to suggest that chloroform was a direct cardiac depressant.[9] Even though this conclusion was generally accepted it still left space for alternative views about the cause of sudden death. Cardiac depression might contribute to this event but other factors might also be at work. A significant publication in this respect was a report published in the *BMJ* of 1902 by E. H. Embley, honourary anaesthetist to the Melbourne Hospital. Embley endorsed the nervous theory of chloroform death. Citing his own experiments on dogs, Embley argued that sudden chloroform death was owing to stimulation of the vagus centre, early in anaesthesia, when high concentrations of the drug increased the cardiac inhibitory action of the nerve to the point where it stopped the heart (reflex inhibition). He noted 'one obvious moral is, use only weak vapour of chloroform (less than 1 per cent) in the early stages [of anaesthesia], until the initial increased excitability of the vagus mechanism has given place to diminished excitability'.[10] One of the results of all these various researches was the attempt to devise inhalers which would limit chloroform concentrations to about 2 per cent, it being generally held that higher concentrations were associated with fatalities whatever the precipitating cause.

Practising anaesthetists of the time were quite familiar with all this experimental work and cited it when explaining sudden death. In his textbook of anaesthesia of 1907, Dudley Buxton explained that chloroform was a direct cardiac depressant, an action which, in excess, produced paralysis. He noted,

> The recent research of Sherrington and Sowton has made it clear that even very small quantities of chloroform act at once upon the heart muscle, but provided that the amount of anaesthetic does not exceed a certain limit the muscle accommodates itself to the chloroform, and its force of beat, although lessened, is not unduly diminished. When, however, the percentage dose is increased, and the limit is a narrow one, the heart muscle becomes paralysed and is irrecoverable.[11]

Respiratory failure, he noted, was secondary to stoppage of the heart. Although Buxton cited Sherrington's work to show that chloroform in increasing dosage caused myocardial depression and paralysis he invoked additional experiments to explain how death occurred in struggling patients soon after induction. The physiologist Leonard Hill had reported that experimental animals, early in induction, often held their breath. Hill suggested that, in the gasping for air which followed this apnoea, a large dose of chloroform suddenly reached the left ventricle. Buxton cited Hill as follows:

> Concentrated vapour of chloroform is presented to the respiratory orifice, the nerve endings of the sensory fibres of the vagus in the respiratory tract are powerfully excited. The animal struggles, the glottis is closed, and by the violent contraction of muscles the intra-thoracic pressure is raised . . . The effect of raising the intra-thoracic pressure is to diminish the output from the right heart, to congest the venous system and lower the arterial tension; the lungs are also compressed and to a great extent emptied of blood. Blood supply to the coronary arteries is diminished . . . The oxygen in the blood is decreased owing to the prolonged holding of the breath. By these means the nutrition of the heart is impaired. Finally, owing to the excitation of the respiratory centres caused by the asphyxial blood, the animal is forced to take two or three deep inspirations. The lungs are immediately surcharged with chloroform vapour, and the blood reaches the coronary arteries carrying a dose of chloroform sufficient to throw the heart into paralytic dilatation.

Buxton then extrapolated to the clinical situation, noting, '[Cardiac] Syncope occurring thus early in the inhalation appears to explain a large number of fatalities under chloroform which have been recorded.' Buxton insisted that quantity of vapour inhaled was unimportant. It was the concentration which mattered. Buxton, however, did not view sudden death as having a single pathological cause, for he also cited Embley's work on the vagus as pertinent. In addition he recognised 'fear-syncope', that is, sudden death of the frightened patient not yet under anaesthetic. He did not explain how this occurred.[12] It might be noted that of all these explanations made it possible to find the cause of chloroform death in the patient's physiology, not the anaesthetist's lack of skill. This was the standard line of defence in coroners' courts where, among all medical deaths, only deaths regarded as being related to anaesthesia were, necessarily, the object of an inquest.[13]

The most scientifically-detailed and comprehensive anaesthetic textbook of the Edwardian era was undoubtedly that of Frederick Hewitt. In the 1907 edition Hewitt reviewed all the experimental evidence on the mechanism of chloroform death. He drew no firm conclusions but cited Embley favourably and noted,

> Owing to the fact that the experimental physiologist cannot reproduce many of the clinical phenomena which play such an important role in the chloroform accidents of practice, we shall not be in a position to complete the consideration of the question before us till we have studied the nature and origin of these clinical phenomena.

Surveying the clinical material Hewitt concluded, '*in a considerable proportion of accidents, overdosage, in the usual sense of the term is conspicuously absent*'. Hewitt employed an explanation similar to Buxton's, stressing the complex combination of circumstances which, in some instances, conspired to bring about death.

> One of the most important physiological phenomena of chloroform inhalation is cardiac dilatation . . . from the direct action of chloroform upon the heart muscle. Supposing, then, that before the full effects of chloroform have been produced . . . any intercurrent asphyxial state arises, not only do we have to reckon with pulmonary engorgement, secondary distension of the right heart, and the widespread effects of non-oxygenated blood, but we have an additional factor to deal with, viz. the continuous absorption of the incarcerated anaesthetic within the lungs and the action of this upon the already embarrassed cardiac muscle. It is hence very easy to see that in certain patients a very slight asphyxial strain under chloroform may cause sudden and fatal syncope, and that, even in the most vigorous subjects, death may take place within a minute or two of respiratory arrest. [14]

Thus Hewitt's explanation allowed for the possibility that a low dosage of chloroform might precipitate syncope, but not a light dose *per se.* It should be noted too that Hewitt's explanation was not exclusive; his approval of Embley's work invited other explanations in other cases.

Alfred Goodman Levy

The second decade of the twentieth century saw a startling intervention into the chloroform debate from the anaesthetist Alfred Goodman Levy. Levy was born in Melbourne in 1866. His parents were English emigrants who returned home. Levy was educated at University College Hospital and qualified MRCS LRCP in 1892. In 1894 he was in Rhodesia acting as a surgeon. He returned to England in 1896. He was a resident anaesthetist at Guy's Hospital 1903–5 and a consultant physician at the London Chest Hospital from 1912–31. He died in 1954.[15] The significant feature of Levy's career here is the period 1910–20 when he was associated with Thomas Lewis at University College Hospital. It is here that Levy's experimental work on chloroform was done.

The first announcement of Levy's views came in January 1911, when he claimed that sudden chloroform death was caused, not by overdosage, but by the action of a small amount of chloroform on the heart, by too light a dosage. This was a position Levy defended in print over the next fifteen years. The claims were based on animal experimentation and, later and increasingly, on clinical evidence. The initial account of his chloroform experiments was made as a preliminary communication to the Physiological Society. Levy reported nine deaths in cats under light (0.5 per cent to 1.5 per cent) chloroform anaesthesia. In two instances blood pressure and respiration were recorded on a kymograph at the moment of death. The tracings showed, he said, that 'The heart failure was absolutely sudden'. At the moment before death the heartbeat (as recorded by the mercury manometer) was 'always rapid'. The respiratory tracing showed, after the heart had stopped, 'a few powerful convulsive gasps'. Levy reported that he had discussed the records with Arthur Cushny, Professor of Pharmacology at University College, London. Cushny had suggested that Levy repeat the experiments and look for ventricular fibrillation. Levy reported three subsequent experimental deaths in which 'I found the ventricles dilated and fibrillating'. He concluded,

'The impression I gained from a review of all the cases was that the heart, under light chloroform administration, may become incapable of accommodation to vascular strain.' This view, he argued, was confirmed when adrenalin was injected under light anaesthesia and similar curves were obtained. Thirteen out of fifteen cats collapsed and in every instance of death (eleven) the ventricles 'were dilated and fibrillating'. Section of the vagi and the subcutaneous injection of atropine did not protect against death but, he concluded, 'Full chloroform anaesthesia appears to be absolutely protective.' He reported that he had been unable to obtain the reaction under ether.[16] On 21 October of the same year Levy made a further communication on the subject. He reported that cats were liable to die from the same cause when recovering from fully established anaesthesia. He concluded, 'By administering a vapour of 2 per cent or thereabouts, *in a perfectly continuous fashion*, cats may be anaesthetized without any risk.'[17]

In 1911 Levy and Thomas Lewis published a lengthy study of chloroform in Lewis's new journal *Heart*. In 1911 Lewis was the recipient of the prestigious Beit Memorial Fellowship and, in his laboratories at University College Hospital, was gradually being acknowledged as a world leader in the new science of electrocardiography. Levy and Lewis used cats exclusively in their experiments. In addition to blood pressure recordings, electrocardiographic (ECG) curves were also obtained. Abnormal tracings, they reported, only occurred with chloroform vapours around 0.5 per cent. The abnormal ECG, they said, showed an 'ectopic rhythm generated in a number of ventricular foci'. They concluded, 'Continued inhalation of percentages exceeding 1.5 per cent usually abolished all irregularity'.[18] On injection of adrenalin in fully chloroformed animals irregularities were recorded but the rhythm returned to normal. However, in light anaesthesia adrenalin injection led to multiple premature contractions followed by fibrillation. The ECG, they said, showed the tachycardia to originate in multiple ectopic beats generated in the heart muscle itself.

It is necessary to note the contemporary significance of this work, which was relatively unimportant for anaesthesia. Levy's experiments were much more significant in the establishment of the 'new cardiology'. This latter was an approach to heart disease which exploited experimental physiology and was orientated to the reduction of symptoms and syndromes to what were construed as objectively reproducible data, for instance ECG traces.[19] Central to the new cardiology was the redefinition of an older medical language and the installation of new pathophysiological entities, such as ventricular fibrillation. It should be noted, then, that Levy's originality lay, not simply in postulating low dosage as the cause of sudden chloroform death, but in his account of the pathological mechanism involved. The heart did not just stop (asystole) or 'fail', it fibrillated. Key figures in the creation of the new cardiology were Thomas Lewis and Arthur Cushny. What was being promoted by Levy and Lewis, therefore, was not merely a finding about chloroform but a whole new approach to disease and an associated range of concepts and techniques. Their work was part of the move by sections of the medical community to effect a laboratory-based, scientific transformation in medicine at large. Significantly Levy's work was announced at the Physiological Society, the cathedral of the basic medical scientists. Most of his papers were published in *Heart*, the bible of the new cardiologists.

Responses

In spite of his startling conclusions Levy's publications seemed to have evoked no immediate response. In November 1911 three chloroform deaths were reported at the Royal Society of Medicine but there was no mention of Levy.[20] In 1912 Levy adopted a tactic he was to use repeatedly over the next fifteen years. After publishing experimental work in *Heart* he gave a more popular account of it in the wider, but serious, medical press. It is a measure of the novelty of this work that Levy regarded his audience as quite unfamiliar with terms such as ventricular fibrillation. In this instance Levy delivered his conclusions to the annual meeting of the BMA and published them in the *BMJ*. Levy first noted that the ECG traces of deeply anaesthetised cats given adrenalin showed what was 'defined technically' as 'multiple extrasystolic ventricular tachycardia', a phrase which he then explained. He described how, if adrenalin was injected into lightly anaesthetised cats, the heartbeat first showed tachycardia and then fibrillation. The effects of fibrillation he catalogued at length. He claimed that the respiratory gasping seen at death was caused by secondary anoxaemia at the respiratory centre, not by chloroform toxicity. He also reproduced the kymographic curves from his first communication to the Physiological Society. Levy then extrapolated to the clinical situation and 'portrayed' the symptomatic effects of adrenalin injection in the patient under light anaesthesia: a rapid pulse which suddenly ceases, respiratory gasping, dilation of the pupils and a possible feeble return of the pulse which then ceases again. In a very few instances, he noted, recovery could occur. Levy then instanced examples from the literature and from his private correspondence which, he claimed, proved this point.[21] The conclusion was obvious. The injection of adrenalin in cases under the influence of *light* chloroform was contraindicated. The *BMJ* also reported the discussion which followed Levy's paper. Dr McCardie reported that he had seen collapse occur immediately after the injection of adrenalin in a septal operation when the patient was fairly *deeply* under a mixture of chloroform and ether. He also reported that Mr Seymour Jones, for whom he gave anaesthetics, insisted on light anaesthesia for septal operations and that he (McCardie) always used chloroform in such cases. It was reported,

> Not uncommonly he found that the pulse became quick, irregular and weak immediately after the injection and the colour paler. On the other hand he himself, when he had had an injection of adrenalin for a septal operation, had had rather a feeling of stimulation. Mr Seymour Jones's, and therefore his experience, was contrary to Dr Levy's experimental results.

The *BMJ* reported 'Dr Levy in reply expressed surprise that Dr McCardie's experience in practice was totally opposed to the results of physiological experiment . . . He considered that Dr McCardie had been extremely lucky'.[22]

Apart from this, Levy's work seems to have made little impression on the anaesthetic literature. Hewitt's textbook of 1912 did not refer to it.[23] In 1913, at the anaesthetic section of the seventeenth International Congress of Medicine in London, Dudley Buxton reviewed recent advances in general anaesthesia. He listed a variety of authors who had contributed to the understanding of the action of chloroform but did not include Levy. He noted,

> The outcome of a very large amount of work done upon

> the influence of chloroform upon the heart and circulation appears to be: blood pressure falls, the heart's action weakens, possibly in part due to dilation (MacWilliam) and the vasomotor control lessens directly as the percentage of chloroform which is in action.

Buxton made it clear that he held overdose to be the cause of death during induction. He noted that 2 per cent chloroform 'will induce anaesthesia . . . while a greater strength will always lessen the activities of respiration and circulation and may at any moment cause cessation of breathing and heart standstill'. Buxton added that, since no suitable device existed for measuring the dose of chloroform administered, the anaesthetist 'is for ever experimenting upon his patients, and the results he obtains depend wholly upon his personal acumen as an experimenter'. Buxton lamented this, 'the system lacks the imprimatur of science and is apt to fail at critical moments'. None the less, he concluded, dosimetric methods (using a graduated inhaler) were the best way of administering the drug 'both from experimental and clinical evidence'.[24]

In the same year, 1913, Levy again published in *Heart.* He reported that all his experiments had been performed on cats although he also observed, 'The reaction in dogs is similar to that in cats.'[25] The grounds for this conclusion were not given. Much of the new material in this paper was devoted to proving that injected adrenalin acted directly at the sympathetic myoneural junction in the heart and that, therefore, sympathetic stimulation of any sort under light chloroform would produce the same effects as adrenalin injection. In other words a suitable stimulus would release natural adrenalin at this junction, injected adrenalin simply magnified the effect. Such stimulation, he argued, could be brought about directly and simply by manipulating the sensory nerves of the skin. Levy also claimed, on experimental grounds, that the effect was produced not only by the sympathetic nerves to the heart but was augmented by the liberation of adrenalin (which acted directly on the heart) from the suprarenal glands, since the sympathetic nerves to that organ were also affected. Levy thus argued that the stimulus of struggling in a barely unconscious, lightly anaesthetised animal produced fibrillation by the same mechanism as adrenalin injection.

Levy then proposed that chloroform deaths in humans were

caused by an identical mechanism; light dosage of chloroform sensitized the heart. Injected adrenalin or the physiological release of the same substance from sympathetic stimulation stopped the heart. Death was not produced by overdosage either directly or, as Embley argued, by means of vagal inhibition: 'Permanent inhibition of the mammalian heart by reflex vagal action is unknown to experimental physiology.'[26] Indeed, Levy's conclusions were diametrically opposed to Embley's. The activity of the vagus, Levy considered, had a stabilising action on the chloroformed heart. Severing the vagi in lightly chloroformed cats, he said, *increased* the possibility of irregularity. Severance removed a beneficial negative stimulus; conversely, stimulating a cut vagus decreased tachycardia. Death from overdosage he argued was quite different. It was characterised by gradual respiratory failure with the heart coming slowly to a standstill. Post-mortem appearances were also different. He concluded 'anaesthesia may be induced with perfect safety with chloroform, provided it is given, *of a full strength* and *in a perfectly continuous manner.*'[27] Most cases of chloroform death in man, he noted, as everyone agreed, occurred during induction. In reports of deaths, he said, it was reapplication of the vapour after its removal or the initial surgical incision which seems to have provoked the incident.

Levy repeated his conclusions in a paper given to the Royal Society of Medicine in May 1914. Once again, addressing an audience less cardiologically sophisticated than the readers of *Heart*, he adopted a popularising tone. He began, 'What is ventricular fibrillation?' After describing it as an experimental phenomenon in cats and how it could be provoked by low chloroform dosage in association with various other circumstances, he turned to what he described as the comparable human condition. Levy analysed the 109 chloroform fatalities found in the Report of the Anaesthetics Committee of the Royal Medical and Chirurgical Society issued in 1864. Only 98 of these cases were amenable to analysis, he said, and 48 per cent of them, Levy considered, showed definite evidence of light anaesthesia. He concluded that there was good evidence that 87 per cent of the total were lightly anaesthetised and he thought the probable total was 92 per cent. In fact, he claimed, there was no definite evidence of overdosage in any instance. Levy then used John Snow's description of sudden death under chloroform – 'cardiac syncope' – to support his view. Once again Levy drew the same practical conclusions. The anaesthetist should ensure continuous administration of vapour rapidly increasing in strength. He warned, 'Should the patient become excited or struggle during the induction, the administration should never, on any account, be remitted, as is at present the practice and teaching.'[28] He observed that the pulse could be a guide to the onset of fibrillation but the condition could occur with startling rapidity. He insisted that the patient with a pale skin, sweating, and a small, rapid pulse was not suffering overdosage and the anaesthetic should not be remitted. If cardiac arrest should occur, he said, artificial ventilation should be instigated and continued for two minutes. If the heart did not recommence beating, the abdomen should be opened and the heart compressed against the diaphragm by the anaesthetist's hand. Levy noted that, although chloroform usage was declining, deaths appeared to be on the increase because of the current insistence on attenuation of the vapour.

In the ensuing discussion the President, Dr Blumfeld, said that Levy's 'laboratory work was of the greatest possible interest to members of the Section, who would naturally criticise it from the point of view of their own clinical experience'. A practising anaesthetist, Richard Gill, raised a number of objections. First he argued that 'Experience drawn from the [surgical] section of vagus in man would . . . seem in conflict with the results of similar operations on the lower animals'. The human heart rate did not increase after section and thus 'it is hazardous to deduce the same results happening in man from those which occur in like operations on the lower animals'. Gill then turned to the question of rapid anaesthetisation and instanced the problem of the frightened patient with a 'quick pulse with small volume and acceleration of respiration'. In such instances, he said, 'Instead of making haste' as Levy's conclusions might indicate, 'we have to proceed slowly'. He argued that in such cases there was danger of overdosage and depression of the vasomotor and respiratory centres. Gill objected to Levy's clinical inferences on the grounds that Levy had correlated only a beginning and an end – an initial vapour concentration and fibrillation – without considering all the intermediate factors, such as 'the condition of the lungs, whether congested and to what extent'. For this reason Levy could not exclude the possibility that fibrillation was the last stage of 'the progressive exhaustion of the cardiac energy from chloroform narcosis – i.e., an overdose of chloroform in the blood'.[29] In other words Levy had no means of knowing what state of narcosis the experimental animals were in when fibrillation appeared. The criticism was a version of the longstanding view that a combination of factors could conspire to bring about local overdosage at the heart or in the brain when, apparently, only a small dose had been given. This was a point never fully explored by Levy's critics. It was taken for granted. Levy himself had admitted, in the technical report of his work, to the difficulty of producing fibrillation during induction. He observed, 'Even in intact animals there is no exact procedure which will *insure* the onset of syncope . . . I have never been able to fathom the particular circumstances attending the success of the experiments . . . a distinct impression is left that the tendency to ventricular fibrillation is one of seasonal incidence'.[30] At any rate Gill took the view that overdosage was the danger. He agreed that 'Experimentalists can acquire information in a way which is denied the practical anaesthetist' but warned that extrapolation to a clinical situation could be misleading.[31]

In 1914 Levy more once published in *Heart.* He reported, 'The whole of the work was again performed solely on cats.' He related that he had investigated the relationship between irregularities of rhythm and the mechanical efficiency of the heart which was, by now, widely agreed to be weakened and dilated by chloroform. Levy injected chloroformed cats with drugs known to have a vasopressor effect. He reported that a rise in blood pressure favoured the appearance of extrasystoles (this was also the case in etherised animals). He concluded that these irregularities, 'pressure, extrasystoles', were of an 'essentially different class' from those produced by chloroform alone because they did not progress to fibrillation. He also concluded, 'Dilation of the ventricles is a condition which is protective against ventricular fibrillation; it is on this ground that the protective action of full doses of chloroform is explained.'[32]

In the same year, in *The Lancet,* came the first published endorsement of Levy's view. Not by an anaesthetist, however, but from the physiologist J. A. MacWilliam. MacWilliam explicitly approved Levy's work, arguing that death in early anaesthesia was owing to low dosage and was caused by fibrillation. Unlike Levy, however, he explained that chloroform overdose caused cardiac enfeeblement and dilatation which might also terminate in fibrillation. There was, he said, 'no shred of evidence for the view' that reflex inhibition of the heart following chloroform stimulation of the vagus centre was the cause of death. MacWilliam also noted that in rabbits chloroform death was associated with enfeeblement but normal rhythm. Man and the cat however, he stressed, had great similarities, notably the 'tendency to excitement and struggling with disturbance of respiration'.[33] Levy, in a juxtaposed article, iterated his conclusions, lamenting that 'The theory of death by overdose has . . . been a most deplorable one for humanity'.[34] MacWilliam's article was to be part of a pattern: the endorsement of Levy's work by those with a direct interest in experimentation as applied to medicine. Thus in the same year Yandell Henderson, Professor of Physiology at Yale, published a review entitled 'Recent experiments defining the dangers of anaesthesia'. Henderson praised Levy fulsomely. He took it as proven that Levy's clinical analyses showed the dangers of light chloroform anaesthesia and, he observed, that human and animal phenomena were interchangeable. He noted, 'These types of cases which Levy has shown are easily reproducible in animals.'[35]

In the following two years Levy's conclusions were challenged in *The Lancet* and the *American Journal of Surgery* by Embley. Embley argued that Levy's extrapolation from cats to humans was not justified. Dogs, he claimed, had an entirely different response to chloroform.

> It is a circumstance of much significance that those experimental physiologists who have worked with dogs in the elucidation of clinical problems, should have reported no observation upon the occurrence of ventricular fibrillation.

In experiments on dogs he had never observed fibrillation, except when the blood pressure had fallen from shock or some other cause. In the dog, he said, chloroform raised the excitability of the vagus mechanism. Death followed from vagal inhibition, depression of the myocardium and exaltation of the vasomotor mechanism. The heart did not fibrillate, it stopped. In clinical situations, he argued, iterating the conventional view, 'syncope from cardio-vascular inhibition is the result of the intake of excessive concentrations of chloroform vapour during normal breathing or too excessive inspirations of concentrations not otherwise too high'. Levy's interpretation was fallacious. The analogies between dog and man, he declared, were strong. Levy's teaching on the relative unimportance of overdosage, he concluded, was 'dangerous'.[36] A leader in *The Lancet* in 1915 endorsed Embley's conclusions, arguing that it was illegitimate to extrapolate from cats to humans.[37]

In 1919 Levy again published in *Heart*. This publication is quite striking for three reasons. First, in it Levy explicitly negated some of his own conclusions. Second, he drew no clinical inferences. Third, neither he, nor any contemporary, nor any historian, ever, to my knowledge, took notice of the work. On the basis of a new series of experiments on cats Levy announced that constant inhalation of low dosage chloroform, '"primary" light anaesthesia' as he called it, did not produce fibrillation.[38] Fibrillation only occurred under light anaesthesia *after* an animal had been more deeply anaesthetised by chloroform. This he observed had been the case in *all* his previous experiments, for the cats had first undergone deep chloroform narcosis in order to prepare them for the experiments. In the new experiments ether was used to prepare the animals.

By now anaesthetists had begun to take note of Levy's views. Stuart Ross, an Edinburgh anaesthetist, even gave them some credit but observed that they had no consequences for the practitioner. Ross noted in his textbook of 1919 that the action of chloroform on the circulatory and respiratory systems 'has been the subject . . . of much embittered controversy'. He employed Embley's model to explain sudden death, observing,

> It is an undoubted clinical fact that there is a risk of sudden arrest of heart's action if the operation is begun before the stage of full anaesthesia is reached. A reasonable explanation of such accidents is furnished by supposing a reflex inhibition acting through the vagal centre already rendered hyper-sensitive by partial chloroformisation.

Ross, however, also recounted Levy's views and added,

> So far as the author understands the views of Dr Levy, his explanation of chloroform syncope need not be taken as introducing any new principle into the administration of

> the drug. Even those who lay most emphasis upon the danger of using vapours of too high a percentage strength would admit the force of Levy's contentions. As usual safety lies in steering between two extremes.

He noted though that, since Levy's work, it was 'the rule has been absolute' that adrenalin must be given before chloroform.[39] Although Levy's conclusions about adrenalin did seem to have been the source of a change in clinical practice, Ross's 'rule' was by no means as absolute as he supposed. In 1930 two University College Hospital anaesthetists observed, 'the injection of adrenalin during chloroform anaesthesia, especially if the anaesthetic is light, is said to have a certain risk, but we have not seen a case where harm has resulted'.[40]

In the second edition of his book in 1923, Ross reconsidered Levy's work. Although Levy had done 'yeoman service' in pointing to the dangers of irregular administration, a practice 'only too prone to appear in . . . inexperienced and nervous administrators', Ross added,

> To the author's mind . . . Levy has gone too far in his attitude that vagal inhibition from the use of vapour strengths of too high percentage, is not to be regarded as a real possibility, or at any rate not a dangerous one . . . in the whole history of the subject one fact stands out clearly, namely that practical anaesthetists and laboratory workers alike were of the opinion that if marked breath-holding, with clenching of the jaw and development of a trace of cyanosis, should occur during any stage of chloroformisation, it was the anaesthetist's duty to intermit the administration, to clear the air-way, and to allow one or two free inspirations of fresh air before continuing the administration. Faced with such an incident, the author would still feel it his duty to follow the old rule.[41]

In contrast to this 'old rule', Levy was teaching that 'A patient who "holds his breath" can generally be induced to inhale freely once more by slightly reducing the strength of the vapour.' During struggling too, he noted, 'it is most essential not to remove the chloroform'. This, he noted, was 'directly contrary to the old teaching'.[42] Neither Ross's 'old rule' nor Levy's 'old teaching' are quite borne out by the literature. In 1901 Probyn

Williams stated 'struggling must be met by an increased dose of chloroform'.[43] Most authors however did not disassociate struggling and breath-holding and did prescribe reducing chloroform if these appeared. Snow did distinguish these events and recommended withdrawing chloroform during breath-holding but during struggling 'The proper course to pursue is to continue the inhalation gently till the struggling and rigidity are subdued'.[44]

In 1920 Levy appeared once more in *Heart*, this time on massage of the ventricles. Massage of the ventricles after abrupt death was a confirmed clinical practice. Levy, who enthusiastically endorsed it, found *experimental* evidence in favour of the practice. He reported experimenting on cats and two dogs in which fibrillation had been produced by light anaesthesia and adrenalin. He said that he had discovered that the cat's heart had a greater capacity to revert to normal rhythm, both spontaneously and with massage, than that of the dog. Clinical evidence, he said, suggested human hearts also had an 'undoubted tendency to spontaneous recovery'.[45] Massage, he considered, was a proper course of action in cardiac syncope. As was Levy's practice after publishing for a specialist audience he spelled out his results for the rank and file. In June 1921 he discussed massage at the section of surgery of the Royal Society of Medicine.[46] Again he iterated his claims about syncope. In November of the same year he repeated his message in *The Lancet*.[47]

In 1922 Levy's monograph, *Chloroform Anaesthesia*, was published. It was a summary of his work of the previous eleven years. The dangers of low dosages of chloroform were reiterated. Significantly, Levy's text had a flag-waving foreword for laboratory science written by Cushny.

> Dr Levy has now shown how much the practice of anaesthesia in man is dependent on the principles of the basal sciences; how the same laws of physics hold in the ward and in the laboratory, and how necessary it is that the anaesthetist should recognize their bearing on his problems . . . We of the laboratory are furnished with a further point of contact with practice and with a further example of the importance of fundamental principles controlling active intervention in disease.[48]

Few practising anaesthetists, however, were convinced. In 1923, Levy's work was given limited recognition in the *Practical Anaesthetics* of the London anaesthetist Charles Hadfield. As with all anaesthetic texts of the time, Hadfield's work valued a scientific basis for practical anaesthetics but equally stressed the importance of the clinician having 'considerable experience'. Hadfield observed that the action of chloroform on the circulation and respiration was controversial but he noted that in most cases respiratory failure, even at an early stage, signalled overdose. He added that in a few cases the heart stopped very suddenly before respiration failed. 'The cause', he observed, 'is somewhat obscure'. He suggested, on familiar lines, that in such instances overdosage had arisen; arising from a combination of anoxia plus sudden inhalation of vapour. He noted, however,

> Another cause of primary cardiac failure under chloroform is due to quite a different train of events, the onset of which proceeds from the administration of too weak rather than too strong a vapour. It is stated by Dr Levy that chloroform, especially in small quantities, acts as an irritant to the cardiac muscle, and tends to induce the dangerous condition of ventricular fibrillation.[49]

This condition, he added, was particularly likely to occur if adrenalin was given although it possibly sometimes followed natural secretion of adrenalin in the lightly chloroformed patient when the operation was begun too early. Another version of the synthetic clinical approach is apparent here; Levy's account might explain *some* of the instances of sudden death.

In 1924 the anaesthetist H. P. Fairlie discussed chloroform in the *Proceedings of the Royal Society of Medicine.* He noted, 'It has been the custom, of recent years, to describe two types of chloroform syncope.' These were the instantaneous sort and the more gradual sort. He doubted, however, whether there was any 'vital distinction' between them. The cardiac failure was of the same type in both, differing only in rapidity of onset. The rapid type was signalled by pallor and dilation of the pupil. Fairlie outlined Levy's findings and conclusions and added, 'I am convinced, from clinical observation, that it [cardiac syncope] results far more often from too much chloroform than from too little.' He observed, 'The theory of reflex vagal inhibition appeals to me as more nearly fitting to the clinical picture.'[50]

In 1926 Arthur Mills, lecturer in anaesthetics at St Andrew's University, discussed chloroform at length in *The Lancet*. He noted that the American Medical Association Committee of Anaesthesia of 1912 had concluded that the use of chloroform was no longer justifiable, except possibly for induction of difficult cases and in alcoholics. Mills stated that he found chloroform a good anaesthetic but one which required care. He claimed that 80 per cent of chloroform deaths occurred during induction. Of the 33 deaths he had investigated, 21 occurred during induction and 12 of these showed extreme excitement followed by collapse. Mills's explanation was a familiar one. Citing the experimental work of Pohl he argued that death in these circumstances was owing to the patient holding his breath, then, in one or two large gasps taking in a large dose of chloroform which affected the left heart. Mills reported that Pohl, experimenting on dogs, in circumstances intended to simulate clinical conditions, had found 2 per cent chloroform in the left ventricle and 0.02 per cent in the right, immediately after death. This was a finding that supported the view that local overdosage could occur under normal circumstances. Mills also recited MacWilliam's and Levy's work and their conclusions at length. But, he observed, 'It is difficult to believe that a low percentage of chloroform in blood can do more harm to the heart than a higher percentage.' He added, 'Levy's work is interesting, and I think of great value, but his manner of application of his results to practical anaesthetics is unfortunate. His teaching is entirely at variance with clinical experience.' The view that death may be due to light chloroform anaesthesia 'conveys . . . the wholly false and dangerous doctrine that safety would have been found in giving more chloroform'.[51]

In 1929, in the *Glasgow Medical Journal*, the anaesthetist W. B. Primrose discussed chloroform anaesthesia in relation to operation risk. Primrose repeated the generally agreed conclusion that induction was the most dangerous period of anaesthesia. He noted that most problems occurred in cases in which the struggling patient ceased to breathe because 'when breathing [re]starts . . . it is very deep and voluminous. If there is any chloroform present it may be rushed into the circulation at a rate that the heart cannot stand.' This longstanding view was confirmed, according to Primrose, by clinical observation. He concluded, 'From observation upon cases under chloroform I think that the relationship of chloroform to the average heart is that the latter will stand a large dosage of chloroform absorbed gradually . . . It cannot stand a sudden increase in the concentration'.[52] Levy's work was not cited.

In 1932 Levy's work was resoundingly endorsed in a paper by Ian Hill. Significantly Hill was not an anaesthetist but a physician and a major second-generation influence in the establishment of the new cardiology. Hill reported putting Levy's theories to the test in an electrocardiographic study of patients undergoing chloroform anaesthesia. Hill took Levy's findings as unequivocal, using such expressions as Levy had 'showed that' such and such was the case. He assumed as a fact 'When cardiac arrest in man occurs under chloroform . . . it is associated with struggling, and with light anaesthesia rather than with overdosage.' Hill asserted that the only problem was to show that death in man was owing to ventricular fibrillation. Hill reported a study of 16 operations under chloroform in which string galvanometric traces were made during induction. The ECGs of eight cases showed no or only minor abnormalities. In the remaining eight, he reported, 'marked disturbances appeared'. In one of these there was 'marked sinus arrhythmia' and in the other seven there were 'multiple ventricular extrasystoles'. In 'some cases' the extrasystoles came from many foci in the ventricles. In six of the cases the extrasystoles arose during induction and in another they appeared under full anaesthesia. In most instances the appearance was transient and the heart settled to a normal rhythm with deep anaesthesia. He observed, 'The appearance of extrasystoles in large numbers was sometimes associated with struggling.' Other anaesthetics, he claimed, did not produce comparable effects. Hill said his records showed 'close correspondence' to Levy's results on cats. The records demonstrated, he said, Levy's 'pre-fibrillation phase' in man.[53]

Hill's work made a definite impression on the anaesthetic literature but anaesthetists were still inclined to a synthetic rather than reductionist position. Langton Hewer, in his prestigious *Recent Advances in Anaesthesia* of 1932, summed up what he saw as the current position. He referred to Levy's work on adrenalin but also noted 'several cases' of 'heart failure' had been reported in which the patient was deeply anaesthetised. He concluded,

> It seems therefore established that chloroform can exert toxic effects in at least four different ways: (i) Vagal stimulation in high concentration, causing primary cardiac failure. In animals under the influence of atropine this effect is not obtained, and it is possible that in man full doses of atropine may give some protection from vagal stimulation. (ii) Ventricular fibrillation due to an intermittent administration or to stimulation before the patient is fully anaesthetized, or to the administration of adrenalin. Recent work with the electrocardiograph seems to show that the site of origin of systole may change from the sinoauricular node to the atrio-ventricular node in the early stages of chloroform anaesthesia, and a definite 'pre-fibrillation phase' has been demonstrated. (iii) Gradual paralysis of the respiratory centre from overdose. (iv) Delayed chloroform poisoning.[54]

Observation (i) was the familiar high dosage theory, in this instance explained by Embley's reflex inhibition hypothesis. Hewer instanced as supporting evidence of position (ii) Hill's *Lancet* paper. This work (and thus Levy's), however, was being accommodated into the longstanding tradition of condemning *intermittent* administration. Hewer does not have to be read as endorsing low dosage as the sole cause of death in all instances.

W. B. Primrose, writing in 1933, referred neither to Levy's nor Hill's conclusions. Primrose took a strikingly teleological view of clinical evidence. The apnoea sometimes seen in induction, he said, was the response of the body to overdosage. He observed,

> the patient *does* actually control the intake of his own anaesthetic, and that he does not take too much, and rarely too little; in fact, when an operation is in progress, he continuously adjusts the depth of the anaesthesia to suit the needs of the operation from beginning to end.[55]

The correct response during breath-holding therefore was to withdraw chloroform, not push on.

In 1940 R. J. Minnitt, one of the leading anaesthetists of the day, cited Embley approvingly and, like Hewer, used Levy's work to condemn intermittent administration.

> Levy appears to have gone too far in his attitude that vagal inhibition from the use of vapour strength of too high percentage is not to be regarded as a real possibility, or at any rate not a dangerous one. At the same time most anaesthetists would agree that the use of very weak vapours during the induction stage is not necessary – probably not desirable – and that to give chloroform intermittently is to give it badly.[56]

Classic experiments?

Surveying the history of Levy's work from the perspective of practising anaesthetists demonstrates both their awareness of it and their guarded view of its applicability to the clinical situation, with the qualified exception of the case of adrenalin. By the 1940s there was by no means general acceptance by practising anaesthetists that cases of sudden death were the result of low dosage and that fibrillation was the pathological mechanism involved. How was it, then, that by the late 1940s and 1950s, Levy's work had become 'classic'? As already suggested the work had another history, that is, among experimentalists. In a variety of contexts Levy's work was paraded as demonstrating the relevance of laboratory work to the clinic. Not surprisingly Levy's experiments appeared prominently in Cushny's textbook of pharmacology. In the 1918 edition Cushny noted Embley's work on chloroform death and added, 'But Levy attributes it to the onset of ventricular fibrillation and has brought a large amount of evidence for his view.'[57] After this the text simply assumed Levy's theory to be correct and Cushny used it to explain the mechanism of syncope.

One of the most striking examples of the dichotomy between practising anaesthetists and experimentalists appeared in the posthumous edition of Hewitt's anaesthetic textbook of 1922. It was edited by an anaesthetist, Henry Robinson. However the chapter on the pharmacology of anaesthesia was written by Cushny's successor in the chair of pharmacology at University College, A. J. Clark. Clark totally endorsed Levy's work and his extension of it to the clinic. He observed,

> These experiments by Levy show, therefore, that sudden cardiac syncope, due to ventricular fibrillation, can be

> produced experimentally in the early stages of chloroform anaesthesia by administration of suprarenal extract or by various procedures which tend to increase the secretion of the suprarenal glands; the results obtained resemble in very striking manner the clinical results observed in cases of deaths in early chloroform anaesthesia, and therefore ventricular fibrillation due to a combination of the action of chloroform and suprarenal extract upon the heart appears to be the most probable cause of the occurrence of deaths in clinical practice in the early stages of chloroform anaesthesia.[58]

The *practical* chapter on chloroform administration, however, presented a very different account. It was written by the new editor, Robinson, senior anaesthetist at the Cancer Hospital, London. Robinson gave his own views on the physiology of sudden chloroform death, emphasising the importance of asphyxia and he concluded,

> Levy claims that there is a special liability to auricular fibrillation in light chloroform anaesthesia. This is quite probably the cause of some of the recorded fatalities; but in the majority there is certainly either overdose or intercurrent asphyxia or both.[59]

Not surprisingly Levy's work was extolled by Thomas Lewis. In 1925 Lewis's major technical text on the heart cited Levy's experiments 'because of their direct practical bearing'. Levy had shown fibrillation to be 'probably the only cause [of death] of moment'. The conclusion was 'upheld by a convincing array of facts and arguments'.[60] Other cardiologists endorsed the work. East and Bain's *Recent Advances in Cardiology* of 1929 cited Levy's experiments as demonstrating that light chloroform anaesthesia definitely caused fibrillation in the cat's heart. They drew the clinical conclusion that 'It is possible that [chloroform deaths] . . . are due to ventricular fibrillation since they occur at the stage at which they would be expected from the experimental evidence'.[61]

In 1937 the Yale physiologist H. E. Hoff discussed the virtues of chloroform and ether. Hoff's article marks a significant turn in the anaesthetic literature. From the very early days of inhalational anaesthesia, practitioners had frequently recounted

Morton's use of ether and the events of the few years subsequent to 1846. No one, however, had ever produced any significant review of the twentieth-century history of anaesthesia. Hoff's article did just that but with his own evaluation of the worth of ether and chloroform. Of chloroform, which he condemned, he noted, quite inaccurately, that it had 'practically been abandoned'. Hoff gave an account of the clinical and experimental work on chloroform prior to 1911 and concluded, 'The final resolution of the problem, harmonizing clinical and experimental findings, was brought about by Levy.' Levy's work was not a debatable topic, or an eye-catching modern contribution, it was an unproblematical historical culmination.[62]

In 1941 the first edition of one of the most widely used textbooks of pharmacology of the twentieth century, 'Goodman and Gilman', transmitted to students and practitioners the apparently uncomplicated finality of Levy's work:

> For many years it was believed that the asystole was vagal in origin, but it is now known that ventricular fibrillation is the cause. The fundamental experiments in this field were performed on animals by Levy who demonstrated that chloroform sensitized the heart so that it is more susceptible to factors precipitating ventricular arrhythmias and fibrillation. He found that fatal ventricular fibrillation could be induced in animals under light chloroform anaesthesia by the injection of epinephrine, and that vagal resection and atropinization were not preventive measures. Levy also demonstrated that deep anaesthesia offered protection against arrhythmia and that ether never precipitated ventricular fibrillation.[63]

In the late 1940s chloroform underwent a massive reappraisal at Wisconsin under the eye of Ralph M. Waters, Director of the Department of Anaesthesia. Chloroform was studied both in the laboratory and in the clinic. One of the workers concluded that animal experiments showed that

> The importance of adequate oxygenation in determining the effects of practically any drug is essential . . . This is especially true with chloroform . . . . It is quite evident from a critical evaluation of many early papers purportedly concerned with an evaluation of chloroform that

> anoxia not only occurred but that the effects attributed to chloroform probably could have been produced by almost any other anaesthetic agent if accompanied by oxygen deprivation.

Dogs were used extensively in the experiments on the grounds that

> there is extensive evidence that in general the canine species responds more like man, particularly insofar as the cardiovascular system functions, than does any other common laboratory animal.

This worker found that, under chloroform, irregularities of rhythm, including fibrillation, were due to 'definite overdosage'.[64] In the clinical evaluation of the effects of chloroform on the cardiovascular system the Wisconsin team used electrocardiography to study 39 major operations. In one patient, breath-holding and deep inspiration were followed by cardiac arrest, but not fibrillation. The authors held that in humans 'ventricular fibrillation is exceedingly rare but that myocardial depression can be very quickly and easily produced'. They observed,

> The results presented herein of the effects of chloroform on the cardiovascular system indicate the ever present possibility of either reflex or direct myocardial depression to cardiac standstill. No evidence of any marked tendency to ventricular tachycardia or ventricular fibrillation was obtained.[65]

The Waters re-evaluation did not endorse Levy's work. However it had no effect on the decline of chloroform use. The agent fell out of favour during the late forties and by the fifties it was gone. New, safer drugs, notably halothane, were being used in its place. There is no evidence that Levy's work was a material influence on the abandonment of chloroform. Not only did the Waters study not challenge the anaesthetists, it did not challenge the experimentalists or the historians either. By the 1950s there was no one left with an interest in questioning Levy's experimental results or their applicability to practice. A consensus now existed; Levy's work was fundamental to modern anaesthesia, it was an unproblematical demonstration of the value of experiments and their relation to practice. Before the 1950s Levy's work was suspect, equivocal and problematical. As long as an interested party (the anaesthetists) had reason to contest it, its status was ambiguous. Put more generally, the evidence of Levy's experiments could not *determine* their acceptance. What constituted sufficient evidence in one setting (the laboratory) was insufficient in another (the clinic). What could be reasonably inferred in one place was unreasonable in another. With the disappearance of one interest group (the chloroform users) only the experimentalists' reading of the evidence remained.

The question of the interests of the experimentalists who promoted Levy's work seems straightforward enough. For the most part the favourable interpretation came from men involved in the promotion of laboratory science in medicine; to them Levy's work was up to date and employed concepts seemingly derived experimentally. For the 'new cardiologists' Levy's experiments illuminated a discipline, cardiology, notoriously immune to physiological understanding. They also demonstrated the clinical relevance of one of their new physiologically derived concepts of heart disease, fibrillation.[66] The interests of the anaesthetists who interpreted Levy's work so differently are less easily explicated. First, they had an accumulated body of clinical skills which they could draw on to deal with and explain untoward situations. It was these they brought to bear on Levy's results. Levy's presentation of these results effectively asked anaesthetists to abandon their perspective as useless, even dangerous, and to admit, overnight, that the wisdom of the community was worthless. As already noted this could have been taken as a confession that most anaesthetic deaths had been produced by errors in administration and not because of a patient's unique physiology. This negative explanation, however, although important, scarcely does sufficient justice to the anaesthetists' perspective. Anaesthetists looked at anaesthetic deaths on a piecemeal basis. Each one was slightly different, each patient arrived at that end point by marginally different routes. A comprehensive theory, requiring a uniform (and completely new) method of administration in all cases ran counter to communal and individual training and experience. Clinical reasoning equipped anaesthetists *to make sense* of an anaesthetic death by combining several pieces of clinical and experimental data to suit a particular case. Levy's results, if they were adopted, were used as just one further possible resource for this activity.

The skills of clinical reasoning in anaesthesia did not disappear along with chloroform. In 1955 the anaesthetist Michael Johnstone reviewed the mechanisms of cardiac arrest during anaesthesia, not just under chloroform. Thoracic surgery, he noted, had shown that arrest was either associated with ventricular fibrillation or 'systole unpreceded by fibrillary phenomena'. He added,

> Many reports of animal experiments have thrown some light on the problem, but the results are controversial. It will be clear to those of us engaged in the practice of clinical anaesthesia that the final solution must inevitably be found through the medium of comprehensive clinical observation. It is doubtful whether the complex pathological and metabolic abnormalities which we regularly encounter in our everyday work will ever be reproduced in the experimental animal.

Johnstone argued that cardiac arrest could not be reduced to a single factor; a variety of mechanisms were at work including potassium intoxication. He acknowledged Levy's work but did not suggest there were any dangers of low chloroform dosage in man. He concluded,

> Writing as an anaesthetist, I should like to emphasize that the majority of cardiac disturbances, which I have described or referred to are due not so much to the anaesthetic agents, as to the manner in which they are used; and they are usually amenable to a physical modification of the anaesthetic technique.[67]

Acknowledgements

Much of the work for this paper was undertaken at the Wood Library of Anesthesia, Chicago, while I was the recipient of a Wood Library Fellowship. I should like to thank the Wood Library Fellowship Committee for their generosity, and the help I received from the Librarian, Mr Patrick Sim.

Notes and references

1. Barbara M. Duncum, *The Development of Inhalation Anaesthesia* (Oxford University Press, London, 1947), p. 620.

2. W. Stanley Sykes, *Essays on the First Hundred Years of Anaesthesia*, 3 vols (Churchill Livingstone, Edinburgh, 1982), vol. II, p. 82; vol. III, p. 136.

3. K. Bryn Thomas, *The Development of Anaesthetic Apparatus* (Blackwell, Oxford, 1975), p. 64.

4. Christopher Lawrence, 'Incommunicable knowledge: science technology and the clinical art in Britain 1850–1914', *Journal of Contemporary History*, vol. 20 (1985), pp. 503–20.

5. John Snow, *On Chloroform and other Anaesthetics* (John Churchill, London, 1858), pp. 109, 217.

6. Duncum, *Development*, p. 396.

7. *British Medical Journal*, vol. ii (1890), pp. 949–50, cited in Duncum, *Development*, p. 443.

8. On the Hyderabad Commission see Duncum, *Development*, pp. 429, 432–5 and Sykes, *Essays*, vol. III, pp. 199–265.

9. On Gaskell see *British Medical Journal*, vol. i (1893), pp. 105–6; on Hill see *British Medical Journal*, vol. i (1897), pp. 958–9. Both cited in Duncum, *Development*, pp. 440–3. C. S. Sherrington and S. C. M. Sowton, 'On the relative effects of chloroform upon the heart and upon other muscular organs', *British Medical Journal*, vol. i (1905), pp. 181–9.

10. *British Medical Journal*, vol. i (1902), pp. 817, 885, 951–61, cited in Duncum, *Development*, pp. 449–50.

11. D. W. Buxton, *Anaesthetics: Their Uses and Administration*, 4th edn (H. K. Lewis, London, 1907), p. 190.

12. Ibid., pp. 192–3.

13. '"Death from anaesthesia properly administered": anaesthesia and the coroner's inquest in late 19th and early 20th century England', Ian Burney, Department of History, University of California, Berkeley (unpublished paper).

14. F. W. Hewitt, *Anaesthetics and their Administration*, 3rd edn (Macmillan, London, 1907), p. 132, 401–3.

15. D. M. Krickler, 'Alfred Goodman Levy – Bulawayo's first doctor', *Central African Journal of Medicine*, vol. 15 (1969), pp. 97–9.

16. Alfred Goodman Levy, 'Sudden death under light chloroform (a preliminary communication)', *Proceedings of the Physiological Society*, vol. 42 (1911), pp. iii–vii.

17. Ibid., 'A further communication', vol. 43 (1911), pp. xviii–xix.

18. Alfred Goodman Levy and Thomas Lewis, 'Heart irregularities resulting from the inhalation of low percentages of chloroform vapour and their relationship to ventricular fibrillation', *Heart*, vol. 3 (1911), pp. 99–112: 101, 103.

19. Christopher Lawrence, 'Moderns and ancients: the "new cardiology" in Britain 1880–1930', *Medical History*, Supplement no. 5 (1985), pp. 1–33.

20. A. M. Browne, J. H. Turnbull and W. A. Mallam, 'Three cases

of death under anaesthesia', *Proceedings of the Royal Society of Medicine* (Anaesthetic Section), vol. 5 (1911–12), pp. 1–9.

21. Alfred Goodman Levy, 'A cardiac effect of adrenalin in chloroformed subjects', *British Medical Journal*, vol. ii (1912), pp. 627–30.

22. Ibid., p. 630.

23. Hewitt, *Anaesthetics*, 4th edn, 1912.

24. D. W. Buxton, 'Recent methods of general anaesthesia', *Transactions of the International Congress of Medicine, London*, vol. vii(b) (1913), pp. 39–47: 41.

25. Alfred Goodman Levy, 'The exciting causes of ventricular fibrillation in animals under chloroform anaesthesia', *Heart*, vol. 4 (1912), pp. 319–78: 331. Levy drew attention to a fatality, reported in the *BMJ*, after adrenalin injection in a patient under light anaesthesia, on p. 333 (*BMJ*, vol. i, 1913, p. 879).

26. Levy, 'Exciting causes', p. 347. Levy was not the only new cardiologist investigating heart rhythms under chloroform. In Edinburgh W. T. Ritchie, collecting cases of auricular flutter, reported on a patient undergoing an operation for osteomyelitis. Using a polygraph he recorded how, thirty minutes into the operation, a normal heartbeat changed into auricular flutter, which three minutes later was followed by cyanosis. The anaesthetic was stopped and artificial respiration was performed. The pulse then became irregular and 'At that time the auricular flutter had apparently passed into fibrillation'. Two minutes later a normal rhythm was re-established. Ritchie drew no conclusions nor referred to Levy's work. 'Auricular flutter', *Edinburgh Medical Journal*, vol. 9 (1912), 485–505. On Ritchie as a new cardiologist see Lawrence, 'Moderns and ancients'.

27. Levy, 'Exciting causes', p. 360, emphasis in original.

28. Alfred Goodman Levy, 'Sudden death under light chloroform anaesthesia', *Proceedings of the Royal Society of Medicine* (Anaesthetic section), vol. 7 (1914), pp. 57–78.

29. Ibid., 'Discussion', pp. 79–84.

30. Levy, 'Exciting causes', p. 361.

31. Levy, 'Sudden death', Discussion.

32. Alfred Goodman Levy, 'The genesis of ventricular extrasystoles under chloroform; with special reference to consecutive ventricular fibrillation', *Heart*, vol. 5 (1914), pp. 299–334: 334.

33. J. A. MacWilliam, 'Cardiac fibrillation and its relation to chloroform anaesthesia', *The Lancet*, vol. ii (1914), pp. 499–501.

34. Alfred Goodman Levy, 'Ventricular fibrillation the cause of death under chloroform', *The Lancet*, vol. ii (1914), p. 502.

35. Yandell Henderson, 'Recent experiments defining the dangers of anaesthesia', *Surgery, Gynaecology and Obstetrics*, vol. 29 (1914), pp. 386–9: 387.

36. E. H. Embley, 'The relation of ventricular fibrillation to clinical chloroform syncope', *The Lancet*, vol. ii (1915), pp. 283–4; *American Journal of Surgery* (Quarterly Anaesthetic Supplement), vol. 30 (1916), pp. 7–10. The papers are virtually identical although in the latter Levy's teaching had become 'dangerous and unreasonable'.

37. *The Lancet*, vol. ii (1915), pp. 295–6.

38. Alfred Goodman Levy, 'Further remarks on ventricular extrasystoles and fibrillation under chloroform', *Heart*, vol. 7 (1919), pp. 105–10.

39. J. Stuart Ross, *Handbook of Anaesthetics* (E. & S. Livingstone, Edinburgh, 1919), pp. 112–13.

40. F. S. Rood and H. N. Webber, *Anaesthesia and Anaesthetics* (Cassell, London, 1930), p. 129, cited in Thomas, *Development*, p. 64.

41. Ross, *Handbook*, 2nd edn (1923), pp. 108–9.

42. Alfred Goodman Levy, *Chloroform Anaesthesia* (John Bale, Sons & Danielsson, London, 1922), pp. 138–9.

43. R. J. Probyn-Williams, *A Practical Guide to the Administration of Anaesthetics* (Longmans, Green & Co, London, 1901), p. 153.

44. Snow, *Chloroform*, pp. 90–1.

45. Alfred Goodman Levy, 'Massage of the fibrillating ventricles', *Heart*, vol. 7 (1920), pp. 175–89, 185.

46. Alfred Goodman Levy, 'Cardiac massage', *Proceedings of the Royal Society of Medicine* (Section of Surgery), vol. 14 (1921), pp. 183–90.

47. Alfred Goodman Levy, 'Cardiac massage', *The Lancet*, vol. ii (1921), p. 949.

48. Levy, *Chloroform*, Foreword.

49. Charles F. Hadfield, *Practical Anaesthetics* (William Wood & Co., New York, 1923) pp. vi, 141, 146, 148.

50. H. P. Fairlie, 'Chloroform anaesthesia', *Proceedings of the Royal Society of Medicine* (Anaesthetic Section), vol. 18 (1924–5), pp. 17–22.

51. Arthur Mills, 'Present position of chloroform', *The Lancet*, vol. ii (1926), pp. 134–7. I have been unable to trace the original work of Pohl.

52. W. B. Primrose, 'Discussion on anaesthesia in relation to operation risk: III Chloroform', *Glasgow Medical Journal*, vol. 112 (1929), pp. 73–82.

53. Ian G. W. Hill, 'Cardiac irregularities during chloroform anaesthesia', *The Lancet*, vol. i (1932), pp. 1139–43. It should be noted that there was a great deal of experimental and clinical work on chloroform and the heart being carried out at this time. I have limited myself here to Levy's publications, the works of anaesthetists which were probably widely read and papers which were often cited and deemed significant at the time or later.

54. C. Langton Hewer, *Recent Advances in Anaesthesia* (J. & A. Churchill, London, 1932), pp. 56–7.

55. W. B. Primrose, 'General anaesthesia', *Glasgow Medical Journal*, vol. 119 (1933), pp. 192–201.

56. R. J. Minnitt, *Handbook of Anaesthetics*, 5th edn (Williams & Wilkins, Baltimore, 1940), p. 188.

57. Arthur R. Cushny, *A Textbook of Pharmacology and Therapeutics*, 7th edn (Lea & Febiger, Philadelphia, 1918), p. 209.

58. Frederick W. Hewitt, *Anaesthetics and their Administration*, 5th edn (Henry Frowde, London, 1922), p. 102.

59. Ibid., p. 364.

60. Thomas Lewis, *The Mechanism and Graphic Registration of the Heart Beat*, 3rd edn (Shaw & Sons, London, 1925), pp. 363, 367.

61. C. F. Terence East and C. W. Curtis Bain, *Recent Advances in Cardiology* (J. & A. Churchill, London, 1929), p. 237.

62. H. E. Hoff, 'Ether versus chloroform', *New England Journal of Medicine*, vol. 217 (1937), pp. 379–92. I suspect, although I cannot substantiate the suspicion, that Hoff's article was an important means by which the picture of Levy's work as 'classic' became an unquestioned tradition in the historiography of anaesthesia.

63. L. S. Goodman and Alfred Gilman, *The Pharmacological Basis of Therapeutics* (The Macmillan Company, New York, 1941), p. 61.

64. Roland Rudolph Liebenow, 'A laboratory re–evaluation of the hepatic, renal and cardiovascular effects of chloroform', MD thesis, University of Wisconsin, 1948. Xerox copy in Wood Library of Anesthesia.

65. Roland R. Liebenow, O. Sidney Orth, Clayton P. Wangeman and Ralph M. Waters, 'A clinical evaluation of the effects of chloroform on the cardiovascular system', typescript in Wood Library of Anaesthesia. See also Ralph M. Waters (ed.), *Chloroform: a Study after 100 Years* (University of Wisconsin Press, Wisconsin, 1951), esp. III.

66. On the vulnerability of cardiology see Christopher Lawrence, '"Definite and Material": coronary thrombosis and the cardiologists in the 1920s', in Charles Rosenberg and Janet Golden (eds), *Framing Disease* (Rutgers University Press, New Brunswick, NJ, 1992).

67. M. Johnstone, 'Some methods of cardiac arrest during anaesthesia', *British Journal of Anaesthesia*, vol. 27 (1955), pp. 566–7.

10

The ambiguous artifact: surgical instruments and the surgical past

Ghislaine Lawrence

Instruments and texts

The literature of the history of medicine is inconsistent on the value of artifacts to the historical enterprise. Henry Sigerist's assertion, in 1951, that the history of medicine was 'to a large extent the history of its tools'[1] was a pronouncement hardly substantiated by work done prior to that date. Subsequent authors have not redressed the balance, but have continued to allude to the potential usefulness of medicine's material remains in reconstructing its past. Nowhere is this ambivalence clearer than in the history of surgery, where many cite old instruments as an important resource but rather few choose to use them as such or indeed to write about them at all. Accounts of instrumentation that do exist still exemplify a concern with discovery and priority which now characterises for many historians an outmoded form of medical history. Many authors still see their prime task as identifying the earliest references to new instrumentation in the literature, or the occurrence in archaeological finds of what we now classify as a forceps or a scalpel, a probe or a lancet. Few consider these artifacts as, for example, the outcome of *processes* of invention or innovation, or as product or commodity. Fewer still question the assumption that old instruments are straightforwardly revealing of the history of surgery – a handy addition to textual sources.

Sigerist himself did little to elucidate the subject further, stating that 'new and improved tools permitted new and more successful operations' while 'new ideas in surgery called for new instruments'.[2] It is indeed as *illustrations* of changing surgical practice that instruments are still used by most authors, even if the titles of their works promise otherwise. A recent North American example, the 1979 monograph *Blood Letting Instruments in the National Museum of History and Technology*, is in fact a historical account of bloodletting, illustrated with photographs of instruments, rather than an account which takes the analysis of instrumentation as its starting point.[3]

Only for the most remote historical periods have authors paid particular attention to the evidence of non-written sources. Discussions of artifactual remains are included in, or form the focus of, many accounts of Roman and pre-Roman surgery. It is archaeological method that has been used to interpret much of this kind of evidence. But archaeologists have recently been subjecting their methods to some close scrutiny. Their questioning has particularly concerned the nature of archaeological evidence and what may acceptably be deduced from it, with an increasing awareness of the role of analogy in the explanation of finds. As one archaeologist recently put it, analysis of the composition, and details of the form of, for example, bronze 'axes', means that 'processes of manufacture will be well understood, some knowledge about the use will be gained from microscopic studies of the working ends, and direct evidence of the transport of the metal over long distances will be available. However, this is definitely the limit of direct inference'.[4] All further deductions, including the designation of these objects as 'axes', rest on analogy with practices and cultures already known to us.

Ian Hodder, also addressing the use of analogy in archaeology, warns 'how dangerous it is to assume that aspects of the material environment are sufficient to define a context', to the exclusion of what he calls 'ideational' factors.[5] Hodder shows how, for instance, theories based on 'discard behaviour' in archaeology rest on the imputation of certain sets of values, regarding what does or does not constitute dirt, as universal – values that demonstrably do not apply, for example, in the complex rituals of Romany culture. Hodder makes further use of gypsy ritual, in this case for burials, to question traditional interpretations of 'grave goods'. He warns that in burial we must expect 'distortions, partial expressions and even inversions of what happens in social life'.[6] Contemporary Romany culture may seem far removed from the history of surgery, but Hodder's general conclusions about the pitfalls of inference from analogy in the absence of any social or ideational context might well be heeded by historians of surgical instruments.

In the interpretation of finds (many of them grave goods) presumed to be medical or surgical, explanation by analogy has been and still is used in a most direct manner. It was, for example, suggested that artifacts taken from a Middle La Tène period grave in 1910 belonged to a surgeon 'because they did not appear strong enough to work wood or metal'.[7] They were considered to have been definitively identified in 1955, when 'a leading London surgeon' provided insights into what could have been done with them surgically.[8] For elucidating the history of surgery, the process has an unpromising circularity – an ancient instrument is surgical if it appears, to modern eyes, capable of performing a surgical procedure – *ipso facto,* ancient surgery is like modern surgery. Equally unenlightening are excursions into 'practical history', or the mechanical testing of instruments. Trepanning skulls with flint scrapers, or showing that the tensile strength of incisions made with obsidian knives is greater than that of incisions made with modern scalpels, adds little to our understanding of a past so remote that we can have little conception of how the category 'surgery' might be separated from categories such as 'wounding', or indeed 'privilege'.[9]

For prehistoric times, written material that would enable us to make more meaningful interpretations is simply not available and Hodder's work should remind us that even for later periods, objects, far from never lying, are the most ambiguous of historical sources. Despite suggestions that they evoke 'the immediacy and the sense of reality' of past surgical practices, looking at old instruments serves largely to evoke the assumptions we already have of the past – in general, or the surgical past in particular. When written sources *are* available to place alongside the 'testimony' of objects, a cursory examination warns us against assuming the similarity of past and present practice, and against evaluations of instrument design, even for the relatively recent past. What are we to make, for example, of the statement in a Surgical Vade Mecum of 1850, that 'the temperature of cutting instruments should be raised to that of the body; since . . . the razor cuts better after being warmed'?[10]

Instruments and pictures

Where actual instruments have not survived, according to one author 'pictures are the next best source'.[11] In constructing the history of surgery, pictures of instruments have indeed been used in much the same way as artifacts. They have been assumed to be uncomplicated sources – so much so that, if none exist in a manuscript, they can be provided by a commentator ten centuries later. Mukhopadhyaya, in his much cited *Surgical Instruments of the Hindus* did just this, on the basis that 'written descriptions of surgical instruments are uninteresting and often fail to convey the true idea which could easily be made evident by the pencil'.[12] According to Mukhopadhyaya, his drawings would be found to tally better with the descriptions given in Sanskrit books than illustrations of previous authors, because, Mukhopadhyaya claimed, his drawings looked '*more like the figures in a modern catalogue of surgical instruments*'.[13] But illustrations are only marginally less ambiguous than artifacts, and such advantages as they do possess – the accompanying context of the manuscript or book in which they occur, and any textual description – must be put against other, less helpful features. These include, for example, the highly conventionalised nature of representation. We have little difficulty in recognising the disembodied hand, depicted in some nineteenth-century drawings of operative surgery, as an illustrator's convention, yet are ready to subject manuscript illuminations of centuries earlier to the most literal interpretation. Peter Jones's survey of medieval medical manuscript illustrations usefully draws attention to instances of copying errors, such as where 'new' instruments have been created by conflating separate items, and acknowledges the stylised nature of many of the illustrations, but still takes a largely realist perspective when it comes to accepting them as indications of accepted surgical practice.[14] The context of illustration production is often unknown. When it is available, it modifies the conclusions we draw about instrument *use*. In the early nineteenth century, perhaps for reasons of economy, the same graphics were re-used many times in different surgical texts, even though the details of the operation they represented may not have remained the same. A century earlier, the exact drawings prepared for de Garengeot's *Nouveau traité des instruments de chirurgie les plus utiles* of 1723 were, according to the author, designed to help young surgeons operate better and might, therefore, be a sound historical source. We know however that de Garengeot was fiercely critical of those instrument makers who claimed priority in instrument design; Garengeot possibly published detailed drawings to establish his own claims.[15]

Pictures, like objects, have largely been used by historians as confirmatory evidence. It has been pointed out, for example, that the most recent, 'definitive' edition of Albucasis' work on surgical instrumentation draws conclusions about instrument design from only two of the available manuscripts, failing to mention that in other versions some depictions are radically different. A discussion of tweezers used to remove foreign bodies from the ear is not supported at all by their depiction in one of the manuscripts that the editors fail to mention. A similar discrepancy exists over illustrations of a tongue depressor.[16]

Both pictures and artifacts can substantiate an almost limitless number of accounts of the past. They are rarely a source of *new* knowledge, despite the claims made for artifacts by the discipline known as material culture studies. Practitioners in this speciality, drawing on such established disciplines as archaeology, anthropology, folklore and folklife studies, aim to produce scholarship based on the 'identification and interpretation of [material culture] data reflecting patterned human behaviour'.[17] In a recent 'state of the art' review, one leading practitioner defined 'material culture'. It consisted of: 1. Art, 2. Diversions (such as books, toys, meals), (3) Adornment (clothing), (4) Modifications of the landscape (architecture, agriculture, etc.), (5) Applied arts (furniture, etc.) and (6) Devices. Revealingly, it is the last category, tools and devices, which is designated as 'the most problematic and, to date, a relatively unproductive range of artifacts for the study of material culture'.[18]

The same author explains that this is so because 'the relationship of the device to the task is so apparently direct as to preclude further analysis'.[19] This statement may well surprise historians of technology, especially if they espouse more recent perspectives in that discipline. By taking function as uncomplicated, the material culturists' construction of the problem of the analysis of tools and devices seems severely limited. Useful information, they claim, can be extracted from 'tools and devices', even such simple ones as hammers, by considering, not their use or function, but their 'style'. Style, however, for the material culturist is largely equated with applied art. Considerably more sophisticated analyses of the 'style' of artifacts are available from historians of technology. One might cite, of several examples, Steven Lubar's work on nineteenth-century North American pin making machinery. If, for the material culturist, 'the configuration of a tool or machine is almost completely dictated by its use', Lubar shows there was no single way for pin machines to look or operate and that 'form need not follow function'. Lubar discusses at length the issue of 'technological style'. The technological style that succeeded for pin machines – rotary form and circular motion – was, he demonstrates, a popular solution to numerous other early nineteenth-century engineering problems and can be convincingly related, not merely to 'technical convenience or precedent', but to such factors as desired labour relations, mechanics' prevailing fascination with cams, and specific features of the pin making industry's rhythm, which traditionally involved workers in short periods of intense concentration followed by long waits.[20]

Surgery and technology

Henry Sigerist had, in 1951, already pointed to the 'general history of technology' as the way forward for the history of surgical instrumentation, writing that it went 'without saying' that the two were closely related and must be studied in relation to each other.[21] It may have gone without saying; it also went without doing, either by historians of technology or of medicine, in Sigerist's day or to any extent since. From at least the 1930s, models existed for historical studies of hand tools which were not, like those of the late nineteenth and early twentieth centuries, primarily anthropological. George Sturt, for example, published what is considered a classic description of the wheelwright's craft in 1934.[22] A recent historian of technology has declared 'serious study' of all craft practices to be inhibited because 'the craftsman's specialist knowledge is not only part of an oral tradition but is organised in categories that are completely alien to modern science'.[23] Undoubtedly, the ways in which surgical knowledge was formerly organised may differ radically from modern ones, despite the fact that the handicraft is still practised, though not by craftsmen. This seems a less likely reason, however, for the neglect of the craft of operative surgery by historians of surgery, many of them medical men. Their interests, until very recently, have demonstrably lain with the biographical and institutional accounts characteristic of professional histories.

Medical tools have further suffered neglect from historians of *technology* since they are not, in the usual sense of the word, production tools, and it has apparently not seemed useful to study them in such contexts as, for example, the mechanisation of craft practice, the division of labour or the breakdown of work-place culture. In fact these might prove insightful avenues to pursue. Surgical instrument design has certainly been affected by the presence or absence of assistants during operations, for example; self-retaining retractors are a case in point. Working practices associated with instrument preparation have changed radically. One Edinburgh surgeon recalls that, as a house officer in the 1930s, his Sunday afternoons were spent in the operating theatre preparing and waxing silk for sutures and ligatures.[24] Studies of this kind, variously characterised as 'from the ground up', 'from the inside out' or as the 'underbelly of technology', have been a prominent theme in the history of technology in recent years and might profitably be attempted in surgery.[25] For surgical tools one might cite particularly everyday practice, and the innovation process, as areas where detailed empirical studies might prove most rewarding. Such studies would inevitably lie within the modern period, for which the detailed sources necessary for reconstructing a context of instrument use are sometimes available. Daybooks, accounts and case records of individual practitioners should prove more revealing than 'classic works' in the history of surgery. The latter are a complex and even anachronistic source for the history of a craft practice. They are regularly cited in articles on surgical instruments, but with little reference to their own context of production. The few studies available which *have* consulted records of everyday surgical practice provide a different account – one that suggests, for example, that instrument use simply did not figure large. Elsewhere in this volume, Lucinda Beier's study of a seventeenth-century London surgeon indicates that his usual practice was more cautious than that implied by contemporary published works. The casebooks of an eighteenth-century country surgeon in France, studied as part of a much vaster survey of medical practice over two centuries, reveal a striking paucity of operative work.[26] The account book and journal of Thomas Hérier, surgeon in the French village of St Christophe de Chalais from 1777 to 1809, include records of only two types of procedure – tooth extraction and vaccination – which presumably required instruments. Undoubtedly, the huge variations in France and elsewhere between practitioners, and between village, provincial and town practice, preclude generalisations from a single case, but Hérier was a qualified master surgeon, apparently with two years, apprenticeship and three years' practical experience to his name, who might have been expected to use more frequently the instruments which we know he once possessed. (Their provision, together with his laundry bills, had been the responsibility of his sponsor when Hérier began his apprenticeship.) We do not, unfortunately, know what instruments these were. Daniel de Moulin, in his history of surgery in the Netherlands, suggests that 'even well-to-do surgeons did not usually possess anything like a trepan or even an amputation saw'.[27] How much this was an idiosyncrasy of Dutch guild practice, where 'loan collections' of instruments were kept for the use of members, is not clear. An account of one such eighteenth-century loan collection, the Rotterdam *Instrumenten-Kasse* of Peter Vink, is striking because of the very *modest* nature of the instruments held in common, presumably too infrequently used to justify purchase by individual surgeons. The first purchase for Vink's collection consisted of 'one screw tourniquet, one pharyngotome, two syringotomes, one wing-probe, one hook and one curved knife', and after this only 'economical purchases or orders on an instrument maker were made'.[28] It is salutary to place this type of information alongside accounts of eighteenth-century instrument use drawn from the works of authors such as Pierre Dionis, Lorenz Heister and Jean Louis Petit, which are profusely illustrated with often complex surgical tools.

From the second half of the nineteenth century, works on operative surgery written and used as textbooks provide an additional source for insights into practice. Throughout the nineteenth century, the amount of surgery performed was such that learning and practising operative technique on the cadaver was apparently the rule, although many operations could not 'readily be performed on the dead subject'. Furthermore it was 'generally the case in England [that] only a small amount of material [was] available for carrying out a course of Operative

Surgery on the dead subject'. The organisation of manuals of operative surgery was directly affected by these constraints, leading one author to explain that the order in which different operations were described might seem 'peculiar' but was necessary if all the procedures were being carried out on the same, presumably dwindling, post-mortem material.[29]

Empirical studies of innovation in surgical tool design and production might provide more insight into surgical instrument *making* than the rather general accounts published to date. Many authors allude to the rise of the specialist instrument maker in the eighteenth and nineteenth centuries, but few look in detail at other aspects of the trade. For earlier periods this necessarily involves examination of the guilds concerned. Boschung briefly touches on the German situation, where the guilds' categorisation of instruments serves to remind us of the disparate origins of surgical instrument making as a craft. In the sixteenth century, 'long' work and 'short' work (that is, of different blade length) was performed by different cutlers, and blade making and handle making by different corporations. By the eighteenth century, engravers, mathematical instrument makers and goldsmiths and silversmiths had gradually encroached on the cutlers' monopoly.[30]

Crawforth has written at length on the day-to-day working of the London guilds. His study, based on the records of fourteen guilds, is part of ongoing research into scientific instrument makers and retailers from 1550 to 1900.[31] Surgical instrument makers are not included, but Crawforth's work challenges many common assumptions about guild practice – an essential part of the context for craft innovation. He suggests, as have others before him, that from about 1720 London guilds were less and less able to control members' activities, but also notes that this relaxation probably included the practice of 'essaying', which was long regarded as a constraint to innovation because of guild insistence on traditional design. A further consequence of relaxed enforcement of regulations – far greater mobility of apprentices and of members, in what seem almost to have been 'nominal' attachments to particular masters or guilds – led to dispersal of different trade skills throughout the guilds.[32] It would be interesting to know where the affinities of cutlers and surgical instrument makers lay (and, incidentally, those of barber-surgeons. In Newcastle the barber-surgeons allied with the wax and tallow chandlers in 1442). Undoubtedly, institutional and political reasons were behind many apparently strange associations but this may not lessen their importance as a source of innovation in technique or design. This theme might be pursued by exploring for cutlers, and later for specialist surgical instrument makers, their other skills and products. A recent listing of London makers entered in trade directories from 1736 to 1811 includes cutlers who were also butchers' tool makers, engraving instrument makers, bookbinders' tool makers and, in one case, a 'plow knife maker'.[33] The relationship of specialist surgical instrument makers with the surgeons they supplied is also relevant to invention and innovation. Boschung's study of the eighteenth-century Paris instrument maker, J. J. Perret, shows this to have been a disputatious area of claim and counterclaim in the matter of priority. (It also, incidentally, shows that we should not assume that new technologies were used in instrument making simply because they were known to have been invented. Of the instrument makers in Paris, only two, said Perret, owned lathes, adding that the metal lathe did in five or six minutes jobs that took three to four hours to do by hand with a file or turner.[34])

When the relationship with instrument makers was not congenial it seems to have been possible for the surgeon to dispense with their services to some extent, even as late as the early decades of the twentieth century. We should not assume that specialist makers, once established, were responsible for all instrument production. Directions for making instruments are to be found in works written for surgeons. In his comprehensive *Text Book on Surgery* of 1888, John Wyeth, 'Professor of Surgery at the New York Polyclinic', advocated the use of absorbable bone wound drains – to be made from 'the bones of young and healthy animals'.[35] The bones were to be cut to size, bored out, turned on a lathe 'round and smooth', and perforated laterally, then decalcified in muriatic acid for twelve hours and stored in a carbolic acid solution. The bones of fowls were particularly to be recommended, but if taken from a cooked chicken, a weaker muriatic acid solution was to be used. The same author advised that almost all the surgeon's requirements for ligatures could be met at the music store, by the purchase of the best quality violin strings – one dozen of each of E and A, six D, and two or three harp strings. The North American context must be taken into account, but specialist surgical instrument makers were certainly well established on the east coast by the late 1880s, and instructions for instrument making also occur in a British textbook of 1915, where the Glasgow surgeon Alexander Maclennan stated that many could be 'quickly made by the amateur'.[36] Maclennan was not referring to minor or peripheral items, but to chisels, periosteal elevators, probes, drills, bone plates and many more; six pages were devoted to a discussion of soldering, brazing and tempering instruments, and a colour chart provided for the degree of tempering of steel required. While it may be hard to believe that many British surgeons of 1915 were forging their own instruments, we should not continue to assume that specialist firms were the only source of instrumentation, even in the present century. Traditional museum practice, with its stress on provenance, particularly maker's names, tends to favour the preservation of instruments which can be attributed over those which cannot.

The vicissitudes of the modern surgical equipment industry have inevitably affected the type of instrument reaching the surgeon's hand. After World War I huge numbers of surplus instruments flooded the British market, and items costing a pound to produce 'were being sold for 6d' even after many hospitals and other institutions had had a free pick of all they wanted.[37] It is possible that many hospitals were able to acquire new instruments in quantity for the first time. It also seems likely that, in order to minimise losses, firms cut back on their ranges, some models disappearing for good. World War II was equally disruptive. In 1939 the British government asked the trade to prepare to devote up to 90 per cent of its output to the war effort if necessary and was prepared to classify its skilled workers as a reserved occupation, pledging that no surgical instrument maker over the age of 23 would be enlisted.[38] The post-war course of the industry to today's position, where only a handful of firms still manufacture in Britain and a very large proportion of the instruments used in British hospitals are made in the Third World, has yet to be charted in detail by any historian, although W. Weston-Davies briefly alludes to this period.[39]

Instrumental diversity

The association between barbering and surgery has frequently been considered as part of the professional history of the latter craft but virtually never as a context for instrument design.

Several successful eighteenth-century surgical instrument makers had been particularly renowned for razor making, going into print on the subject in at least two cases – Savigny of London produced a *Treatise on the Use and Management of a Razor*, in its fourth edition by 1786.[40] Perret in Paris had published a similar pamphlet.[41] Did this affect the form of surgical knives? Authors who do discuss changing forms in instrumentation are more likely to perceive diachronic continuity between the designs illustrated by subsequent surgical authors than to examine the wider context for innovation. This must include not only other 'flesh-working' tools, such as domestic cutlery, weapons, veterinary and butchering implements, but razors, domestic and craft equipment of all types. This wider context is virtually ignored in historical accounts of surgical instruments. A few interesting exceptions occur in discussions of needle design, where, for some reason, authors more readily perceive the potential relevance of the non-surgical realm. Kirkup refers to the use of glovers', sailmakers' and leather workers' needles by surgeons, to the eyeless 'larding needle' used for suturing by Petit, and to an atraumatic needle patented by superintendents of the Birmingham School for the Blind in 1891 to overcome the difficulties of the sightless in threading eyed needles.[42]

Clearly the design of new instruments did not occur *in vacuo*, nor, presumably, was surgical instrumentation without influence on other types. According to a note in *The Lancet* for 1866, 'the principal [*sic*] of passing and arresting the thread' in the Singer sewing machine was taken from a surgical instrument invented in 1836 for closure of recto-vaginal or vesico-vaginal fistulae.[43] A single example of international transfer of surgical technology – that of Charrière's locking ratchet for artery forceps – is widely quoted by historians. Of more general differences in instrument design or use between countries we know very little. According to the anonymous author of a work entitled *To the Medical Profession: Modern Surgical Instruments Chiefly of France and Germany*, published in London in 1844, most of the tools he described were 'comparatively unknown in this country'.[44] Historians of hand tools identify national styles in, for example, the handles of tenon saws.[45] Presumably similar influences may be detected in the design of surgical saws and perhaps in surgical tools of all kinds. Questions of this nature about design raise other questions about use. They are questions which historians of surgical instruments have singularly failed to address, notably for the material culturists' reason: because the relation between design and use appears so direct. It is precisely the relationship of the surgical device to the surgical task that is hardest to discuss; the apparently empirical nature of cutting defies analysis, making it infinitely easier to talk about the percussion hammer than the surgical mallet. Those who write on medical and surgical instrumentation have employed various strategies, from evasion to diversion, to avoid getting to grips with this problem.

In a recent large history of medical instrumentation the author chooses to 'emphasise the attitude of the physician toward his implements and largely omit the evolution of surgical instruments', although she gives no reason for the omission.[46] Those who set out specifically to write on surgical instruments have also circumvented the problem, most opting to discuss areas such as instrument making, or the development of aseptic technique, rather than to address specifically the way surgical instruments are designed or used to perform surgical tasks. The author of the *Encyclopaedia Britannica* entry on surgical instruments for 1911 devoted well over half his article to 'three great principles – the use of anaesthetics, the use of antiseptic or aseptic methods and the surgical uses of electricity' – rather than the use of instruments to cut flesh.[47] The history of operative surgery has almost exclusively been perceived as the history of the attempted cure of morbid anatomical conditions. But did surgeons cut like barbers – or, for that matter, like butchers, or cooks, or carpenters? Does flaying or boning or jointing relate to what has come to constitute operative technique? There are certainly national styles in butchering, are there national styles in operating? Within a given period, surgeons themselves have been aware of divergent 'styles' of operating, though not necessarily between nations. George Heuer, a protégé of W. S. Halstead, moved from Johns Hopkins to the relative wilds of Cincinnati in 1921 and encountered surgeons who likened their operative technique to 'fixing an old road, by filling potholes, straightening curves, reducing grades.'[48] Surgeons have also been aware that operating 'styles' might directly influence decisions about appropriate surgery. The popularity of paravertebral sympathectomy, frequently performed for peripheral vascular disease in the 1920s and 1930s, has been attributed to the fact that it was 'a dissection' and 'attractive to anatomically minded surgeons'.[49]

Prospects

Unquestionably, surgical instruments must embody surgical knowledge. Until we have an account of the social construction of that knowledge, however, tackling the social construction of surgical tools remains problematic. Rewarding new perspectives in the history and sociology of technology have found far greater scope in the complex choices involved in machine design rather than in the apparent simplicity of tool configuration. Ultimately, these approaches *should* have something to offer in analysing hand tools. The distinction between machines and tools has, after all, proved extremely difficult for historians of technology to agree upon.[50] When surgical theory is quite obviously embodied in instrumentation, and for periods when that theory is still controversial, the potential for a social constructivist account is readily seen. Historians of all persuasions note that the eventual acceptance of 'aseptic technique' resulted in surgical instruments of an all-metal construction. Clearly, however, the change did not serve the interests of all groups. The preface to Brady and Martin's instrument catalogue of 1897 referred to Lister's work as 'one of the most beneficent resolutions of modern surgery' and offered instruments with aseptic [metal] handles as alternatives to ivory or ebony, but added that experience did not lead them 'to think that the universal adoption of metal handles for every instrument is near at hand'.[51] British manufacturers went on offering instruments with non-metal handles until the 1930s. Asepsis served different interests among the makers and users of instruments. Surgeons who adopted the wearing of rubber gloves in the 1910s and 1920s required larger handled and therefore more expensive instruments to obtain a secure grip. More generally, the adoption of distinctive, all-metal (usually steel) instrumentation by surgeons while physicians continued to use tools with wooden, brass or ivory parts, emphasised that surgery was different, and independent, from medical specialities.[52]

For if old instruments prove, anachronistically, a rather difficult source for the past *practice* of operative surgery, what we do know of their use may yet offer insights into the institutional and professional history of the discipline. To control access to instruments was to control practice. Where surgical tools were held in common, as by the Dutch barber-surgeons, the guild limited access to them to its members. During the late eighteenth century, the Filles de la Charité of St Vincent de Paul, nursing sisters attached to a hundred and seventy-five French hospitals, adopted the practice of sending their members to new establishments 'fully equipped with boxes of syringes and other surgical instruments'. This has been interpreted as a strategy to prevent increasing loss of control of ward procedures, as the surgical students of Revolutionary France entered the hospitals for the first time.[53] It has been suggested that the adoption of complex apparatus and techniques for local anaesthesia in the 1930s and 1940s was a move by surgeons to resist the growing influence of anaesthetists with their own specialist tools. In recent years, at least one surgeon-inventor has tried to restrict supply of an innovatory device (the Charnley hip prosthesis) to surgeons who also adopted his particular operative technique.[54]

In these professional disputes, having or using instruments conferred status or was a means of retaining power. But in that larger professional confrontation, which occupied surgeons for much of the eighteenth and nineteenth centuries, having anything much to do with instruments was a distinct disadvantage. The rise of the surgeons, to achieve equal footing with physicians, has been examined by several authors. Gelfand in particular has described how the strategy of the surgeons of the Paris Académie Royale de Chirurgie involved a public distancing from the empiricism of craft practice. In the process, Gelfand shows, these French surgeons had almost to denigrate operative surgery, and the use of instruments. 'The art of operating . . . which most impresses common people is only a single point in the cure of diseases', wrote François Quesnay, Secretary of the Académie in 1743, and 'the time of the operation is only an instant in the cure of the patient', echoed a contemporary surgeon.[55] 'The success of major operations is truly the surgeon's triumph, but this very triumph can be surgery's shame. Why should it not be possible for us to count our successes only by the operations which we are able to prevent?' wrote Antoine Louis in 1749, and he incorporated these views in the surgical entries which he was commissioned to write for the *Encyclopédie* of Diderot and D'Alembert. In Quesnay's view, those who, when they did operate, blindly followed procedures learned by habit were 'mere labourer[s] bound to a miserable routine, often pernicious for the patients and always harmful to the progress of the Art'.[56]

As Gelfand points out, condemnations of operations were not limited to France. John Hunter called them a 'tacit acknowledgement of the insufficiency of surgery' and apparently said, 'to perform an operation is to mutilate a patient we cannot cure'. Gelfand does not omit to mention that the context for Hunter's remarks must include his vitalist perspective, but taken *out* of context, such remarks were useful to subsequent British surgical authors, who placed them prominently on the flyleaves and in the introductions to works on operative surgery.[57] The opening quotations in Bryant's *Surgery* of 1879 contained a typical example: 'Surgery consists in curing a disease rather than the removal of it by mechanical means. But so differently do most think upon this subject that a surgeon who performs most operations and gives most pain is commonly thought the best. John Hunter, MS. Lectures, 1787'.[58] The proper balance between the manual and the theoretical aspects of surgery, between the 'art' and the 'science', preoccupied surgical authors throughout the nineteenth century. With few exceptions, 'art' was given inferior connotations. 'It will be impossible to make an accomplished operator except the art and science of surgery are both united', wrote the English surgeon John Hunt in 1801. He added, 'Dexterity may be acquired by habit; but the most accomplished address on the management of instruments will be inadequate to the purpose, except it is accompanied with scientific information to direct the knife.'[59] By the twentieth century former surgery could be regarded as 'an art dangerous, barbarous and almost repulsive' which had been transformed into 'a scientific procedure, beautiful in its details and beneficent in its results'.[60] Whereas Celsus' definition of surgery had been that which treats by the hand, nineteenth-century surgical authors preferred 'that primary division of medicine which has for its object the care or relief of morbid conditions of the body, in a corresponding division of Pathology'.[61] It is perhaps in this context that a remark of the surgeon James Syme should be heard. After the International Exhibition of 1862 he wrote, 'If you only saw the outrageous increase in the way of surgical instruments that have been submitted for our approval. I sometimes think of taking down a bagful to laugh at.'[62]

Syme was speaking of new instruments, and excess in instrumentation was still anathema to the medical world of the 1860s.

By the 1870s in Britain, however, other bagfuls of instruments were being re-opened in the very heart of the surgical establishment, not to be laughed at, but to be displayed with pride. Contemporary practitioners, increasingly distanced from craft associations, now used *obsolete* instruments as evidence of a long and honourable lineage for surgery. The Royal College of Surgeons of England established a formal historical instrument collection in the early 1870s, displayed in a separate room of their museum, and by 1910, 806 items had been collected.[63] From the late Victorian era onwards, craft origins and guild customs were no longer shunned, but provided material for surgical iconography and ceremonial. Antiquated robes were worn with pride and fleams were favoured as decorative devices. Surgical institutions in Britain and elsewhere are now to the fore in preserving and displaying obsolete instruments. Here their function is clearly to represent skill and achievement in surgery. Surgeons cannot, by and large, display the work done *with* their tools; the eviscerated organ preserved in a bottle is but a partial record of a successful operation, even for a medical audience, although A. F. McGill of Leeds is said to have presented a line of old men, each holding his own prostate in a bottle, to a British Medical Association meeting in 1889.[64] Unlike production crafts, and perhaps even more than in other 'service' professions and industries, the commemorative options for surgery are limited. (Histories of barbering and hairdressing, for example, largely describe and illustrate not details of instrumentation but the hairstyles achieved.[65])

The curator C. J. S. Thompson made an attempt to distil and preserve the 'essence' of surgical skill in the 1920s when he arranged for plaster casts of the hands of eminent surgeons to be made. At least one – that of James Syme – was evidently still valued enough in 1950 to warrant replacing after the original had been destroyed in the bombing of 1941.[66] This disembodied hand, holding an example of the amputation knife which Syme devised, epitomises the commemorative use of old surgical instrumentation, and it is individual prowess, and innovation, that are being commemorated. A history of surgery more concerned with the everyday practice of users and makers may well prove more productive when the complexity of old instruments as historical sources is recognised.

Notes and references

1. H. Sigerist, *A History of Medicine: Primitive and Archaic Medicine*, 2 vols (Oxford University Press, New York, 1951), vol. 1, p. 19.
2. Ibid.
3. A. Davis and T. Appel, *Blood Letting Instruments in the National Museum of History and Technology*, Smithsonian Studies in History and Technology no. 41 (Smithsonian Press, Washington, 1979).
4. E. W. MacKie, *Science and Society in Prehistoric Britain* (Paul Elek, London, 1977), p. 8.
5. I. Hodder, *The Present Past* (B. T. Batsford, London, 1982), p. 24.
6. Ibid., p. 145.
7. H. A. Reid, 'Zur Prähistorischen Chirurgie', *Archiv. für Anthropologie*, New Series, vol. xii (1913), pp. 225–7.
8. J. M. de Navarro, 'A doctor's grave of the Middle La Tène period from Bavaria', *Proceedings of the Prehistoric Society*, no. 23 (1955), pp. 231–74: 242.
9. T. Wilson Parry, 'The art of trephining', reprinted from *Journal of the British Archaeological Association*, March 1916, pp. 31–7; B. A. Buck, 'Ancient technology in contemporary surgery', *Western Journal of Medicine*, vol. 136 (1982), pp. 265–9.
10. R. Druitt, *The Surgeon's Vade Mecum*, 5th edn (John Churchill, London, 1851), p. 566 (quoting Malgaigne's *Operative Surgery*, trans. F. Brittan, London, 1846).
11. A. B. Davis, 'Historical studies of medical instruments', *History of Science*, vol. xvi (1978), pp. 107–33: 111.
12. G. Mukhopadhyaya, *The Surgical Instruments of the Hindus*, 2 vols (Calcutta University, 1913), vol. 1, p. xvi.
13. Ibid., p. xvii, my emphasis.
14. P. M. Jones, *Medieval Medical Miniatures* (The British Library in association with the Wellcome Institute for the History of Medicine, London, 1984); see, for example, pp. 28, 105–7.
15. U. Boschung, 'Chirurgiemechanik im 18. Jahrhundert – Der chirurgishce Instrumentenmacher', *Medita*, vol. 10 (1980), p. iv.
16. E. Savage-Smith, 'Some sources and procedures for editing a medieval Arabic surgical tract', *History of Science*, vol. 14 (1976), pp. 247–8, reviewing M. S. Spink and G. L. Lewis, *Albucasis on surgery and Instruments* (Wellcome Institute for the History of Medicine, London, 1973).
17. T. J. Schlereth, *Material Culture Studies in America, 1876–1976* (American Association for State and Local History, Nashville, Tenn., 1982), p. xvi.
18. J. D. Prown, 'Mind in matter: an introduction to material culture theory and method', *Winterthur Portfolio*, vol. 17, no. 1 (1982), pp. 1–19: 12–15.
19. Ibid., p. 14.
20. S. Lubar, 'Culture and technological design in the 19th-century pin industry: John Howe and the Howe Manufacturing Company', *Technology and Culture*, vol. 28 (1987), pp. 253–82: 267 and 276.
21. Sigerist, *History of Medicine*, vol. 1, p. 19.

22. G. Sturt, *The Wheelwright's Shop* (Cambridge University Press, Cambridge, 1934).

23. A. Pacey, 'The history of technology', in P. Corsi and P. Weindling (eds), *Information Sources in the History of Science and Medicine* (Butterworths, London, 1983), pp. 44–60: 50.

24. J. A. Ross, *The Edinburgh School of Surgery after Lister* (Churchill Livingstone, Edinburgh, 1978), p. 62.

25. See, for example, D. A. Hounshell, 'Commentary: on the discipline of the history of American technology', *Journal of American History*, vol. 67, no. 4 (1981), p. 863.

26. E. H. Lemay, 'Thomas Hérier, a country surgeon outside Angoulême at the end of the XVIIIth century: a contribution to social history', *Journal of Social History*, vol. 10, no. 2 (1976), pp. 524–37.

27. D. de Moulin, *A History of Surgery* (Martinus Nijhoff, Dordrecht, 1988), p. 259.

28. M. J. van Lieburg, 'The instrument collection of Peter Vink: a chapter in the development of the surgical profession in the Netherlands during the 18th century', *Janus*, vol. 67 (1980), pp. 207–19: 212.

29. H. J. Waring, *Manual of Operative Surgery*, 3rd edn (Henry Hodder & Stoughton, London, 1909), p. ix.

30. Boschung, 'Chirugiemechanik', p. iv.

31. M. A. Crawforth, 'Instrument makers in the London guilds', *Annals of Science*, vol. 44 (1987), pp. 319–77, part of Project SIMON (Scientific Instrument Making, Observations and Notes).

32. Ibid., p. 328.

33. D. Wright, 'An index of London surgical and scientific instrument makers, 1736–1811, compiled from the Guildhall Library Trades Directories', unpublished MS.

34. Boschung, 'Chirurgiemechanik', p. xi.

35. J. A. Wyeth, *A Text-Book on Surgery* (Swan Sonnenschein & Co., London, 1888) pp. 7–8.

36. A. MacLennan, *Surgical Materials and their Uses* (Edward Arnold, London, 1915), p. 203.

37. Surgical Instrument Manufacturer's Association, *Report of the Annual General Meeting, October 27, 1939* (London, 1939), p. 10.

38. Ibid., p. 11.

39. W. H. Weston-Davies, 'The surgical instrument maker: an historical perspective', *Journal of the Royal Society of Medicine*, vol. 82 (1989), pp. 40–3.

40. J. H. Savigny, *Treatise on the Use and Management of a Razor*, 4th edn (London, 1786).

41. Boschung, 'Chirugiemechanik', p. v.

42. J. Kirkup, 'The history and evolution of surgical instruments V: Needles and their penetrating derivatives', *Annals of the Royal College of Surgeons of England*, vol. 68 (1986), pp. 29–33.

43. Referred to in W. E. Thompson, 'Historical surgical instruments in the museum of the Royal College of Surgeons of England', *Journal of Bone and Joint Surgery*, vol. 36-B, no. 1 (1954), pp. 135–9, 135.

44. Anonymous, *To the Medical Profession: Modern Surgical Instruments Chiefly of France and Germany* (London, 1844).

45. A. Jackson and D. Day, *The Complete Book of Tools* (Michael Joseph, London, 1978), p. 74.

46. Davis, 'Historical studies', p. 124.

47. *Encyclopaedia Britannica*, 11th edn, 29 vols (Cambridge University Press, London, 1910–11), vol. 26, pp. 132–6.

48. E. C. Cangi, 'Abraham Flexner's philanthropy: the full-time system in the department of surgery at the University of Cincinnati College of Medicine, 1910–1930', *Bulletin of the History of Medicine*, vol. 56 (1982), pp. 160–74: 170.

49. M. M. Ravitch, 'The reception of new operations', *Annals of Surgery*, vol. 200 (1984), pp. 231–45: 243.

50. D. Mackenzie, 'Marx and the machine', *Technology and Culture*, vol. 25, no. 3 (1984), p. 486.

51. Brady and Martin, *Surgical Instrument Catalogue* (Newcastle upon Tyne, 1897), p. viii.

52. On surgeons' perceptions of their being apart from the rest of medicine see Daniel M. Fox and Christopher Lawrence, *Photographing Medicine: Images and Power in Britain and America since 1840* (Greenwood Press, New York, 1988), pp. 49–50.

53. C. Jones, essay review, '"Professionalizing modern medicine" in French hospitals', *Medical History*, vol. 26 (1982), pp. 341–9: 345.

54. W. Waugh, *John Charnley: the Man and the Hip* (Springer-Verlag, London, 1990), p. 129.

55. T. Gelfand, 'Empiricism and eighteenth century French surgery', *Bulletin of the History of Medicine*, vol. 43 (1969), pp. 40–53: 51.

56. Ibid., p. 52.

57. Ibid., see also Jacyna, this volume.

58. T. Bryant, *Manual for the Practice of Surgery*, 3rd edn, 2 vols (J. & A. Churchill, London, 1879), vol. 1.

59. J. Hunt, *Historical Surgery* (S. Adams, Loughborough, 1801), p. vii.

60. A. Carlees, *Rose and Carlees's Manual of Surgery*, 9th edn (Baillière, Tindall & Cox, London, 1917), p. 271.

61. F. J. Gant, *The Science and Practice of Surgery*, 2 vols. (Baillière, Tindall & Cox, London, 1886), vol. 1, following frontispiece.

62. R. Paterson, *Memorials of the Life of James Syme* (Edmonston & Douglas, Edinburgh, 1878), p. 143.

63. A. Keith, *Illustrated Guide to the Museums of the Royal College of Surgeons, England* (London, 1910), pp. 106, 118. Keith states the instrument collection was formed in 1875, but his successor as Museum Conservator, Alban Doran, dates this to 1871 in the preface to his typescript catalogue of the surgical instrument collection of 1924.

64. Lord Brock, 'Advances in general surgery', in W. C. Gibson (ed.), *British Contributions to Medical Science* (Wellcome Institute for the History of Medicine, London, 1971), p. 167.

65. See, for example, M. Louis, *Six Thousand Years of Hair Styling* (1939).

66. W. E. Thompson, 'Historical surgical instruments in the museum of the Royal College of Surgeons of England', *Journal of Bone and Joint Surgery*, vol. 35-B, no. 2 (1953), pp. 298–308: 298–9.

Index

For Product Safety Concerns and Information please contact our EU representative GPSR@taylorandfrancis.com Taylor & Francis Verlag GmbH, Kaufingerstraße 24, 80331 München, Germany

Batch number: 10725800

Printed by Printforce, the Netherlands